Register Now for to Your

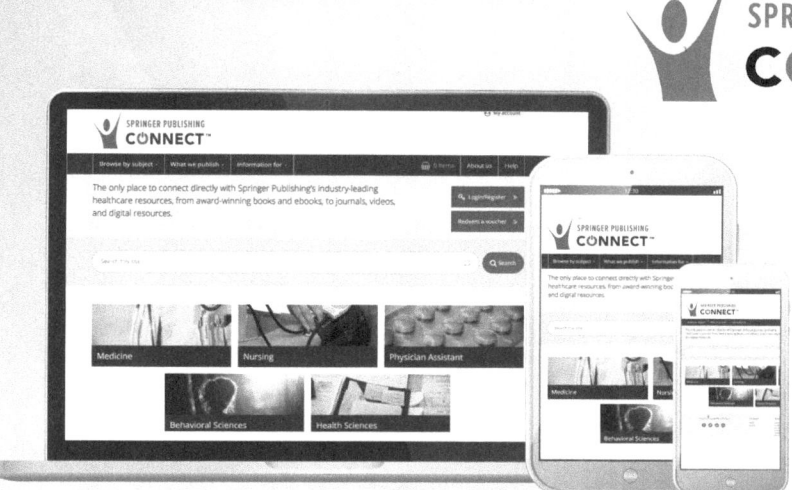

Your print purchase of *Population Health Management: Strategies, Tools, Applications, and Outcomes* **includes online access to the contents of your book**—increasing accessibility, portability, and searchability!

Access today at:
http://connect.springerpub.com/content/book/978-0-8261-4427-0
or scan the QR code at the right with your smartphone. Log in or register, then click "Redeem a voucher" and use the code below.

7U6KU859

Scan here for quick access.

Having trouble redeeming a voucher code?
Go to https://connect.springerpub.com/redeeming-voucher-code

If you are experiencing problems accessing the digital component of this product, please contact our customer service department at cs@springerpub.com

The online access with your print purchase is available at the publisher's discretion and may be removed at any time without notice.

Publisher's Note: New and used products purchased from third-party sellers are not guaranteed for quality, authenticity, or access to any included digital components.

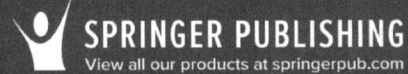

Population Health Management

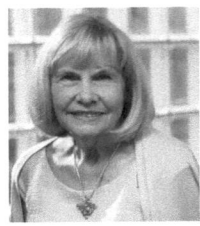

Anne M. Hewitt, PhD, MA is Acting Chair for the Department of Interprofessional Health Sciences and Health Administration and Professor at Seton Hall University. She also serves as Director of the Elizabeth A. Seton Institute for Community and Population Health. Dr. Hewitt's academic career began with a doctoral dissertation grant from the American Lung Association and has continued with grants from federal and state agencies and national nonprofit agencies such as RWJ Foundation. She regularly publishes in health-related peer-reviewed journals and is currently on the *Journal of Health Administration Education* editorial board. Dr. Hewitt also contributes book chapters on diverse topics such as online learning, population health management, virtual healthcare, and the sociology of health. Her service activities include appointments on state nonprofit and public health advisory boards. As part of a multiyear consulting relationship with the New Jersey Department of Health, she completed a sabbatical working with the Division of Community Health and Aging. Dr. Hewitt recently served as faculty for the New Jersey Healthcare Executive Leadership Academy sponsored by the NJ Medical Society, NJ Hospital Association, and NJ Association of Health Plans. Her honors include Distinguished Service Awards from professional health executive organizations such as the American Lung Association, the Healthcare Planning and Marketing Society of NJ, and the Association of Healthcare Executives of New Jersey. Dr. Hewitt founded *Mountainside Associates* in 2006 and retains an active consulting role with numerous health sector clients.

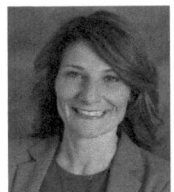

Julie L. Mascari, MHA, a healthcare executive with over 20 years of experience, is currently the Regional President of Humana. Julie's responsibilities include managing the overall performance, development, and expansion of Humana's business presence and financial success in the northeast region. She has broad responsibilities in the areas of strategic growth, clinical operations, network expansion, provider engagement, risk adjustment, and product development. Prior to Humana, Julie served as the Medicare leader for EmblemHealth, Horizon Blue Cross Blue Shield of New Jersey, and Optum Care, a subsidiary of UnitedHealth Group. She oversaw performance and strategic direction in a highly regulated and complex environment and continually developed and implemented population health management programs for at-risk populations. Julie obtained her MHA from Seton Hall University and her BA in Political Science from Rider University and has published/contributed to numerous health management books and industry abstracts. She is an Adjunct Professor at Seton Hall University's MHA program, Rutgers University School of Pharmacy, and for Hackensack Meridian's School of Medicine. She serves on the boards of Seton Hall University's President's and Dean's Advisory Group and the Southern Maine Agency on Aging. She is a member of CHIEF and the Women Business Leaders of the U.S. Healthcare Industry Foundation. Julie believes passionately in the providing of outstanding healthcare services in a manner that serves both the customer and the company in a sustainable, mutually beneficial environment.

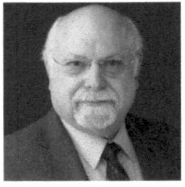

Stephen L. Wagner, PhD, FACHE, LFACMPE has been active in the healthcare field for more than 45 years, focusing on the U.S. system and its ongoing transformation. He has extensive experience as a textbook author, researcher, and healthcare executive with a long career in medical practice administration. Dr. Wagner served as an executive at the Carolinas Healthcare System (CHS) for 20 years until retiring in 2015. He was instrumental in the creation of the Sanger Heart and Vascular Institute (formerly the Sanger Clinic) where he served as Chief Nonphysician Executive. During his last five years at CHS, he was Director of Organization Development where he was responsible for their change management strategy. He is devoted to educating future leaders in the field and is the executive in residence/assistant professor for the Master of Healthcare Administration program in the School of Health and Medical Sciences at Seton Hall University. He has taught in the program for over 20 years, including courses such as strategic planning, health management, health economics, and emergency management. Dr. Wagner received his master's degree in Healthcare Fiscal Management from the Wisconsin School of Business (Madison) and his doctorate in Healthcare Public Policy Analysis from the University of Louisville College of Business.

Population Health Management

Strategies, Tools, Applications, and Outcomes

Anne M. Hewitt, PhD, MA
Julie L. Mascari, MHA
Stephen L. Wagner, PhD, FACHE, LFACMPE

Editors

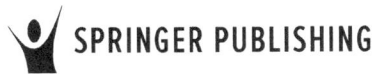

Copyright © 2022 Springer Publishing Company, LLC
All rights reserved.

No part of this publication may be reproduced, stored in a retrieval system, or transmitted in any form or by any means, electronic, mechanical, photocopying, recording, or otherwise, without the prior permission of Springer Publishing Company, LLC, or authorization through payment of the appropriate fees to the Copyright Clearance Center, Inc., 222 Rosewood Drive, Danvers, MA 01923, 978-750-8400, fax 978-646-8600, info@copyright.com or at www.copyright.com.

Springer Publishing Company, LLC
11 West 42nd Street, New York, NY 10036
www.springerpub.com
connect.springerpub.com/

Acquisitions Editor: David D'Addona
Compositor: Amnet Systems

ISBN: 978-0-8261-4426-3
ebook ISBN: 978-0-8261-4427-0
DOI: 10.1891/9780826144270

Podcasts are provided that illustrate the key points of each chapter. These podcasts can be accessed by visiting: https://connect.springerpub.com/content/book/978-0-8261-4427-0/front-matter/fmatter7

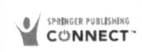 A robust set of instructor resources designed to supplement this text is located at http://connect.springerpub.com/978-0-8261-4427-0. Qualifying instructors may request access by emailing textbook@springerpub.com.

Instructor's Manual: 978-0-8261-4428-7
Test Bank: 978-0-8261-4429-4
PowerPoint Slides: 978-0-8261-4431-7
Sample Syllabus: 978-0-8261-4432-4

22 23 24 / 5 4 3 2

The author and the publisher of this Work have made every effort to use sources believed to be reliable to provide information that is accurate and compatible with the standards generally accepted at the time of publication. The author and publisher shall not be liable for any special, consequential, or exemplary damages resulting, in whole or in part, from the readers' use of, or reliance on, the information contained in this book. The publisher has no responsibility for the persistence or accuracy of URLs for external or third-party Internet websites referred to in this publication and does not guarantee that any content on such websites is, or will remain, accurate or appropriate.

Library of Congress Cataloging-in-Publication Data

Names: Hewitt, Anne M., editor. | Mascari, Julie L., editor. | Wagner,
  Stephen L., 1951- editor.
Title: Population health management : strategies, tools, applications, and
  outcomes / editors, Anne M. Hewitt, Julie L. Mascari, Stephen L. Wagner.
Other titles: Population health management (Hewitt)
Description: New York, NY : Springer Publishing Company, LLC, [2022] |
  Includes bibliographical references and index.
Identifiers: LCCN 2021021490 (print) | LCCN 2021021491 (ebook) | ISBN
  9780826144263 (paperback) | ISBN 9780826144270 (ebook)
Subjects: MESH Population Health Management | Outcome Assessment, Health
  Care | United States
Classification: LCC RA418.5.P66 (print) | LCC RA418.5.P66 (ebook) | NLM W
  84 AA1 | DDC 362.10973—dc23
LC record available at https://lccn.loc.gov/2021021490
LC ebook record available at https://lccn.loc.gov/2021021491

Contact sales@springerpub.com to receive discount rates on bulk purchases.

Publisher's Note: New and used products purchased from third-party sellers are not guaranteed for quality, authenticity, or access to any included digital components.

Printed in the United States of America by Gasch Printing.

To Bob, whose everlasting support and perceptive humor sustained and enabled all my dreams.

Contents

Contributors ix
Preface xi
Acknowledgments xiii
Podcast List xv
Introduction: Framing the Need for Population Health Management Skills and Competencies xvii

I. POPULATION HEALTH MANAGEMENT

1. Population Health Management: A Framework for the Health Sector 3
   Anne M. Hewitt

2. Public Health Foundations for Population Health Managers 21
   Rosemary M. Caron

3. Assessing Population Health: Community Health Needs Assessments 39
   Anne M. Hewitt and Don Dykstra

4. Social Determinants of Health: Health Promotion for Diverse Populations 55
   Rhonda BeLue, Teaniese Davis, and Michaila Dix

   Appendix A: PRAPARE: Protocol for Responding to Assessing Patient Assets, Risks, and Experiences 71

II. POPULATION HEALTH MANAGEMENT STRATEGIES AND TOOLS

5. Health Data Analytics for Population Health Management 79
   Nalin Johri

6. Population Health Decision-Making: Risk Segmentation, Stratification, and Management 103
   Julie L. Mascari and Anne M. Hewitt

7. Population Health Models—Part I 121
   Anastasia Miller

III. POPULATION HEALTH MANAGEMENT APPLICATIONS

8. Alternative Payment Systems: Volume- to Value-Based Care 139
   Anastasia Miller and Thomas B. Woodard

9. Population Health Models—Part II: Care Coordination Continuum, Behavior Change, Patient Engagement, and Telehealth 155
   Anne M. Hewitt

10. Consumerism: Population Health Marketing Applications — 173
Julie L. Mascari, Moses O. Salami, and Anne M. Hewitt

IV. POPULATION HEALTH MANAGEMENT: OUTCOMES AND ACCOUNTABILITY

11. Population Health Management: Quality Outcomes and Accountability — 191
Stephen L. Wagner

12. Collaborations and Coproduction of Health — 211
Stephen L. Wagner and Anne M. Hewitt

13. Leadership for the Future Health Sector: Transformation, Innovation, and Change for Population Health Managers — 229
Stephen L. Wagner, Patrick D. Shay, and Edward J. Schumacher

V. POPULATION HEALTH MANAGEMENT CASES

14. Case Studies — 253

Case Study 1. Coproduction of Health: *Baby's First* — 255
Anne M. Hewitt

Case Study 2. Implementing a Population Health Data Analytics Platform: A Multispecialty Group Case Study — 263
Ashish Parikh, Jamie L. Reedy, and Nalin Johri

Case Study 3. A Case Study on Population Health Addressing Health Equity During a Crisis: Flattening the Curve of Hispanics With COVID-19 in Somerset County, New Jersey — 273
Paula A. Gutierrez and Serena Collado

Case Study 4. Coproduction Leadership for the Future Health Sector — 279
Patrick D. Shay and Edward J. Schumacher

Glossary — 283
Index — 291

Contributors

Rhonda BeLue, PhD
Professor and Chair, Department of Health Management and Policy, College for Public Health and Social Science, Saint Louis University, St. Louis, Missouri

Rosemary M. Caron, PhD, MPH
Professor, Department of Health Management and Policy, Master of Public Health Program, College of Health and Human Services, University of New Hampshire, Durham, New Hampshire

Serena Collado, MS
Director, Community Health, Robert Wood Johnson University Hospital Somerset, RWJBarnabas Health, Somerville, New Jersey

Teaniese Davis, PhD, MPH
Assistant Professor, Department of Psychology, Morehouse College, Atlanta, Georgia

Michaila Dix
Department of Health Management and Policy, College for Public Health and Social Justice, Saint Louis University, St. Louis, Missouri

Don Dykstra
Director, Planning and System Development, Atlantic Health System, Morristown, New Jersey

Paula A. Gutierrez, MHA
Director, Diversity & Inclusion, Robert Wood Johnson University Hospital Somserset, RWJBarnabas Health, Somerville, New Jersey

Nalin Johri, PhD, MPH
Acting Program Director, Master of Healthcare Administration Program, Department of Interprofessional Health Sciences and Health Administration, School of Health and Medical Sciences, Seton Hall University, Nutley, New Jersey

Anastasia Miller, PhD
Assistant Professor, Department of Healthcare Administration, Texas Woman's University, Dallas, Texas

Ashish Parikh, MD
Chief Quality Officer, Summit Health, Berkeley Heights, New Jersey

Jamie L. Reedy, MD, MPH
Chief Population Health Officer, Summit Health,
Berkeley Heights, New Jersey

Moses O. Salami, MHA
Director, Marketing Communications, Marketing and Public Relations Department, Holy Name Medical Center, Teaneck, New Jersey

Edward J. Schumacher, PhD
Professor, Department of Healthcare Administration, Trinity University, San Antonio, Texas

Patrick D. Shay, PhD, MS
Associate Professor, Department of Healthcare Administration, Trinity University, San Antonio, Texas

Thomas B. Woodard, MBA
Executive Director, Primary Care Partners, Atlantic Health System, Morristown, New Jersey

Preface

Opportunities often arrive in the form of new challenges or final chances to fulfill a special goal. The nexus for this text, *Population Health Management: Strategies, Tools, Approaches, and Outcome,* arises after more than 25 years of teaching experience that coalesced and aligned with a unique body of knowledge known as population health management (PHM). After many semesters of patching together various chapters and sections from an eclectic group of health-related texts, I discovered that other health faculty were also searching for a PHM text appropriate for educating future health managers and professionals. My opportunity finally aligned with the serendipity of both circumstance and timing!

Population health, an approach closely aligned with many public health strategies, enjoys strong general awareness and popularity among health professionals. Although *population health* books are abundant, a smaller number of PHM texts exist, and these vary considerably depending on the writers' background, field of expertise, and perspective. It is not easy to bridge concepts from community, public, and global health and then align them with the essential applications of health management. Combining these interrelated perspectives is the primary goal for the textbook. By melding together fundamental strategies, approaches, and tools from these diverse health-related disciplines, students learn to provide quality care and efficient health services and produce successful outcomes that are sensitive to the needs of diverse populations.

Current experts and critics often suggest that PHM is an enormous topic. I agree that creating a complex, interprofessional approach to PHM requires attention to topic, scope, and depth. Several expert health management faculty and practitioners serve as chapter authors to ensure academic rigor, relevant applications of concepts, and student-friendly learning.

Today's students are bright, articulate, and quick to see diverse ways for defining and solving health sector problems and challenges. My wish is this book provides them with the knowledge, skills, and intentional mind-set to jettison the past in order to transition successfully for today and transform the future of PHM. As healthcare management faculty face daily new teaching challenges, some as consequential as the recent COVID-19 pandemic, the imperative and need is clear.

Anne M. Hewitt, PhD, MA

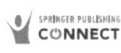 A robust set of instructor resources designed to supplement this text is located at http://connect.springerpub.com/978-0-8261-4427-0. Qualifying instructors may request access by emailing textbook@springerpub.com.

Acknowledgments

Just as nature and nurture form the individual, experience and learning collaborate to inform an author's viewpoint. Beginning with an undergraduate teacher's special guidance, I have benefited from amazing mentors and colleagues who willingly shared their tremendous expertise and provided unselfish support. They all have contributed to the vision for this text. *Population Health Management: Strategies, Tools, Applications, and Outcomes* represents a culmination of years of graduate instruction focused on aligning three interprofessional disciplines, community health, public health, and health administration.

Special thanks to the many faculty colleagues at Seton Hall University, especially Dr. Nalin Johri, who consistently provided wisdom, welcomed humor, and understanding. I also owe great appreciation to the hundreds of graduate students over the years who endured with patience multiple versions of a population health management (PHM) course without this comprehensive text to guide them.

Developing an interdisciplinary text requires expert and informed perspectives from both current faculty and industry professionals. I am extremely grateful to all the contributing chapter and case study authors from across the country and especially the two section editors, Dr. Stephen Wagner and Julie Mascari, MHA, who never say "no" and delivered exceptional individual chapters and edited text sections.

The unwavering support and assistance from both David D'Addona and Jaclyn Shultz of Springer Publishing provided me with motivation, affirmation, and excitement to ensure an enjoyable development process.

And to my family cheerleaders, to my sister Beth for her candid quips and proofreading, and to my daughter Christine, Dan, Peter, and Tommy, a million heartfelt thank-yous for all your love.

Anne M. Hewitt, PhD, MA

To my husband, John, for always encouraging me to exceed my potential and having my back when things work out or not. I love you and our beautiful children, Joe and Jillian, with all my heart.

Julie L. Mascari, MHA

I would like to acknowledge my colleagues of many years, Dr. Anne Hewitt, Dr. Nalin Johri, and Julie Mascari, MHA, for being so supportive and who have helped shape my philosophy of teaching. I would also like to acknowledge the support of my family, especially Cindy, who has provided me with good counsel, perspective on the human condition, and unwavering commitment to what is right. For that I am eternally grateful. Finally, for the many students who I have had the opportunity to work with over the years. I know that they will seek to make our healthcare system better and to improve the health of the people they will serve.

Stephen L. Wagner, PhD, FACHE, LFACMPE

Podcast List

Organized by chapter, the *Population Health Management* podcasts are available as support and provide explanatory information. The majority of chapters include two podcasts. The first presented podcast, the author anecdote, helps place the chapter content into perspective and is narrated by the chapter author. The second podcast, the practitioner perspective, generally applies the chapter information using real-world examples to provide important context. Readers would benefit from listening to the author anecdote first followed by the practitioner perspective. You can access the podcasts by following this link to Springer Publishing Company Connect™: http://connect.springerpub.com/content/book/978-0-8261-4427-0/front-matter/fmatter7

Chapter 1
   Podcast 1.1. What Is Population Health Management?
   Author Anecdote with Anne M. Hewitt

   Podcast 1.2. HRAs, HEDIS, and STARS
   Practitioner Perspective with Julie L. Mascari

Chapter 2
   Podcast 2.1. How Does Public Health Relate to Population Health Management?
   Author Anecdote with Rosemary M. Caron

Chapter 3
   Podcast 3.1. Why Does a Hospital Need to Demonstrate Community Benefit?
   Author Anecdote with Anne M. Hewitt

   Podcast 3.2. Who Needs a Community Health Needs Assessment?
   Practitioner Perspective with Don Dykstra

Chapter 4
   Podcast 4.1. The Impact of Social Determinants of Health-on-Health Outcomes
   Author Anecdote and Practitioner Perspective with Rhonda BeLue and Rocco Gonzalez

Chapter 5
   Podcast 5.1. What Happens When Technology Enables the Health Sector to Move Beyond Only Clinical Data?
   Author Anecdote with Nalin Johri

   Podcast 5.2. Data Analytics as the PHM Challenge
   Practitioner Perspective with Ashish Parikh and Jamie L. Reeder

Chapter 6
Podcast 6.1. Can You Risk Stratify?
Author Anecdote with Anne M. Hewitt

Podcast 6.2. Moving Onto Risk Decision-Making
Practitioner Perspective with Julie L. Mascari

Chapter 7
Podcast 7.1. QUICK: Define IDS, ACO, and PCMH
Author Anecdote with Anastasia Miller

Podcast 7.2. Why Doesn't One Size Fit All for Our Patients?
Practitioner Perspective with Shannon Huggins

Chapter 8
Podcast 8.1. What Do You Know About Risk and Financial Incentives?
Author Anecdote with Anastasia Miller

Podcast 8.2. Have ACOs Changed Over Time?
Practitioner Perspective with Thomas B. Woodard

Chapter 9
Podcast 9.1. Could You Identify Four New Patient-Centered Care Strategies?
Author Anecdote with Anne M. Hewitt

Podcast 9.2. Virtual Care or Telehealth?
Practitioner Perspective with Harshal Shah

Chapter 10
Podcast 10.1. How Did You Find Your Doctor?
Author Anecdote with Julie L. Mascari

Podcast 10.2. Think of the Last Item You Purchased – Why Did You Buy It?
Practitioner Perspective with Moses O. Salami

Chapter 11
Podcast 11.1. What Is the Real Purpose of Quality Improvement?
Author Anecdote with Stephen L. Wagner

Podcast 11.2. Moving to Become a High Reliability Organization
Practitioner Perspective with Ishani Ved

Chapter 12
Podcast 12.1. Isn't Cooperation the Same as Collaboration?
Author Anecdote with Stephen L. Wagner

Podcast 12.2. Collaborators and Not Competitors
Practitioner Perspective with Paschal Nwako

Chapter 13
Podcast 13.1. Understanding Design Thinking
Author Anecdote with Patrick D. Shay and Edward J. Schumacher

Podcast 13.2. From Transactions to Transformations: Innovation at Work
Practitioner Perspective with John E. Hornbeak

Introduction: Framing the Need for Population Health Management Skills and Competencies

Despite years of federal health task forces and reports, various philanthropic foundations' initiatives, countless health professional organizations' recommendations, and legislative and regulatory mandates, the American healthcare system remains complex, inconsistent, and costly (Tikkanen & Abrams, 2020). With the passage of the Patient Protection and Affordable Care Act (PPACA, 2010), a new policy and regulatory framework helped speed up the greatly needed transformation of the health sector's triple aim focus on quality, cost, and access to care (Berwick et al., 2008). Responding to these demanding challenges and innovative policy pathways, population health emerged as an alternative strategy to the traditional medical model of taking care of one patient at a time accompanied by a fee-for-service payment system. Population health management (PHM) is now a viable approach to transform U.S. healthcare. Current health management students will need PHM strategies and tools to effectively visualize the next 10 years and move toward a management care model that ensures optimal health for all populations.

ENSURING POPULATION HEALTH MANAGEMENT LEARNING AND COMPETENCIES

Regardless of a student's discipline and/or background experience, the PHM career pathway requires mastery of an integrated population management perspective. Both faculty and students recognize that knowledge can be only the first marker of managerial excellence and that the second step requires skill development. As presented in this text, both these learning processes result in the successful attainment of student competencies.

Each of this book's four sections integrates a scaffolding framework that begins with PHM fundamentals and introductions to innovative strategies/tools, moves to problem-based applications, and culminates with integrated skill outcomes. Written by experts in their respective disciplines, each chapter is relatable for students from diverse health-related programs such as health management, public health, social work, clinical degrees, and other health professions (see Figure 1).

These four sections align with the industry standard's Population Health Alliance (PHA) PHM Framework (Population Health Alliance, n.d.) as a visual step-by-step process model applicable to all health professions (see Figure 2).

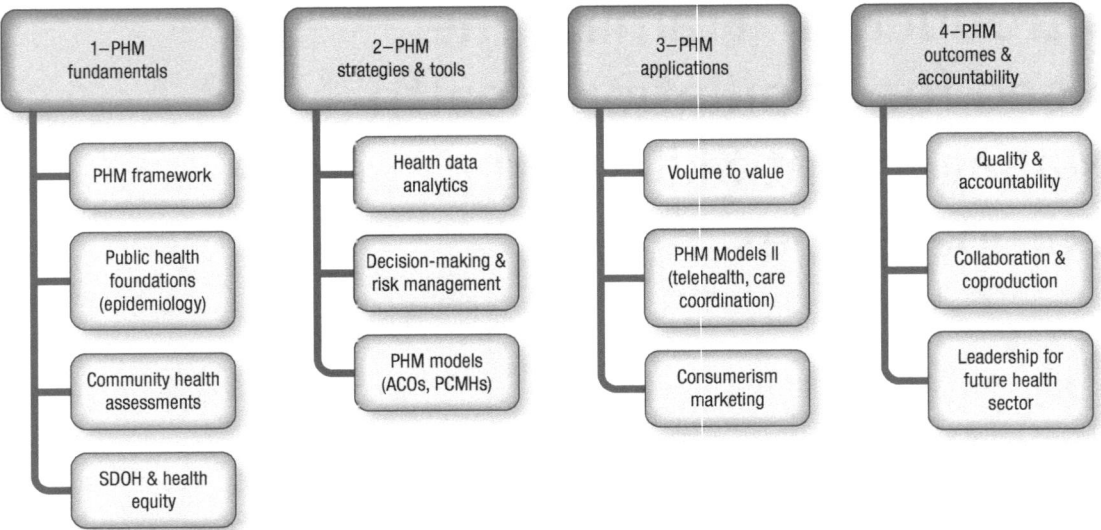

FIGURE 1 Population Health Management Topic Outline by Sections and Chapters

SECTION I—POPULATION HEALTH MANAGEMENT FUNDAMENTALS

To frame Section I, which presents PHM fundamentals, the first chapter introduces important health management frameworks, recent policy impact factors, and contemporary, implementation models that now guide healthcare delivery. This chapter also provides a clear explanation of differences and commonalities between PHM and public health (PH). Chapter 2 presents essential public health strategies and skills including applications of basic and managerial epidemiology (rates, prevalence, incidence, and risk ratios). Chapters 3 and 4 further describe PHM approaches via explanations of community health needs assessment protocols and applications, and the importance of social determinants of health, the role of health equity and equality, and health promotion principles and tools for diverse populations.

SECTION II—POPULATION HEALTH MANAGEMENT STRATEGIES AND TOOLS

Section II reviews current and emerging PHM technology options and innovative decision-making techniques. Chapters 5 through 7 present and discuss strategies and useful tools that emphasize the roles of information technology (data analytics, predictive models, and artificial intelligence) as well as the crucial steps involved in PHM decision-making efforts for risk segmentation and stratification. The final chapter in this section covers three essential PHM models: Accountable Care Organizations, Patient-Centered Medical Homes, and the Chronic Condition Care Management Model.

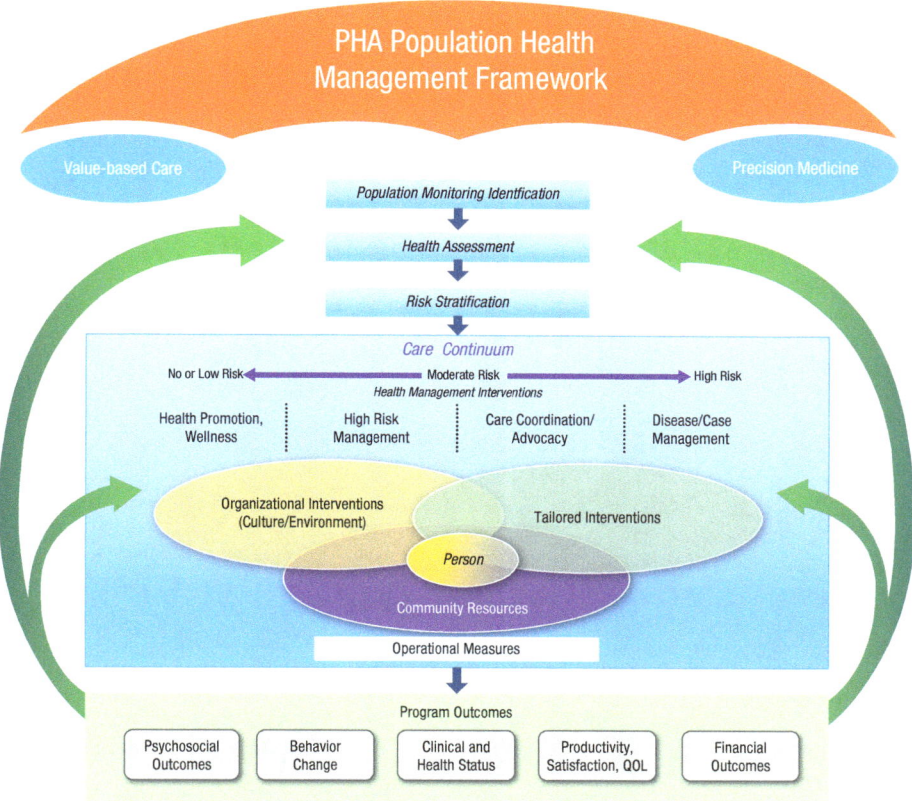

FIGURE 2 Textbook Section Alignment With PHA Population Health Management Framework

PHA, Population Health Alliance.

Source: Population Health Alliance. (n.d.). *PHA—Population health management framework.* Population Health Alliance. Reprinted with permission © PHA PHM Framework 2010 PHA–PMH Umbrella for VBC 2018 RMaljanian. https://population healthalliance.org/research/understanding-population-health/

SECTION III—POPULATION HEALTH MANAGEMENT APPLICATIONS

Building on the skills developed in the previous chapters, Section III provides management application examples. As most PHM applications emphasize cost analysis, Chapter 8 describes and explains volume to value management models and includes the essential financial risk continuum. Chapter 9 introduces emerging Population Healthcare Delivery Models including Telehealth/Virtual Care/Remote Care Monitoring and patient engagement pathways. Chapter 10 reviews the current roles of consumerism and behavioral economics, along with both marketing and social marketing applications as important PHM components.

SECTION IV—POPULATION HEALTH MANAGEMENT: OUTCOMES AND ACCOUNTABILITY

Healthcare managers remain continually focused on improving quality and safety while reducing cost. Chapter 11 describes essential quality

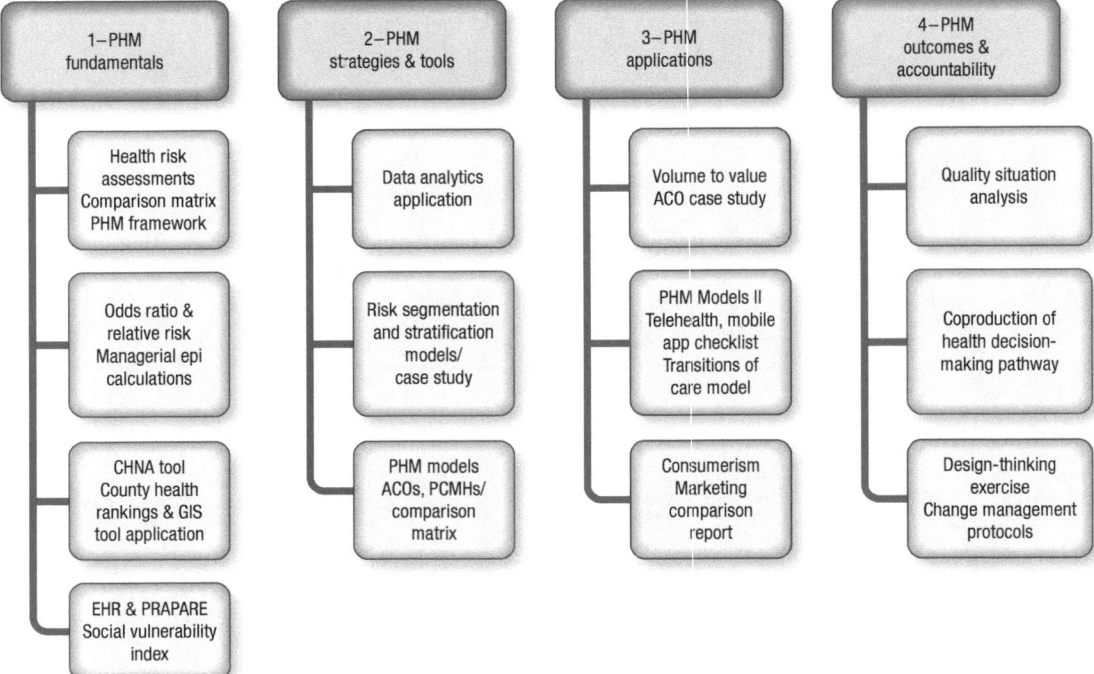

FIGURE 3 Population Health Management Tools and Applications by Sections and Chapters

management approaches and the importance of comparative effectiveness research as applicable to PHM. In Chapter 12, the emerging coproduction of health process introduces models for partnering with new community partners, other innovative organizations, and even converting current competitors to collaborators. The authors of Chapter 13 share a contemporary perspective on strategic planning skills with an emphasis on systems design, innovation, and change management as vital for improving future population health outcomes.

POPULATION HEALTH MANAGEMENT STRATEGIES AND TOOLS APPLICATIONS

To ensure that strategies, techniques, and tools adequately translate into skills and competencies, each chapter includes various models, frameworks, checklists, sample calculations, mini case studies, or simulations to ensure students' proficiency in utilizing PHM concepts (Figure 3).

POPULATION HEALTH MANAGEMENT CASE STUDIES

Recognizing the importance for students to apply and synthesize the PHM chapter concepts, four diverse case studies (Section V) for integrated learning, critical thinking, and strategic analysis are included:

- Coproduction of Health: *Baby's First*
- Implementing a Population Health Data Analytics Platform: A Multispecialty Group Case Study

- A Case Study on Population Health Addressing Health Equity During a Crisis: Flattening the Curve of Hispanics with COVID-19 in Somerset County, New Jersey
- Coproduction Leadership for the Future Health Sector

Each case study features opportunities for integrative PHM strategic and critical thinking.

POPULATION HEALTH MANAGEMENT TEXT COMPETENCY ALIGNMENT

This textbook's content, objectives, and competency statements support established guidelines from national taskforces and/or professional accrediting organizations including the Health Leadership Competency Model 3.0 (NCHL, 2018) and the Competencies for Population Health Professionals (CPHP) (Public Health Foundation, 2019). A matrix aligning each chapter's objectives with the corresponding CPHP and NCHL competencies is available in the Instructor's Manual. To meet requirements, competency building activities were integrated using multidisciplinary approaches that emphasize interprofessional education perspectives as recommended by the Association of Schools and Programs of Public Health (ASPPH) in their publication, *Population Health Across All Professions* (ASPPH, 2015).

INSTRUCTOR RESOURCES

All PHM text chapters include key terms, learning objectives with aligned student competencies, and mini case studies/examples, tables and figures, discussion questions, and suggested resources. The Instructor's Manual also provides examples of classroom activities and teaching tips. Other resources include PowerPoints and a Test Bank. Each chapter introduces a skill-building tool and includes an applied activity to demonstrate student mastery. Podcasts are available for all chapters. This text enables students to develop a strong toolkit of new skills and capabilities to solve contemporary PHM problems.

SUMMARY

As major PHM transformations continue to evolve in the workplace, health management educators recognize the immediate need to design curriculums, introduce new skill-building approaches and tools, and enhance student competencies to meet the challenges and find solutions for a future healthscape that achieves the quadruple aim of access, cost, quality, and patient experience.

REFERENCES

Association of Schools and Programs of Public Health. (2015). *Population health across all professions expert panel report.* www.aspph.org/ftf-reports/population-health-in-all-professions/

Berwick, D., Nolan, T., & Whittington, J. (2008). The triple aim: Care, health, and cost. *Health Affairs, 27*(3), 759–769. https://www.healthaffairs.org/doi/full/10.1377/hlthaff.27.3.759

National Center for Healthcare Leadership. (2018). *Health Leadership Competency Model 3.0.* https://www.oha.com/Documents/NCHL%20Health%20Leadership%20Competency%20Model.pdf?utm_medium=email&utm_campaign=October%202%20-%20HR%20Leadership%20Program&utm_content=October%202%20-%20HR%20Leadership%20Program+Preview+CID_8723ddd7c9948150198964a92e7f520a&utm_source=CampaignMonitor#:~:text=A%20health%20leadership%20model%20adds,clinical%20practice%2C%20and%20to%20faculty.&text=The%20NCHL%20Health%20Leadership%20Competency,to%20the%20unique%20health%20environment

Patient Protection and Affordable Care Act. (2010, March 23). *The patient protection and affordable care act (PPACA)*, Pub. L. No. 111-148, 124 *Stat.* 119.

Public Health Foundation. (2019, March). *Competencies for Population Health Professionals.* http://www.phf.org/resourcestools/Pages/Population_Health_Competencies.aspx

Population Health Alliance. (n.d.). *PHA—Population health management framework.* Population Health Alliance. https://populationhealthalliance.org/research/understanding-population-health/

Tikkanen, R., & Abrams, M. (2020, January 30). U.S. Health Care from a Global Perspective, 2019: Higher spending, worse outcomes? *The Commonwealth Fund.* https://www.commonwealthfund.org/publications/issue-briefs/2020/jan/us-health-care-global-perspective-2019?gclid=CjwKCAiAsaOBBhA4EiwAo0_AnHHtGcdzhQYmbJO4US49IMIQ_aDx2tmwoWyS9JN7svwI30j32hqZBRoCqSAQAvD_BwE

PART I

Population Health Management

CHAPTER 1

Population Health Management: A Framework for the Health Sector

Anne M. Hewitt

KEY TERMS

Community Health
Components of Health
Culture of Health
Global Health
Health
High-Level Wellness
Population Health

Population Health Alliance Framework
Population Health Management (PHM)
Public Health
Spectrum of Health
Triple/Quadruple Aim
Wellness

LEARNING OBJECTIVES

1. Define population health management (PHM).
2. Identify at least five major factors that contributed to the need for new healthcare delivery models in the 21st century.
3. Describe the importance of Healthy People 2020.
4. Compare and contrast public, community, global, and population health.
5. Discuss the various population health models and frameworks (Pathways to Population Health [P2PH], the Four Pillars of Health, and the National Priorities Partnership [NPP]).
6. Describe the Population Health Alliance's PHM Framework.

> Podcasts that exemplify the content of this chapter are available at Springer Publishing Connect™
>
> Podcast 1.1. What Is Population Health Management?
> Podcast 1.2. HRAs, HEDIS, and STARS

Access the podcast online at http://connect.springerpub.com/content/book/978-0-8261-4427-0/part/part01/chapter/ch01

INTRODUCTION

"Population"—"health"—"management." Three well-known words, but when combined they represent a 21st-century unique approach to health. This chapter introduces and defines PHM, provides examples of supporting frameworks and models, describes useful strategies, and highlights future challenges.

PHM, coupled with rapid technological and genetic advances, represents the most influential healthcare administrative challenges for the near future.

To better understand the importance of PHM, consider a single example that represents one of the biggest health challenges for America to date. Compare the two photographs in Figure 1.1 before reading the narrative explanation.

More than a century ago, the world suffered a major influenza pandemic that cost an estimated 500 million lives (CDC, 2019). Although global epidemics have emerged in recent years, such as SARS, MERS, Ebola, and Zika (Vass, 2020), no one expected the catastrophic COVID-19 (SARS-2) pandemic with its disastrous human and economic impact. Similarities between the previous pandemic and the universal health disaster of COVID-19 exist, but the U.S. health system response differed significantly to mitigate the number of lives lost (Mineo, 2020). All components of the nation's health sector transformed within a span of a few weeks to fulfill the medical needs of the population. The concepts of PHM were essential and applicable to help the health sector meet this incredible challenge. Health managers, administrators, and other health professionals in leadership positions rapidly addressed the crisis issues of care coordination, availability of first responders, lack of personal protective equipment (PPE), surge capacity for intensive care unit (ICU) beds and ventilators, and even conducting parking-lot, drive-by tests, and screenings. All the fundamental components of basic management and administration (Olden, 2019) were utilized to secure the *health* and safety of the American people. This single example frames the importance of PHM as a strategic skill and competency for all health professionals.

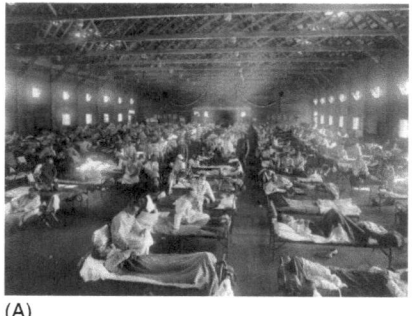
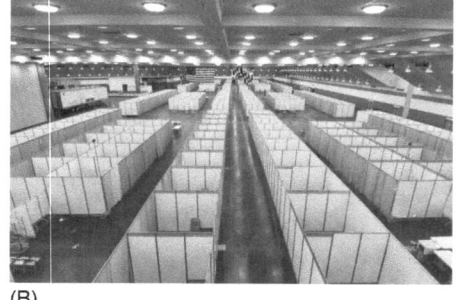

(A) (B)

FIGURE 1.1 Comparison of Pandemic Field Hospitals 1919–2020. (A) Emergency hospital in the midst of the influenza epidemic, Camp Funston, Kansas, circa 1918 (NCP 1603). OHA 250 New Contributed Photographs. Otis Historical Archives, National Museum of Health and Medicine. Reprinted by permission. (B) 2020 COVID-19 Field Hospital. Courtesy of Maryland GovPics

Aligning Health and Wellness With Population Health Management

PHM is a blending of three disciplines and to fully examine the relationships between these concepts. We begin by discussing the operational meanings of "health," followed by a review of population definitions, and finally a synthesis of emerging management roles and responsibilities. See Box 1.1.

What Is Health?

Most clinical, public health, and other health profession students recognize the WHO definition of **health**—"a state of complete physical, mental and social well-being and not the merely the absence of disease or infirmity" (WHO, 1946). Why was this definition so important? Because it challenged the established medical model that stated you were healthy if you were not sick. For centuries, the medical (disease-focused) model had served as the foundation for most practiced medicine. But the WHO definition neglected to include a "spiritual" or an "emotional" component, and it was not until Canadian health promotion and community health experts developed the "wellness" model that a more holistic definition of health was introduced to the medical establishment (Ottawa, 1986). Today, the concept of wellness has expanded exponentially as individuals define personal wellness on a continuum based on their perceptions, goals, and healthy activities.

Table 1.1 presents the five components of individual health, and Figure 1.2. depicts **high-level wellness** as a desirable balance and integration between the five **components of health**.

Wellness is visually expressed as a balanced state of the five interrelating components.

The idea of personal health and wellness being defined by the individual serves as a foundation for current health promotion and disease prevention activities. Today, these concepts guide us as an accepted framework for contemporary American healthcare and policy. We all seek to live a long and healthy life and the compression of morbidity is the idea that the length of time a person spends sick or disabled can be reduced, so that maximum life span is achieved (Stibich, 2019).

The WHO defines quality of life as an individual's perception of their position in life in the context of the culture and value systems in which they live and in relation to their goals, expectations, standards, and concerns (WHO, 1995).

But health status is not just determined by the five personal factors described earlier as we all live, work, and play in different circumstances, and these also impact our health status. Experts have determined that diverse external

BOX 1.1 Conceptual Progression for Population Health Management (PHM)

What is health?
What is population health?
What is PHM?
What is the role of PHM?
How does it differ from previous health management approaches?
How do we implement PHM?
What have been the major impacts of PHM?

TABLE 1.1 Components of Individual Health

Component	Definition
Physical health	Ability to perform daily tasks without undue fatigue, refers to the biological integrity of the individual.
Social health	Ability to interact well with people and the environment. Having satisfying interpersonal relationships.
Mental health	Ability to learn, one's intellectual capacity.
Emotional health	Ability to control emotions so that one feels comfortable expressing them when appropriate and does not express them inappropriately.
Spiritual health	Belief in some unifying force. For some, it is nature; for others, it is scientific laws, and for others, it is a godlike force.

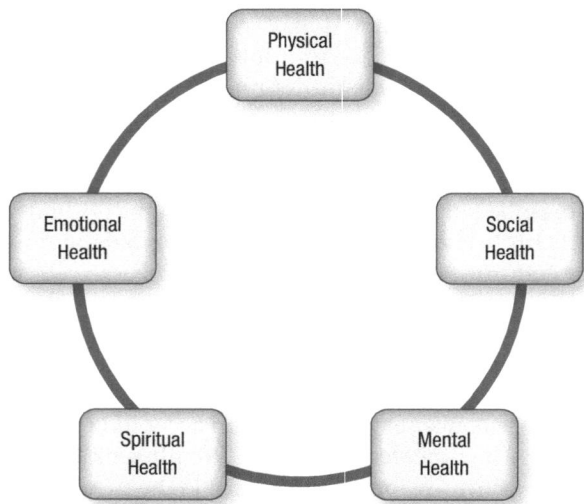

FIGURE 1.2 High-Level Wellness: Total Alignment of Health Components

factors affect our health and determine our quality of life, and because these external factors affect more than just "groups of individuals," we refer to those affected as populations. The commonly mentioned external factors are environmental, socioeconomic (SEC) status, health behaviors (lifestyle), and quality of healthcare.

In Figure 1.3, notice the population health factor with the highest percent impact on health status refers to SEC factors (40%) and not healthcare (Short & Mollborn, 2015). The concept of SEC factors, an important component of assessing a population's health risk, has been expanded to be more inclusive and replaced by the social determinants of health (SDOH), which is much more than just assessing income and educational levels. SDOH are especially important for managing a population's health. Also note that the second largest impact factor contributing to health status relates to basic lifestyle behaviors! Over 70% of our health status can be attributed to our lifestyle choices and SDOH. This finding represents one of the primary challenges for population health managers.

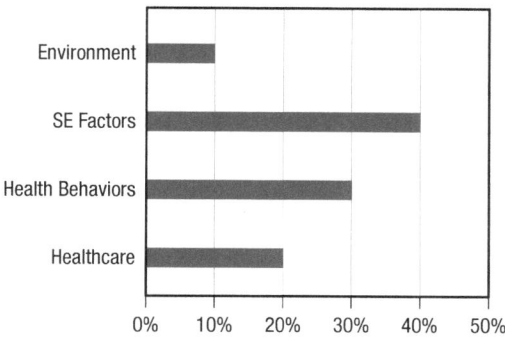

FIGURE 1.3 Population Health Status Factors

What Is Population Health?

Today, the wellness model, with an emphasis on quality of life, serves as a framework for individual, public, community, and global health as well as population health. The term **population health** was defined early in the 21st century as "the health outcomes of a group of individuals, including the distribution of such outcomes within the group" (Kindig & Stoddart, 2003). Population health focuses on groups and not the individual and expands and enhances previous health approaches such as public, community, and global health.

DID YOU KNOW?

Understanding Community, Public, Global, and Population Health Approaches

Review the four types of health approaches and perspectives explained and placed in context in the following videos.
What is community health?
www.youtube.com/watch?v=vSkCc5coS7c
What is public health?
http://www.youtube.com/watch?v=Bpu42LmLo4U
What is global health?
https://vimeo.com/14017971, https://vimeo.com/55371178
What is population health?
https://www.youtube.com/watch?v=Ik2DszDb1Eg
https://www.youtube.com/watch?v=O5WtS_q4_zI&feature=youtu.be

Notice the *differences* and similarities between these types of health approach definitions as presented in Table 1.2.

As you watched these videos and then compared them with the corresponding definitions, the various perspectives toward quality of life and health should have been evident. Each of these approaches refers to a specific group—meaning a defined and distinct set of people. In the United States, **public health's** three-pronged mandated focus, which includes assessment, policy development, and assurance (safety net services), encompasses everyone. Sometimes, public health and population health are used interchangeably although they are not identical.

TABLE 1.2 Definitions for Public, Community, Global, and Population Health

Type of Health Approach	Definition
Public health	"Science and art of preventing disease, prolonging life, and promoting physical health and efficiency through organized community efforts" (Winslow, 1920).
Community health	"Refers to the health status of a defined group of people and the actions and conditions, both private and public (governmental), to promote, protect, and preserve their health" (McKenzie et al., 2005).
Global health	"Collaborative trans-national research and action for promoting health for all" (Beaglehole & Bonita, 2010).
Population health	"The health outcomes of a group of individuals, including the distribution of such outcomes within the group" (Kindig & Stoddart, 2003).

A community is "a group of people who have common characteristics," but communities can be defined by location, race, ethnicity, age, occupation, education, interests, and other diverse characteristics. Often, a community priority population is based on geographic area, but the location and size determine a group as in the case of a municipality, as compared with public health, which includes all within a national boundary. **Global health** has no physical boundary.

DID YOU KNOW?

Culture of Health: An Exemplary Model for Population Health

The Culture of Health model, developed in 2013, combines essential components of community, public, global, and population health approaches. The Culture of Health: Action Framework emerged from a collaboration between the Robert Wood Johnson Foundation and Rand Corporation (Chandra et al., 2017). The 10 principles provide a foundation for four action steps (Figure 1.4).

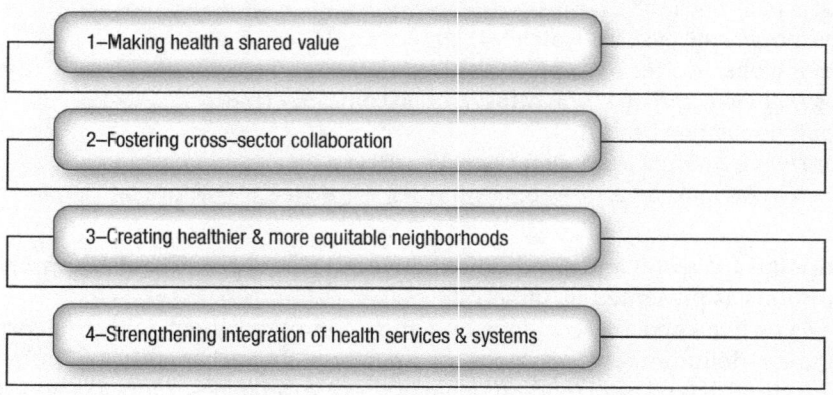

FIGURE 1.4 Culture of Health: Action Framework

This widely adopted national model focuses on improving community health outcomes and emphasizes the elimination of health disparities, which reinforces and aligns with Healthy People's 2020 ongoing goal to reduce health inequities (CDC, 2020a).
A **culture of health** and wellness is also characterized by these activities:
- Makes it easier and more rewarding to select lifestyles that foster health
- Cultivates the appropriate use of healthcare services
- Leverages all population health strategies
- Provides and tracks the progress of risk reduction programs
- Assures that participants have easy access to healthcare services
- Fosters the use of evidence-based clinical guidelines
- Promotes health throughout the workplace environment
- Assess and improves its program regularly

Several of the 10 principles rely on PHM activities that do not occur in community health or public health initiatives, including the focus on delivery care models and risk reduction monitoring.

Population health differs from public health because of its continuum of care approach and the capability to provide comprehensive health services. And yet, both health approaches regularly incorporate health promotion strategies. Population health significantly expanded health services by emphasizing health outcomes and moving away from individual acute care as the primary healthcare focus (Faulk, 2014). A huge misunderstanding of the definitions of public, population health, and PHM still exists, and this text presents important discussion about healthcare administrators' roles and responsibilities for each of these categories.

The Two Key Questions for Population Health Managers
Who is defining the population?
Who is paying for the population's healthcare?

These are the two most important issues for population health managers, and their impacts go beyond defining populations by geographic and demographics parameters.

Defining the Role of Population Health Management

PHM has been characterized as gathering and analyzing data to solve problems and/or a variety of approaches developed to foster health and quality of care improvements while managing costs. **Population health management** also refers to the process of improving clinical health outcomes of a defined group of individuals through improved care coordination and patient engagement supported by appropriate financial and care models (AHA, n.d.). But the clearest definition of PHM stresses the functions and operations of healthcare delivery, the importance of a system approach, and optimal health outcomes that are also cost efficient. PHM has to do with the organization and management of the healthcare delivery system in a manner that makes it more clinically effective, cost-effective and safer. PHM means "the proactive application of strategies and interventions to defined groups of individuals across the continuum of care to improve the health of the individuals within the group at the lowest necessary cost" (Burton, 2015; Caron, 2017).

Regardless of the definition, PHM implements and integrates the various strategies, models, and approaches and has become the touchpoint for new innovations in delivering care, not just for one individual at a time, but for defined populations, to achieve a cross-sector coordinated system instead of unconnected silos of healthcare.

How Does Population Health Management Differ From Previous Health Approaches?

The answer is found within the question "Who defines the population?" In PHM, a health system chooses to provide healthcare to a specific population made up of its consumers and patients and defines the population based on its own criteria. This differs significantly from public health and other federal government health initiatives. Healthcare systems are also impacted by payers whether they be public, private, or state, regional, national, and international in size. These financing organizations directly influence a health system's choice of priority populations. PHM helps to develop a partnership between providers and the patient community built on mutual trust and effort to generate better outcomes for everyone involved in the process of care (Bresnick, 2015). Some experts suggest that PHM may refer to an arbitrarily designated group of individuals that may not even define themselves as a community.

In summary, PHM is concerned with who, where, and when health services are provided, the appropriate cost of the service, and population health outcomes. Given that PHM provides the necessary operational expertise to ensure the desired outcomes of a specific healthy population, the next question is, "How do we implement PHM?"

Population Health Management Approaches and Frameworks

There has been no lack of population health approaches in the 21st century to address the challenges of providing quality healthcare, but fewer models emerged specific to PHM. The initial population health models and frameworks formed a foundation for PHM to evolve and be adopted by healthcare organizations and systems. Figure 1.5 is a brief timeline that frames this model's development progress over time.

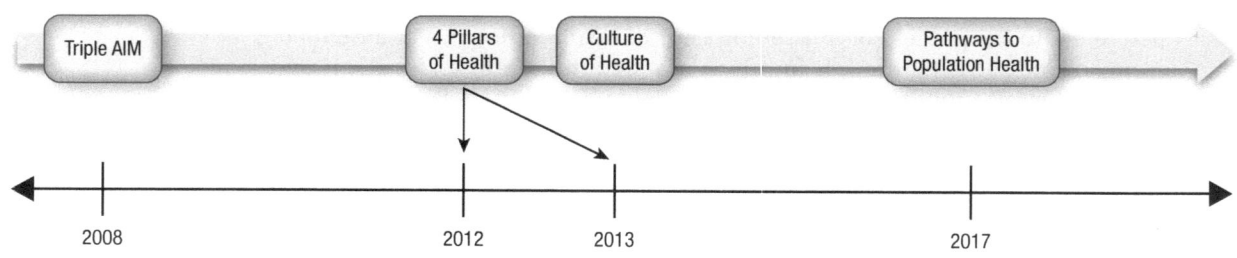

FIGURE 1.5 Timeline of Population Health Frameworks and Models
Source: Adapted from Triple Aim (Berwick et al., 2008), Pillars of Health (2012–2013); Culture of Health: Action Framework (Institute for Health Improvement [IHI], n.d.); P2PH (Chandra et al., 2017).

These PH frameworks included the Triple Aim, the Culture of Health, P2PH, and the Four Pillars of Health. Why were new models needed? While the Affordable Care Act of 2010 served as a catalyst for change, no definitive strategies were clearly outlined in the lengthy document and healthcare experts began to identify underlying conceptual ideas, frameworks, and approaches for implementing population health. Although concepts of population health were borrowed from public health strategies, the healthcare industry relied on a few major frameworks for guidance to transition the healthcare sector, such as the Healthy People initiatives. Healthy People 2020 serves as cornerstone for addressing population health issues.

DID YOU KNOW?

The Role of Healthy People 2020

Healthy People 2020 serves as the latest national health strategy that provides goals, objectives, baselines, and future targets to serve as a unifying strategy and accountability pathway to improve every American's health status. The current Healthy People 2020 is based on the accomplishments of four previous Healthy People initiatives (Office of Disease Prevention and Health Promotion [ODPHP], n.d.).
- 1979 Surgeon General's Report: *Healthy People: The Surgeon General's Report on Health Promotion and Disease Prevention*
- *Healthy People 1990: Promoting Health/Preventing Disease: Objectives for the Nation*
- *Healthy People 2000: National Health Promotion and Disease Prevention Objectives*
- *Healthy People 2010: Objectives for Improving Health*

Every 10 years, the Healthy People goals are updated by a diverse group of individuals, organizations, and experts. Healthy People 2020 major goals include the following:
1. Attaining high-quality, longer lives free of preventable disease, disability, injury, and premature death
2. Achieving health equity, eliminating disparities, and improving the health of all groups
3. Creating social and physical environments that promote good health for all
4. Promoting quality of life, healthy development, and healthy behaviors across all the stages (CDC, 2020a)

Achieving health equity and creating positive social and physical environments remain a major challenge for the federal government, states, municipalities, and local public health offices. Preparations began for Healthy People 2030 on August 18, 2020 (CDC, 2020b). Healthy People 2020 served as a cornerstone for addressing population health issues.

The Triple Aim

The original idea for a tripart health sector framework was articulated by Berwick et al. in 2008 and later validated by the Institute for Healthcare Improvement (IHI). The **Triple Aim** underlined three important and sometimes lacking aspects of healthcare: access, cost, and quality. Today, population health initiatives routinely evaluate success by these criteria. These three goals remain difficult to implement in a systematic way and require continuous quality initiatives and innovations to reduce waste and streamline the care delivery model. The Triple Aim, one of the most referenced population health models, articulated a clear requirement that all three factors be pursued simultaneously, which necessitated a new approach— not one based on the medical model of one person at a time healthcare with fee for service. This approach also emphasized the cost factor needed to be a central consideration, and the current fee structures were unsustainable. Now, the Triple Aim has become the Quadruple Aim, with the fourth focus point being either the "joy of work" or "pursuing health equity" (Feeley, 2017). Given the health industry's focus on quality, this model appeals strongly to both public and private sectors.

The NPP: In 2008, an elite group of approximately 50 national healthcare organizations issued four major healthcare challenges for population health (National Priorities Partnership [NPP], 2008). As individual healthcare providers and organizations were encouraged to transition away from the medical model, it was just as vital for professional organizations to support the population health movement. These four goals became aligned with institutional strategic plans:

- Eliminating harm
- Eradicating disparities
- Reducing illness
- Removing waste

This model integrated concepts from other previous frameworks but also added a primary emphasis on eliminating harm. Two earlier national reports, *To Err Is Human* (NAM, 2000) and *Crossing the Quality Chasm: A New Health System for the 21st Century* (NAM, 2001), served as catalysts to reduce the number of harmful errors in the health system and to focus on both quality and safety.

The Four Pillars of Health: Another popular population health approach provided a unique view that integrated management issues (quality and safety) with public health and policy (Nash, 2012). See Figure 1.6.

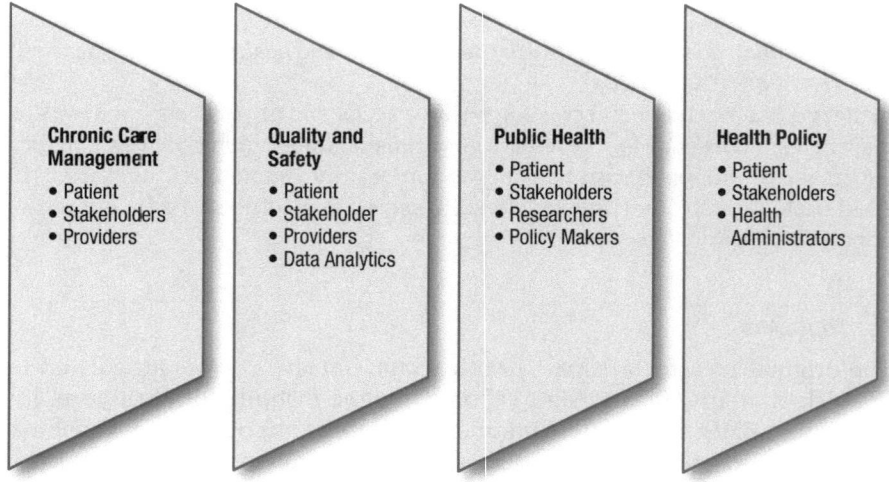

FIGURE 1.6 The Four Pillars of Health

This framework provided an opportunity for beginning transitions in healthcare that involved the entire health sector. Each of the four topics could be operationalized to include which parties were responsible and accountable, as well as aligning the drivers of health, (need) appropriate locations and sites of care, and timing of care (Fabius, 2021).

P2PH: A more recent collaboration between the American Hospital Association (AHA) and the IHI along with other major stakeholders produced the P2PH framework in 2017 (IHI, n.d.). This framework focuses on four portfolios of population health that help healthcare entities organize their work leading to sustainable advances in population health. The four portfolios consist of multiple steps and pathways to achieve specific goals, including the following:

P1: Physical and/or Mental Health

P2: Social and/or Spiritual Well-Being

P3: Community Health and Well-Being

P4: Communities of Solutions (Saha et al., 2017)

The unique feature of this popular P2PH framework is the design capability to align with community coalitions, municipalities, and hospitals.

For a comparison view of these population health models and frameworks, see Table 1.3.

All these models and pathways provide population health frameworks for implementation purposes. But they do not completely address PHM, as the enterprise system view is missing. Population health managers need to function as cross-sector integrators.

How Do We Implement Population Health Management?

The Population Health Alliance (PHA) conceptual model for PHM pragmatically envisions the various functions and roles to effectively operate in today's health environment. The PHA's **PHM Framework** was developed by

TABLE 1.3 Comparison of Population Health Models and the PHA–PHM Framework

Culture of Health	Triple/ Quadruple Aim	NPP	P2PH	Four Pillars of Health	PHA–PHM Framework
Making health a shared value	Access to healthcare	Eliminating harm	Physical and/or mental health	Chronic care management	Assessment
Fostering cross-sector collaboration	Cost of healthcare	Eliminating disparities	Social and/or spiritual well-being	Quality and safety	Stratification
Creating healthier and more equitable neighborhoods	Healthcare quality	Reducing illness	Community health and well-being	Public health	Person-centered intervention
Strengthening integration of health services and systems		Reducing waste	Communities of solutions	Health policy	Impact evaluation

the industry's multistakeholder professional and trade association and conceptualizes healthcare delivery systems implementation activities for quality health outcomes (PHA, n.d.). See Figure 1.7.

NPP, National Priorities Partnership; PHA, Population Health Alliance; PHM, population health management; P2PH, Pathways to Population Health.

The PHM Framework simplifies administrative processes into four operational action steps: Assessment (knowing your population), Stratification (identifying risk level), Person-Centered Intervention (aligning patient's needs using available resources and tailored plans), and Impact Evaluation (assessing health status, effectiveness, and efficiency). Aligned with the overarching process umbrella are two important and relatively new impact factors: value-based care and precision medicine.

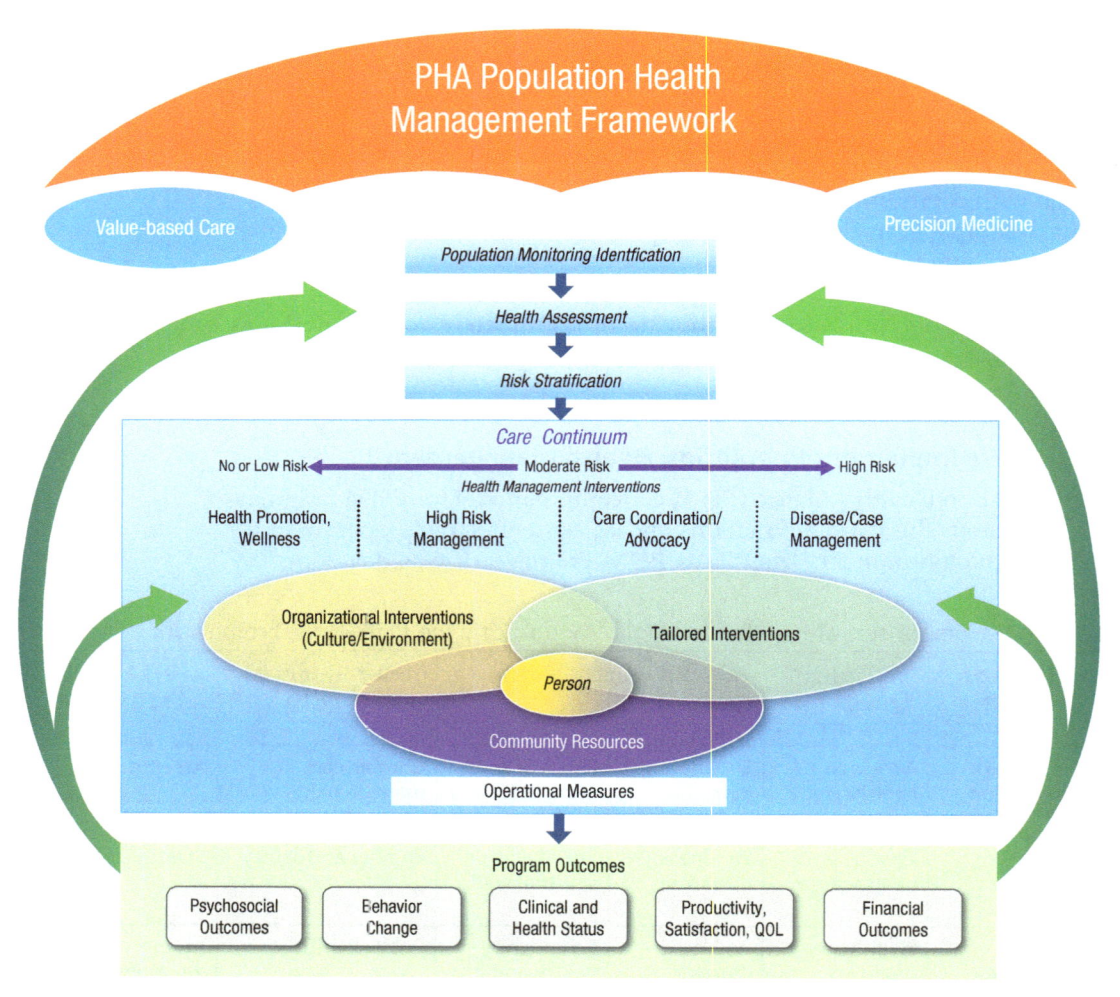

FIGURE 1.7 PHA Population Health Management Framework

PHA, Population Health Alliance.

Source: Population Health Alliance. (n.d.). *PHA—Population health management framework.* Population Health Alliance. Reprinted with permission © PHA PHM Framework 2010 PHA–PMH Umbrella for VBC 2018 RMaljanian. https://population healthalliance.org/research/understanding-population-health/

DID YOU KNOW?

PHM Framework

The PHM Framework's primary strength is that it addresses the health needs at all stages along the **continuum of health** and wellness. As presented in the framework, the Care Continuum includes multiple segments: Health Promotion/Wellness, Health Risk Assessment, Care Coordination and Advocacy, and Disease/Case Management. Notice the two-way flow of information showing a reciprocal relationship between all components for the framework. Healthcare managers and administrators can apply these conceptual ideas by aligning and completing identified operational tasks with each process stage. The PHA framework introduced an administrative process perspective and continued the PH priorities for community partnerships, patient-centered care, cultural inclusion, expanded program outcome scope and breadth, and accountability. Most importantly, because the person remains central to all processes, the framework can be applied and adapted to multiple populations whether they are determined by geographic area, health status, or insurance affiliation.

Recent healthcare challenges may serve as catalysts for revisions to the current population health and PHM models, frameworks, and pathways presented, just as the PHM Framework was recently updated to include value-based care and precision medicine.

Population Health Management: Impact and Outcomes

At the beginning of the 21st century, and even preceding that, three major health sectors—the public (consumers), private and nonprofit healthcare institutions, and government (public health)—began to recognize the limitations of the current fragmented healthcare system. Primary stakeholders, such as business employers, insurance companies, and financial institutions, also voiced dissatisfaction with unacceptable health outcomes and unsustainable healthcare costs. The Affordable Care Act passed in 2010 became the catalyst that precipitated the adoption of new population approaches and led directly to necessary changes for improved access to healthcare and increased accountability for delivery and services.

DID YOU KNOW?

Patient Protection and Affordability Care Act and Population Health Management

Experts compare the significance of the Patient Protection and Affordability Care Act of 2010 to the major health industry legislation of the 1960s that introduced the concepts and funding for both Medicare and Medicaid. At the time of enactment, the act itself only outlined the strategies and outcomes with no complete frameworks or guidance of the healthcare industry to follow. The law offered three primary goals:
- Make affordable health insurance available to more people. The law provides consumers with subsidies ("premium tax credits") that lower costs for households with incomes between 100% and 400% of the federal poverty level.

- Expand the Medicaid program to cover all adults with income below 138% of the federal poverty level. (Not all states have expanded their Medicaid programs.)
- Support innovative medical care delivery methods designed to lower the costs of healthcare generally.

Although these were the immediate goals, the law's impact affected individual consumers, the delivery of care, the cost of care, and the availability for many Americans. Why was it so significant? Because healthcare leaders recognized that the current health delivery system was unsustainable, and costs were spiraling out of control reaching almost 20% of the Gross National Product (GNP) (Cordani, 2020).

The ACA's impact along with healthcare delivery mandates immediately challenged managers, administrators, and all other health professionals who organize, deliver, or insure the nation's populations. New population health terminology and concepts such as accountable care organizations and patient-centered medical homes entered the vocabulary of healthcare managers. Health providers and administrators quickly learned the importance of innovative business strategies: risk segmentation and stratification based on data analytics, and alternative payment mechanisms. In response to the COVID-19 pandemic, health systems reported telemedicine visits expanded by incredible percentages and even as high as 600% in only a few months (NYU Langone Health, 2020). Today, the health sector is integrating SDOH into electronic medical records, adopting behavior change models, and factoring in consumer behavior and social media communication options throughout the healthcare sector (Cantor & Thorpe, 2018).

Another important consequence of addressing the needs of populations has been the expansion of the continuum of care. The continuum of care refers to care over time and was commonly thought of in terms of the phases of illness (HIMSS, 2014; NCI, n.d.). Now, the continuum of care framework is more than primary care and acute care. Healthcare services expanded in both directions to encompass preventivecare (health promotion, disease prevention) and postacute care (rehabilitation, home care, palliative, and hospice) services. Most importantly, we can add the concept of virtual care to the continuum. See Figure 1.8.

This expansion focuses on increasing services across the continuum of care and responding to the patient's, consumer's, and population's health needs beyond the treatment phase.

The new PHM strategies also sought to address the ever-increasing cost of health, and the traditional fee-for-service payment system began transitioning to a value over volume and payment risk perspective based on accountability for patient outcomes. The very foundations of the healthcare exchange system, previously centered on single interactions with patients, shifted to focus on managing and sharing risk for identified populations. But to characterize PHM as simply value over volume financial implications misses the significance of the transformation. The healthcare system emerged as the healthcare sector where chronic care, virtual care (telemedicine), and health disparity issues became managerial equivalents to formerly traditional medical business lines such as oncology and cardiology. Independent hospitals merged into healthcare systems and began seriously partnering with public health entities, technology and innovation entrepreneurs, for-profit patient engagement companies, and local nonprofit health agencies to coproduce services and ensure positive health outcomes for their populations.

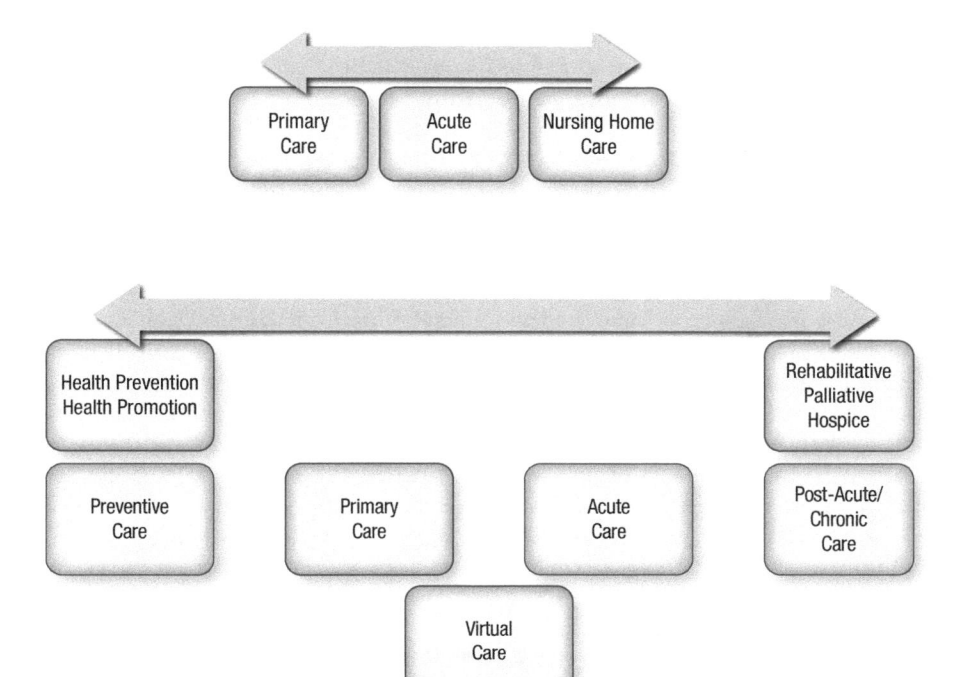

FIGURE 1.8 Comparison of the Initial and Expanded Continuum of Care

The impact of government alternative payment policies nudged current healthcare providers toward a risk-sharing portfolio of services and expanded the potential configurations for not only how healthcare was delivered, but by who, when, where, and how the service had occurred. The "right care, right time, right place, right health provider" mantra infiltrated the very foundations of the healthcare management environment.

Challenges for Population Health Management

PHM encompasses a new way of doing business based on multiple frameworks but ultimately remains committed to improving the quality of life for populations with the individual patient remaining centric in the process. As the healthcare sector continues to adopt and refine PHM processes and approaches, additional changes and transformations will evolve in quicker time frames with positive impacts on the overall quality of health.

PHM challenges include finding solutions to these reoccurring questions while achieving accessible, effective, and efficient quality of care.

- Who has access to healthcare?
- Who delivers healthcare?
- Who is the payer?
- Where is care delivered?
- How is the care is delivered?
- When is care available?
- Who bears the risk for the cost of healthcare?

PHM continues to transform the role of the health manager. The promising news is that the past 10 years yielded successful models and approaches to healthcare that can inform and guide future innovations.

SUMMARY

The often-quoted phrase "The only constant is change" (Singer, 2018) certainly describes the emergence and adoption of PHM in the past 20 years. PHM encompasses a new way of doing business based on multiple frameworks but ultimately focuses on improving the quality of life for identified populations. This chapter discusses the operational definitions of health and populations before presenting multiple models, frameworks, and pathways for population health and PHM. The informative distinction between public, community, global, and population health underscores the role and importance of PHM with the emphasis on quality, cost, meeting the needs of populations and integrated delivery systems that span cross-sector relationships. The pace of future challenges will be accelerated as new models emerge to address technological and clinical advances as well as innovative frameworks for risk-sharing and alternative payment systems and collaborative relationships.

DISCUSSION QUESTIONS

1. Identify at least five major factors that contributed to the need for new healthcare delivery models in the 21st century.
2. Why is Healthy People 2020 seen as a foundation document for PHM?
3. Discuss how the concept of a culture of wellness became essential for the alignment of public, community, and population health.
4. Describe the differences between public heath, population health, and population health wellness.
5. Analyze the similarities and differences between the P2PH, the Four Pillars of Health, and the NPP.
6. Explain the role and responsibilities of PHM.
7. Provide ideas for future enhancements of the continuum of care.

Toolkit Competency Application
Mini Case Study: Mountain Orthopedics

Jayson is the office director (coordinator) for five office locations that comprise Mountain Orthopedics. This specialty practice sees a wide-age range of patients—from high school athletes (sports medicine) to senior patients needing joint replacements, and adults with complex spine conditions requiring pain management. While the health outcomes, patient experience, and satisfaction of the younger population are more than satisfactory, the adult and senior population's surgical health outcomes and rehabilitative patient engagement rates are below benchmarks.

Jayson was recently introduced to the *PHA–PHM Framework* and feels that organizing the practice to focus on the subpopulation of seniors would provide an opportunity for the health providers, patients, and other health practitioners to achieve higher level quality outcomes.

The *PHA–PHM Framework* is used to develop a project outline, based on the four administrative action steps: Assessment, Stratification, Person-Centered Intervention, and Impact Evaluation.

REFERENCES

American Hospital Association (AHA). (n.d.). *What is population health management?* Retrieved May 18, 2021, from https://www.aha.org/center/population-health-management

Beaglehole, R., & Bonita, R. (2010). What is global health? *Global Health Action, 3.* https://doi.org/10.3402/gha.v3i0.5142

Berwick, D., Nolan, T., & Whittington, J. (2008). The triple aim: Care, health, and cost. *Health Affairs, 27*(3), 759–769. https://www.healthaffairs.org/doi/full/10.1377/hlthaff.27.3.759

Bresnick, J. (2015, April 29). Is there a true definition of population health management? *Health It Analytics.* https://healthitanalytics.com/news/is-there-a-true-definition-of-population-health-management

Burton, D. (2013, September 30). Population health management: Implementing a strategy for success. *HealthCatalyst.* https://www.healthcatalyst.com/whitepaper/PopulationHealthManagement

Cantor, M., & Thorpe, L. (2018, April). Integrating data on social determinants of health into electronic health records. *Health Affairs, 37*(4), 585–590. https://doi.org/10.1377/hlthaff.2017.1252

Caron, R. (2017). *Population health: Principles and applications for management.* Health Administration Press.

CDC. (2019). *1918 Pandemic (H1N1 virus).* Centers for Disease Control and Prevention. https://www.cdc.gov/flu/pandemic-resources/1918-pandemic-h1n1.html

CDC. (2020a). *Healthy people 2020.* National Center for Health Statistics. https://www.cdc.gov/nchs/healthy_people/hp2020.htm

CDC. (2020b). *Healthy people 2030.* National Center for Health Statistics. https://www.cdc.gov/nchs/healthy_people/hp2030/hp2030.htm

Chandra, A., Acosta, J., Carman, K. G., Dubowitz, T., Leviton, L., Martin, L. T., Miller, C., Nelson, C., Orleans, T., Tait, M., Trujillo, M., Towe, V., Yeung, D., & Plough, A. L. (2017). Building a national culture of health: Background, action framework, measures, and next steps. *Rand Health Quarterly, 6*(2), 3. https://www.ncbi.nlm.nih.gov/pmc/articles/PMC5568157/

Cordani, D. (2020, February 29). Healthcare is on an unsustainable trajectory, requiring a renewed push for transformation. *Modern Healthcare.* https://www.modernhealthcare.com/opinion-editorial/healthcare-unsustainable-trajectory-requiring-renewed-push-transformation

Fabius, R. (2021). The population health promise. In D. Nash, A. Skoufalos, R. Fabius, & W. Ogelesby (Eds.), *Population health: Creating a culture of wellness* (3rd ed.). Jones and Bartlett Learning.

Faulk, L. H. (2014, July 30). What is population health and how does it compare to public health? *Health Catalyst.* https://www.healthcatalyst.com/what-is-population-health/

Feeley, D. (2017, November 28). *The triple aim or the quadruple aim? Four points to help set your strategy.* IHI. http://www.ihi.org/communities/blogs/the-triple-aim-or-the-quadruple-aim-four-points-to-help-set-your-strategy

Health Information Management System Society (HiMSS). (2014). *Definition: Continuum of care.* http://s3.amazonaws.com/rdcms-himss/files/production/public/2014-05-14-DefinitionContinuumofCare.pdf

Institute for Health Improvement (IHI). (n.d.). *Resources: Pathways to population health.* Retrieved May 18, 2021, from http://www.ihi.org/Topics/Population-Health/Pages/Resources.aspx

Kindig, D., & Stoddart, G. (2003). What is population health? *American Journal of Public Health, 93*(3), 380–383. https://doi.org/10.2105/ajph.93.3.380

McKenzie, J., Pinger, R., & Kotecki, J. (2005). *An introduction to community health* (p. 5). Jones and Bartlett Publishers.

Mineo, L. (2020, May 19). The lesson is to never forget. *Harvard Gazette*. https://news.harvard.edu/gazette/story/2020/05/harvard-expert-compares-1918-flu-covid-19/

Nash, D. B. (2012). The population health mandate: A broader approach to care delivery. In *The four pillars of health* (Special Edition). Boardroom Press. http://populationhealthcolloquium.com/readings/Pop_Health_Mandate_NASH_2012.pdf

National Academy of Medicine (formerly the Institute of Medicine) (NAM). (2000). *To err is human: Building a safer health system*. National Academy Press.

National Academy of Medicine (formerly the Institute of Medicine) (NAM). (2001). *Crossing the quality chasm: A new health system for the 21st century*. National Academy Press.

National Priorities Partnership. (2008). *National priorities and goals: Aligning our efforts to transform America's Healthcare*. National Quality Forum. http://www.qualityforum.org/Setting_Priorities/National_Priorities_Partnership_-_Call_for_Organizational_Nominations.aspx

NCI Dictionary of Cancer Terms. (n.d.). *Continuum of care*. NCI Dictionary. Retrieved May 18, 2021, from https://www.cancer.gov/publications/dictionaries/cancer-terms/def/continuum-of-care

NYU Langone Health / NYU School of Medicine. (2020, April 30). Telemedicine transforms response to COVID-19 pandemic in disease epicenter. *ScienceDaily*. https://www.sciencedaily.com/releases/2020/04/200430150220.htm

Office of Disease Prevention and Health Promotion (ODPHP). (n.d.). *History and Development of Healthy People 2020*. Updated June 23, 2021. Retrieved July 28, 2021 from https://www.healthypeople.gov/2020/About-Healthy-People/History-Development-Healthy-People-2020

Olden. (2019). *Chapter 1 – Management of healthcare organizations: An introduction* (3rd ed., pp. 1–28). Health, Healthcare, and Healthcare Organizations.

Ottawa, C. (1986). *Ottawa charter 1986*. World Health Organization. https://www.who.int/publications/i/item/ottawa-charter-for-health-promotion. http://www.who.int/healthpromotion/conferences/previous/ottawa/en/

Population Health Alliance. (n.d.). *PHA – Population health management framework*. Population Health Alliance. Retrieved May 18, 2021, from https://populationhealthalliance.org/research/understanding-population-health/

Saha, S., Loehrer, S., Cleary-Fisherman, M., Johnson, K., Chenard, R., Gunderson, G., Goldberg. R., Little, J., Resnick, J., Cutts, T., & Barnett, K. (2017). *Pathways to population health: An invitation to health care change agents*. 100 Million Healthier Lives, convened by the Institute for Health Improvement. http://www.ihi.org/Topics/Population-Health/Documents/PathwaystoPopulationHealth_Framework.pdf

Short, S. E., & Mollborn, S. (2015). Social determinants and health behaviors: Conceptual frames and empirical advances. *Current Opinion in Psychology, 5*, 78–84. https://doi.org/10.1016/j.copsyc.2015.05.002

Singer, J. (2018). The only constant is change. *PsychCentral*. https://psychcentral.com/lib/the-only-constant-is-change

Stibich, M. (2019, November 25). *Compression of morbidity and reducing suffering*. Verywellhealth. https://www.verywellhealth.com/compression-of-morbidity-2223626#:~:text=Reducing%20Age%2DRelated%20Suffering&text=Compression%20of%20morbidity%20is%20a,means%20%22being%20unhealthy%22

Vass, A. (2020, March 2). Pandemics of the 21st century preceding coronavirus. *Hungary Today*. https://hungarytoday.hu/pandemics-of-the-21st-century-preceding-coronavirus/

Winslow, E. (1920). The untilled fields of public health. *Science, 51*(1306), 23–33. https://doi.org/10.1126/science.51.1306.23

World Health Organization (WHO). (1946). *Constitution of the World Health Organization*. https://www.who.int/about/who-we-are/constitution

World Health Organization (WHO). (1995). *WHOQOL: Measuring quality of life*. https://www.who.int/healthinfo/survey/whoqol-qualityoflife/en/

CHAPTER 2

Public Health Foundations for Population Health Managers

Rosemary M. Caron

KEY TERMS

Attack Rate
Case Definition, Report, Investigation, Series
Case Fatality Rate
Chain of Transmission
Clinical and Randomized Controlled Trial
Cohort Study—Prospective, Retrospective
Crude, Age-Specific, Cause-Specific, and Adjusted Rates
Distribution and Determinants
Endemic, Epidemic, Pandemic
Epidemiology—Analytic, Descriptive, Managerial
Frequency Measures of Disease
Incidence and Prevalence Rates
Isolation and Quarantine
Morbidity and Mortality Rate
Odds Ratio and Relative Risk (Risk Ratio)
Population Medicine
Prevention—Primary, Secondary, Tertiary
Proportional (Population) Mortality Ratio
Prospective and Retrospective Cohort Study
Public Health—Core and Essential Functions
Standardized (Morbidity/Mortality) Ratio
Social Determinants of Health
Study—Cross-Sectional, Experimental, Observational,
Surveillance—Active, Passive

LEARNING OBJECTIVES

1. Define and describe the role, function, and essential services of the public health system.

> 🔊 Podcasts that exemplify the content of this chapter are available at Springer Publishing Connect™
>
> Podcast 2.1. How Does Public Health Relate to Population Health Management?

Access the podcast online at http://connect.springerpub.com/content/book/978-0-8261-4427-0/part/part01/chapter/ch02

2. Identify how public health metrics serve as indicators of population health status.
3. Explain how descriptive epidemiological calculations, prevalence, and incidence relate to population health management (PHM).
4. Provide application examples of analytical epidemiological rate calculations (crude, specific).
5. Show alignment between analytical rate calculations and their importance in assessing a population's health outcome.
6. Demonstrate epidemiological risk calculations (odds ratio and relative risk).

INTRODUCTION

As described in Chapter 1, one's health status considers the mental, physical, and social state and is not defined by the absence of disease (WHO, 1946). To assure this state of health for populations across the globe, the public health and healthcare systems must work collaboratively.

The integration of primary care and public health can enhance the capacity of both sectors to carry out their respective missions and link with other stakeholders to catalyze a collaborative, intersectoral movement toward improved population health.

—Health and Medicine Division, National Academies of Science, Engineering, Medicine (2020)

These systems use the basic science of public health known as epidemiology to help assess the health needs of a community, and this information can then be used to develop interventions that promote health and prevent disease. This chapter will examine the fields of public health and population health and how they utilize epidemiology to manage the health of populations.

Public Health Defined

Charles Edward Amory Winslow, a public health leader and founder of the Yale School of Public Health, defined **public health** as "the science and art of preventing disease, prolonging life, and promoting health through the organized efforts and informed choices of society, organizations, public and private communities, and individuals" (Winslow, 1920).

The National Academy of Medicine, formerly the Institute of Medicine, defined the public health mission as "fulfilling society's interest in assuring conditions in which people can be healthy" (Institute of Medicine [IOM], 1988). Turnock (2001) further described that the public health mission could be completed via community efforts that are organized to identify and prevent public health threats. This mission of promoting health and preventing disease among populations by way of a collaborative approach requires the expertise of a public health professional (IOM, 1988). Representative examples of professions that implement a public health approach include medicine, nursing, dentistry, social work, allied health professionals, pharmacy, law, engineering, public administration, and journalism (IOM, 1988).

The Public Health System

The Centers for Disease Control and Prevention (CDC) described the public health system as "all public, private, and voluntary entities that contribute to the delivery of essential public health services within a jurisdiction" (CDC, 2014). Representative entities that are considered part of the public health system include, but are not limited to, local and state governmental public health departments, healthcare providers, environmental agencies, public safety organizations, education organizations, and so forth (CDC, 2014).

A community's **public health system** should undertake the following essential public health services, which provide a framework for addressing myriad public health issues (CDC, 2014):

1. Assess and monitor population health status, factors that influence health, and community needs and assets.
2. Investigate, diagnose, and address health problems and hazards affecting the population.
3. Communicate effectively to inform and educate people about health, factors that influence it, and how to improve it.
4. Strengthen, support, and mobilize communities and partnerships to improve health.
5. Create, champion, and implement policies, plans, and laws that impact health.
6. Utilize legal and regulatory actions designed to improve and protect the public's health.
7. Assure an effective system that enables equitable access to the individual services and care needed to be healthy.
8. Build and support a diverse and skilled public health workforce.
9. Improve and innovate public health functions through ongoing evaluation, research, and continuous quality improvement.
10. Build and maintain a strong organizational infrastructure for public health (CDC, 2014).

Figure 2.1 illustrates the essential public health services and how they align with the **core functions of public health** (CDC, 2014):

Assessment: The public health system must continuously and systematically assess the health of the populations to determine the baseline of morbidity (illness) and mortality for communities. The assessment core function helps us to establish what is a "normal" health status for a community.

Policy development: The public health system must work with the community to identify, educate, and solve health problems via a policy approach based in science.

Assurance: The public health system must evaluate the effectiveness of its interventions and assure a competent workforce to carry out the public health mission.

The services provided by the public health system are based in research findings, which provide the foundation for evidence-based practice.

THE 10 ESSENTIAL PUBLIC HEALTH SERVICES

To protect and promote the health of all people in all communities

The 10 Essential Public Health Services provide a framework for public health to protect and promote the health of all people in all communities. To achieve optimal health for all, the Essential Public Health Services actively promote policies, systems, and services that enable good health and seek to remove obstacles and systemic and structural barriers, such as poverty, racism, gender discrimination, and other forms of oppression, that have resulted in health inequities. Everyone should have a fair and just opportunity to achieve good health and well-being.

Assessment
- Assess and monitor population health
- Investigate, diagnose, and address health hazards and root causes

Policy Development
- Communicate effectively to inform and educate
- Strengthen, support, and mobilize communities and partnerships
- Create, champion, and implement policies, plans, and laws

Assurance
- Utilize legal and regulatory actions
- Enable equitable access
- Build a diverse and skilled workforce
- Improve and innovate through evaluation, research, and quality improvement
- Build and maintain a strong organizational infrastructure for public health

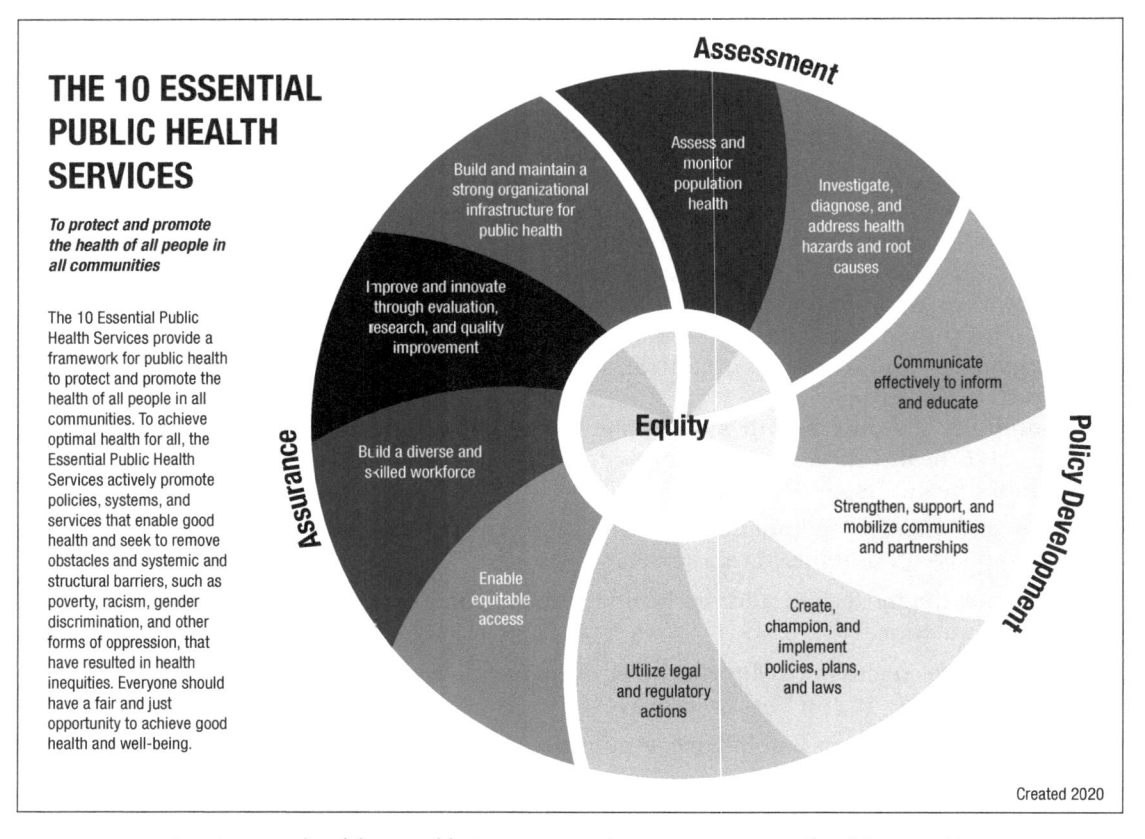

Equity

Created 2020

FIGURE 2.1 Ten Essential Public Health Services and Core Functions of Public Health
Source: 10 Essential Public Health Services Futures Initiative Task Force. 10 Essential Public Health Services. February 2, 2021. https://phnci.org/uploads/resource-files/EPHS-English.pdf

---

❓ DID YOU KNOW?

Common Public Health Required Activities

The essential public health services are a road map for the public health system to conduct the following representative public health activities:
- Prevent outbreaks, epidemics, and pandemics.
- Protect against exposure to environmental hazards.
- Prevent injuries in the workplace setting.
- Promote and encourage healthy behaviors and lifestyles.
- Respond to communities in need from natural and anthropogenic disasters.
- Assure the quality and accessibility of healthcare services (CDC, 2014).

Do you know where your local public health office is located? Find their webpage and the population health services they provide.

Integration of Public Health and Healthcare Prevention Approaches

Public health and healthcare professionals share the common mission of working to improve health. However, the focus of public health is to improve health for a population, whereas healthcare is concerned with improving health at the individual level. The "treatment" approach implemented by public health professionals includes interventions that could be policy based or educational, for example. In contrast, healthcare professionals focus on the classic diagnosis and treatment paradigm. Population health management (PHM) ensures that both important healthcare functions are delivered in an efficient and effective manner.

As previously stated, the public health mission is focused on promoting health and preventing disease. **Prevention** occurs via three approaches described as the following:

- **Primary prevention:** Acting prior to the occurrence of an adverse health effect. Vaccination is an example of a primary prevention method.
- **Secondary prevention:** Screening prior to the earliest detection of disease, usually prior to the onset of signs and symptoms. Mammography and colonoscopy are examples of secondary prevention methods.
- **Tertiary prevention:** "Managing disease post diagnosis to slow or stop disease progression through measures such as chemotherapy, rehabilitation, and screening for complications".

Public health and healthcare work mainly in the areas of secondary and tertiary prevention. Yet, they do overlap in the area of primary prevention when working to prevent the initiation of disease. Prevention approaches, also known as health promotion, represent an area where the public health and healthcare systems can integrate more effectively.

Population Health Defined

Population health refers to the health of a population that is influenced by the social, physical, and biological environments, lifestyle, and healthcare access. It focuses on the interrelationship of those factors that influence health over one's life and implements actions and policies that are focused on improving the overall health of populations (Public Health Agency of Canada, 2013).

The Public Health Agency of Canada makes the case to invest upstream, which refers to addressing those determinants of health that influence health outcomes. A population health approach focuses effort on the root causes of adverse health effects and directs resources to those areas that hold the greatest potential to positively influence a population's health status (Public Health Agency of Canada, 2013).

Population Medicine

Population medicine is a term used to describe the role of the healthcare system with respect to influencing health in a comprehensive approach. It considers the role of multisector partnerships and their effort to positively influence health via healthcare determinants (Kindig, 2012).

A component of population medicine is PHM, which involves utilizing care coordination and patient engagement models to improve the clinical health outcomes of a specified population (American Hospital Association [AHA], 2020). The next section will discuss how we use the basic science of public health, epidemiology, to assess the population's health.

Epidemiology Defined

The basic science of public health, **epidemiology**, is defined as the study of the distribution of determinants and their associated health outcomes in a population and the application of this basic public health science to control and prevent adverse health outcomes (Last, 2001). This science aims "to promote, protect, and restore health" (Last, 2001). Thus, the tools epidemiology provides via descriptive and analytic epidemiology approaches contribute to fulfilling the public health mission and a PHM approach.

Taking a closer look at this definition, **distribution** focuses on the pattern of health events in a population and their frequency of occurrence (CDC, 2012) and refers to conducting an analysis that examines the person, place, and time characteristics of the affected people (Last, 2001). Examining health events based on person, place, and time characteristics are descriptive epidemiology actions (CDC, 2012).

Determinants are factors that may be biological, social, cultural, physical, and behavioral in nature that have the potential to influence health (Last, 2001). Epidemiologists assume that illness occurs when the appropriate health determinants exist to result in illness (CDC, 2012). Epidemiologists use analytic studies to answer "how" and "why" health outcomes occur. Epidemiologists assess why certain groups experience different rates of disease based on their demographics, genetic composition, environmental exposures, and other potential risk factors (CDC, 2012). The results from analytic epidemiology studies provide evidence for the development, implementation, and evaluation for effective public health control and prevention efforts (CDC, 2012).

The following questions may be addressed, via an interdisciplinary approach, by epidemiology (Friis & Sellers, 2014):

- How do determinants influence health outcomes?
- How do demographic and geographic information contribute to describing disease variation?
- Based on the community's disease status, what should the appropriate responses be on the part of the public health and healthcare systems?
- How applicable are the findings from epidemiologic investigations across communities?

Epidemiology may be used in public health practice to conduct public health surveillance, field investigations, analytic studies, evaluation and linkages, and policy development (Tyler & Last, 1992).

⁇ DID YOU KNOW?

COVID-19 Epidemiology

The following excerpt from Public Health England (2020) provides an epidemiological update on COVID-19. Can you identify the epidemiological features in this update?

> On 31 December 2019, the World Health Organization (WHO) was informed of a cluster of cases of pneumonia of unknown cause detected in Wuhan City, Hubei Province, China.
>
> On 12 January 2020 it was announced that a novel coronavirus had been identified in samples obtained from cases and that initial analysis of virus

genetic sequences suggested that this was the cause of the outbreak. This virus is referred to as SARS-CoV-2, and the associated disease as COVID-19.

As of June 1 2020 (10:00 am CET), over 6.1 million cases have been diagnosed globally, with more than 371,000 fatalities (European Centre for Disease Prevention and Control, situation update worldwide).

Managerial Epidemiology

Managerial epidemiology is described as the application of epidemiology to healthcare decision-making (Fleming, 2013). Healthcare and public health professionals need to know the characteristics of the populations they serve; the health and nonhealth areas of need; why certain healthcare services are utilized; and the implications of acting (and not acting) to improve a population's health (Oleske, 2001).

Managerial epidemiology allows for the following questions to be explored (Oleske, 2001):

- Who does the healthcare setting serve and what is their health status?
- What are the needs of the population the healthcare setting serves?
- What services should the healthcare setting offer to address the population's health needs?

Managerial epidemiology can assist healthcare managers in implementing a population health approach by examining the interrelated conditions and factors that affect the health status of populations over a life course and variations in the occurrence of adverse health outcomes and implementing policies and actions to improve the population's health (Public Health Agency of Canada, 2013).

Frequency of Disease

A key attribute of epidemiology is that it determines the rate of occurrence, or frequency, of a health condition, such as an infectious or chronic disease (Friis & Sellers, 2014). The following terms are used to describe the frequency of disease:

Epidemic: A sudden increase in the number of disease cases above what is normally expected in a geographic area (CDC, 2012).

Example: Severe Acute Respiratory Syndrome (SARS)

Outbreak: Same definition as above but typically refers to a geographic area that is limited (CDC, 2012).

Example: Measles

Cluster: A group of cases oriented in place and time and are greater than what is expected (which may be unknown) (CDC, 2012).

Example: Leukemia cancer cluster in Woburn, MA

Endemic: Constant prevalence of disease in a population residing in a specific geographic area (CDC, 2012).

Example: Malaria in Africa

Pandemic: An epidemic that has spread to several countries or continents (CDC, 2012).

Example: Spanish Flu of 1918

Surveillance and Infection Control Measures

One way to monitor the frequency of disease is via surveillance, which is the continuous collection, analysis, interpretation, and communication of health data that is used to inform decision-making and action with respect to public health issues (CDC, 2012). Information gathered from surveillance activities can demonstrate the patterns of disease and inform investigation, control, and prevention measures (CDC, 2012).

The surveillance cycle illustrated (see Figure 2.2) highlights that information (e.g., mortality, morbidity, disease registry, health survey) is systematically collected from the public health and healthcare systems, evaluated, and disseminated through a feedback look for the development of effective disease control and public health decision-making (CDC, 2012).

Should surveillance data indicate the presence of an infectious disease, the public health and healthcare systems may recommend **infection control measures** to reduce or prevent the spread of a communicable illness. The two main infection control measures implemented are quarantine and isolation. **Quarantine** measures "separate and restrict the movement of people who were exposed to a contagious disease to see if they become sick" (CDC, 2017). **Isolation** measures separate those who are infected and sick with a communicable disease from those who are not infected (CDC, 2017).

Descriptive Epidemiology

The science of epidemiology is comprised of two branches: descriptive epidemiology and analytic epidemiology. **Descriptive epidemiology** works to determine the answers to questions including the following (CDC, 2012): Who (person) is affected? Where (place) were they affected? When (time) were they affected? Why (risk factors) were they affected?

The epidemiologist observes the exposure and disease status of the study participant in an observational study design, which is used in descriptive

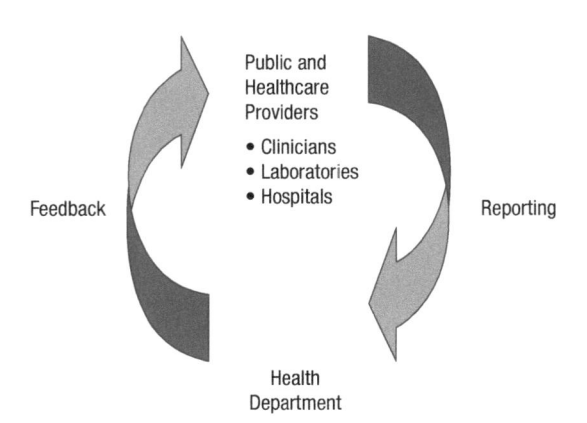

FIGURE 2.2 The Surveillance Cycle (CDC, 2012)

TABLE 2.1 Descriptive Epidemiologic Studies

Case Report (or Count)	Case Series	Cross-Sectional Study
• Based on a case of illness' uniqueness or magnitude, a case report describes a patient or event that could warrant further investigation • Submitted by healthcare and/or laboratory professionals to the health department so patterns of disease occurrence regarding person, place, and time may be examined • Useful when examining notifiable diseases, which are mandated to be reported to the local and state public health system by healthcare professionals • Confidential; no comparison group; useful in surveillance	• A summary of characteristics for a listing of patients from one or more healthcare settings • Confidential; no comparison group; useful in surveillance	• Exposures and health outcomes are measured simultaneously • Assesses prevalence of disease or health outcome at some point in time; does not consider duration • *Measure of Association Between Exposure and Disease*: Prevalence rate • *Strength*: Used to determine prevalence of health outcomes, behaviors, states in a community; survey technique • *Limitation*: Cannot determine incidence • *Application*: Assist in planning for type of health services

epidemiology (CDC, 2012). There are three common types of descriptive epidemiologic approaches (see Table 2.1): **case reports** (or **counts**), **case series**, and **cross-sectional study** (CDC, 2012).

Measures of Disease Frequency

Representative **frequency measures of disease** include prevalence, incidence, crude rate, specific rate, and adjusted rate (see Box 2.1). The **prevalence rate** is the proportion of the population that has a health condition of interest at a specific point in time (CDC, 2012). The **incidence rate** is the proportion of new cases of disease, injury, or new deaths that occur in a population over a specific period of time (CDC, 2012). Synonyms include the attack rate and cumulative incidence (CDC, 2012).

Crude Rate

Crude rates are raw in the sense that they are calculated by dividing the total number of cases by the total number of persons in the population in a specified period of time (Boston University School of Public Health [BUSPH], 2016).

Specific Rate

Specific rates are summary measures based on a particular subgroup of the population. The subgroups may be defined in terms of age, race, or gender, or a single illness or cause of death (Friis & Sellers, 2014).

Adjusted Rate

Adjusted rates are a summary measure that involves statistical procedures to account for differences in the composition (e.g., age or gender) of populations. Rates are often adjusted for age to allow for comparisons within a diverse population. Rates may be adjusted via direct or indirect procedures (Friis & Sellers, 2014).

BOX 2.1 COMMON MEASURES OF DISEASE FREQUENCY

1. Age-specific rate (e.g., mortality rate)

Number of deaths among a specific age group of the population during a specific time period / number of persons who comprise that age group during the same time period; answer is expressed per number at risk (e.g., per 100,000).

2. Attack rate

An alternative form of the incidence rate that is used when the nature of a disease or condition is such that a population is observed for a short time period. The attack rate is calculated by the following formula: ill / (ill + well) × 100 (during a time period).

3. Case fatality rate

Number of deaths due to disease "X" during a given time interval / number of new cases of that disease reported during the same time interval; answer is expressed as a percent (%).

4. Cause-specific rate (e.g., cause-specific death or mortality rate)

Number of deaths assigned to a specific cause during a year / estimated population size; answer is expressed per number at risk (e.g., per 100,000).

5. Crude birth rate

Number of live births within a given period / population size; answer is expressed per number at risk (e.g., per 1,000).

6. Crude mortality rate

Number of deaths during a given year / reference population; answer is expressed per number at risk (e.g., per 100,000).

7. General fertility rate

Number of live births within a year / number of women aged 15 to 44 years during the midpoint of the year; answer is expressed per number at risk (e.g., per 1,000).

8. Incidence rate

Number of new cases during a time period / total population at risk during the same time period; answer is expressed per number at risk (e.g., per 100,000).

9. Infant mortality rate

Number of infant deaths under 1 year of age (0–365 days) during a year / number of live births reported during that same year; answer is expressed per number at risk (e.g., per 1,000).

10. Interrelationship between prevalence and incidence

Prevalence (P) of a disease is proportional to the incidence rate (I) times the duration (D) of the disease.

11. Maternal mortality rate

Number of deaths assigned to causes related to childbirth during a year / number of live births during the same year; answer is expressed per number at risk (e.g., per 100,000).

12. Prevalence

Number of existing cases during a time period / total population during the same time period; answer is expressed per number at risk (e.g., per 1,000) or as a percent (%).

13. Proportional (population) mortality ratio (PMR)

Mortality (number of deaths) due to a specific cause during a year / mortality (total deaths due to all causes) due to all causes during the same year; answer is expressed as a decimal or a percent (%).

14. Standardized morbidity (or mortality) ratio (SMR)

Number of observed cases (or deaths) / expected number of cases (or deaths); answer is expressed as a decimal or a percent (%).

> **DID YOU KNOW?**
>
> **Calculating COVID-19 Rates**
>
> There are 8,701 COVID-19 laboratory-confirmed cases in the past 2 weeks in New York. The population of New York is 8,400,000 people. There have been 372,000 COVID-19 cases in New York and 23,959 deaths attributed to COVID-19 in New York to this point in the pandemic.
> Calculate the following:
>
> *Incidence rate* for the past 2 weeks =
>
> *COVID-19-specific mortality rate* =
>
> *COVID-19 case fatality rate* =
>
> These rates are used to help determine the magnitude of the public health issue, which is necessary to assist with developing a PHM approach.
>
> Which rate would you use to determine the percentage of COVID-19 deaths that comprise the total death rate?

Analytic Epidemiology

As previously discussed, descriptive epidemiology addresses the person, place, time, and why aspects of health outcomes. **Analytic epidemiology** builds on this work by focusing on the "how" and "why" or causes and effects of health events. An important feature of analytic epidemiology is that it attempts to quantify the association between exposure and outcomes and test hypotheses that are generated by the descriptive epidemiologic approaches described earlier. Analytic epidemiologic studies also utilize a comparison group, which makes these types of studies more rigorous (and more expensive) than descriptive epidemiology approaches (CDC, 2012).

There are three types of analytic epidemiologic studies that attempt to demonstrate a causal relationship between exposure and health outcome (see Table 2.2): **case–control study, cohort (prospective and retrospective) study**, and **experimental study**. The case–control and cohort studies are observational in nature, whereas the epidemiologist intervenes in an experimental study. Please note that these two study types are more common when conducting population health analysis, as randomization is often impossible to attain when examining health phenomenon for defined population groups.

Measures of Association Between Exposure and Disease

Case–control studies and cohort studies are important observational study designs that allow for the association between exposure and disease to be

TABLE 2.2 Analytic Epidemiologic Studies

Case–Control Study	Cohort Study

• *Cases*: People who have the disease under study.
• *Controls*: Comparison group; people without the disease of interest; provide baseline or expected amount of exposure.
• Exposures between the two groups are compared.
• *Matching*: It is important to match the cases and controls so they are as similar as possible with the exception of having the health outcome of interest.
• *Confounding*: The importance of matching cases and controls is to assist in reducing the effect of a confounder. Confounding is defined as "the distortion of the association between an exposure and a health outcome by a third variable that is related to both" (CDC, 2012).
• *Measure of association between exposure and disease*:
Odds ratio:
$$\frac{\text{Number of exposed cases} \times \text{Number of }\underline{\text{unexposed controls}}}{\text{Number of exposed controls} \times \text{Number of unexposed cases}}$$
• *Strengths*:
  • Useful for studying rare diseases.
  • Cost efficient.
• *Limitations*:
  • Not useful for rare exposures.
  • Unable to provide a direct estimate of risk.
• *Application*:
  • Infectious disease outbreak.
• *Example*: A case–control study was performed (2015–2017) to identify risk factors for acute HEV in the Netherlands.
Highlights of the study include the following:
• "A large patient–control study identified traditional Dutch dry raw sausages, called "cervelaat," "snijworst," and "boerenmetworst"as the main transmission routes for HEV to the general population of the Netherlands.
• The prevalence and cause of HEV contamination in these sausages of raw pork muscle meat require further investigation.
• Strong, yet rarely reported risk factors for acute HEV were direct contact with pigs and working with a septic tank.
• Host risk factors were preexisting liver disease, diabetes, and use of immunosuppressants or gastric acid inhibitors.
Reference: Tulen et al. (2019)
	• *Prospective*: Study participant's exposure history is taken and is followed over time to determine if the disease or health outcome of interest develops; length of follow-up varies.
	• *Retrospective*: Study participant's disease or health outcome of interest has occurred, and they are questioned about previous exposures.
	• *Measure of association between exposure and disease*:
	Relative Risk or Risk Ratio
	$$\frac{\text{Attack rate (risk)}}{\text{Attack rate (risk)}}\text{ in exposed group}\atop\text{in unexposed group}$$
	• *Strengths*:
	  • Useful for studying rare exposures.
	  • Provides strong evidence for exposure–disease relationships.
	• *Limitations*:
	  • Lengthy to conduct.
	  • Attrition of participants.
	• *Application*:
	  • Study of chronic disease.
	• *Example*: The Framingham Heart Study began in 1948 (with funding from the National Heart Institute, which is known today as the National Heart, Lung, and Blood Institute) to identify risk factors and characteristics of cardiovascular disease. This study has followed participants over three generations in Framingham, MA. Findings from this cohort study have provided important information about blood pressure, cholesterol, triglycerides, age, gender, and psychosocial issues; see https://framinghamheartstudy.org/fhs-about (Framingham Heart Study, 2020).

measured. An important tool used in both study designs for this purpose is the **2 × 2 table** (see Exhibit 2.1).

Odds Ratio

The odds ratio is a measure of association between frequency of exposure and frequency of outcome for a case–control study. The formula is (AD)/(BC) (see Exhibit 2.2). The value represents the odds that an outcome will

	Disease Status		
	Yes	No	Total
Exposure Status Yes	A	B	A+B
Exposure Status No	C	D	C+D
Total	A+C	B+D	

A = Exposure and disease is present
B = Exposure present but disease is not present
C = No exposure but disease is present
D = No disease and no exposure
A+C = Total number with disease
B+D = Total number without disease
A+B = Total number exposed
C+D = Total number with no exposure
Disease Status Yes = People with disease
Disease Status No = People without disease
Exposure Status Yes = Exposure present
Exposure Status No = No Exposure

EXHIBIT 2.1 2 × 2 Table

occur depending on a particular exposure in those with cases of a disease or health condition relative to the control group. Odds ratios compare the relative odds of the occurrence of the outcome of interest given exposure to the variable of interest. The odds ratio can be used to determine whether a particular exposure is a risk factor for a particular outcome (Szumilas, 2010). An odds ratio of 1.0 indicates the cases and controls have equal odds of exposure to the disease so, in this case, the exposure of interest is not a risk factor for the disease under study. A protective effect is implied for an odds ratio that is less than 1.0 (Friis & Sellers, 2014). Thus, the odds ratio is useful when developing a PHM approach that requires information about the relationship between an exposure and an outcome of interest (e.g., relationship between depression and suicide). It is important to consider the size and composition of the population that was studied and other confounding variables when developing a PHM approach (Szumilas, 2010).

Relative Risk

Relative risk is a measure of association between frequency of exposure and frequency of outcome for a cohort study. The ratio of the risk of disease or death among the exposed to the risk among the unexposed. The formula used is $(A/A+B)/(C/C+D)$. The value represents the incidence of disease in the exposed group divided by the incidence of disease in the nonexposed group. A relative risk of 1.0 indicates that the risk of disease among the exposed group is no different from the risk among the nonexposed group. A relative risk less than 1.0, for example, 0.5, indicates that the risk among the exposed is half that of the nonexposed group (Friis & Sellers, 2014). Thus, the relative risk is useful when developing a PHM approach that must consider the incidence of an outcome. The relative risk is most often reported in studies that involve the outcome of a clinical treatment regimen (daily aspirin use and heart attack risk, for example).

> **? DID YOU KNOW?**
>
> **Calculating Relative Risk**
>
> In an outbreak of varicella (chickenpox) in Oregon in 2002, varicella was diagnosed in 18 of 152 vaccinated children compared with 3 of 7 unvaccinated children. Calculate the risk ratio.
>
> **TABLE 2.3** Incidence of Varicella among Schoolchildren in Nine Affected Classrooms—Oregon, 2002
>
> | | Varicella | Noncase | Total |
> | --- | --- | --- | --- |
> | Total | 21 | 138 | 159 |
> | Vaccinated | a = 18 | b = 134 | 152 |
> | Unvaccinated | c = 3 | d = 4 | 7 |
>
> Data from Tugwell, B. D., Lee, L. E., Gillette, H., Lorber, E. M., Hedberg, K., & Cieslak, P. R. (2004). Chickenpox outbreak in a highly vaccinated school population. *Pediatrics, 113*(3 Pt 1), 455–459. http://doi.org/10.1542/peds.113.3.455
>
> Risk of varicella among vaccinated children = 18/152 = 0.118 = 11.8%
>
> Risk of varicella among unvaccinated children = 3/7 = 0.429 = 42.9%
>
> Risk ratio = 0.118/0.429 = 0.28
>
> The risk ratio is less than 1.0, indicating a decreased risk or protective effect for the exposed (vaccinated) children. The risk ratio of 0.28 indicates that vaccinated children were only approximately one-fourth as likely (28%, actually) to develop varicella as were unvaccinated children.
>
> Source: Reprinted from CDC (2012).

Experimental Study

An **experimental study** allows for direct intervention on the part of the epidemiologist who determines, in a controlled environment, the exposure for the study participants and then tracks the participants to determine the effect(s) of the exposure (CDC, 2012). A **clinical trial** is an example of an experimental study where a test regimen, often involving a prevention or treatment intervention, is evaluated for its effectiveness and safety (CDC, 2012).

The most rigorous type of experimental study design in analytic epidemiology is the **randomized controlled trial** (RCT), which involves testing a hypothesis by randomly assigning an experimental procedure or intervention to the study group and not the control group and comparing the outcomes from the two groups (Porta, 2014).

Features that make an experimental study considered to be scientifically rigorous include the assignment of participants via a random (by chance) process to the study or control group while assuring both groups are comparable except in the study regimen being tested (Porta, 2014). In addition, implementing a **blinding** approach helps to make the participants unaware as to whether they have been assigned to the test group or the control group (single blinded study). In a double-blind study, both the epidemiologist and the study participants do not know who has been assigned to which group (Porta, 2014). This direct intervention approach must be conducted in an ethical fashion where **informed consent** is incorporated into the study and each participant is made aware and understands the study and potential risks and can withdraw their participation at any time (Porta, 2014).

SUMMARY

The public health system serves the entire American population by preventing disease, prolonging life, and promoting health by providing the safety net of the 10 essential public health services. Primary public health activities include assessment, policy development, and assurance. Public health regularly focuses on primary, secondary, and tertiary prevention throughout every community. The opportunities for increased collaboration between public health and population health are many.

Managerial epidemiology, as a specific type of epidemiology, adapts and applies epidemiological approaches and tools to the population health decision-making process and may include prevalence and incidence rate calculations, relative risks, and odd ratios in addition to computing standard rates of mortality and morbidity. An excellent example of managerial epidemiology is COVID-19 and the collaboration between multiple health sectors.

DISCUSSION QUESTIONS

1. Describe how the essential public health services serve as the core functions of public health?
2. How do the essential public health services contribute to fulfilling the public health mission?
3. Describe the levels of prevention and how the public health and healthcare systems engage in preventing disease.
4. Provide an example of how public health and healthcare systems can work together.
5. Define population health and the role for population medicine in improving community health.
6. Describe the utility of descriptive and analytic epidemiology.
7. Discuss the types of studies implemented in descriptive and analytic epidemiology and describe the strengths and limitations for each study.
8. Describe the challenges that can be encountered in a disease outbreak investigation and the importance of surveillance.

Toolkit Competency Application

Managerial Epidemiological Applications for Population Health

Background: Outbreak Investigation

On February 11, 2020, the WHO announced COVID-19 as a new disease, caused by a novel coronavirus that has not previously been seen in humans.

People with COVID-19 have had a wide range of symptoms that may appear any time between 2 and 14 days after exposure. Representative symptoms include the following:

- Fever or chills
- Cough
- Shortness of breath or difficulty breathing

- Fatigue
- Muscle or body aches
- Headache
- New loss of taste or smell
- Sore throat
- Congestion or runny nose
- Nausea or vomiting
- Diarrhea

COVID-19 transmission is direct from person to person via respiratory droplets that are released following the sneeze or cough from an infected person that land in the mouth or nose, or are inhaled by nearby people.

COVID-19 spreads via community transmission (CDC, 2020b). Basic public health strategies and epidemiologic steps for responding to a pandemic include a fieldwork investigation outbreak step-by-step checklist (CDC, 2016). For additional information, review this CDC tutorial: https://www.cdc.gov/csels/dsepd/ss1978/lesson6/section2.html. A recent CDC posting applied both the outbreak investigation steps and contact tracing protocols using COVID-19 as an example (CDC, 2020d): https://www.cdc.gov/coronavirus/2019-ncov/php/contact-tracing/contact-tracing-plan/investigating-covid-19-case.html.

Population Health Management Perspective: COVID-19 Mini Case Study

See the following coronavirus reports.

Novel Coronavirus Report from the *Morbidity and Mortality Weekly Reports* (*MMWR*) produced by the CDC:

1. Patel, A., Jernigan, D. B. (2020). Initial public health response and interim clinical guidance for the 2019 novel coronavirus outbreak—United States, December 31, 2019–February 4, 2020. *Morbidity and Mortality Weekly Report, 69*, 140–146. http://doi.org/10.15585/mmwr.mm6905e1

Novel Coronavirus Report from the *MMWR* produced by the CDC:

2. Jernigan, D. B. (2020) Update: Public health response to the coronavirus disease 2019 outbreak—United States, February 24, 2020. *Morbidity and Mortality Weekly Report, 69*, 216–219. http://doi.org/10.15585/mmwr.mm6908e1

3. Coronavirus Disease 2019 (COVID-19) Situation Summary, CDC, https://www.cdc.gov/coronavirus/2019-nCoV/summary.html

4. Coronavirus, World Health Organization, (WHO), https://www.who.int/health-topics/coronavirus

CASE STUDY QUESTIONS

After reviewing the aforementioned reports, respond to the following questions and consider the factors mentioned:

1. Compare the public health and clinical response to this novel virus. How might the responses be integrated via a population health approach?

2. Identify representative stakeholders from the public health and healthcare systems who should be involved in the response to this pandemic.
3. Provide examples of the three types of prevention approaches that may be useful in such pandemic.
4. Describe why the social determinants of health (SDOH) are important to consider in the respective communities impacted by the pandemic.
5. How is the MMWR a valuable tool to public health and healthcare professionals?
6. Explain which analytical epidemiology study design would be most helpful in providing useful information about the association between exposure and disease.
7. Which measure of association would be most useful?
8. Calculate the case fatality rate for COVID-19 for your state and/or the nation? Which data source(s) did you use? Why is this value important?
9. This novel pandemic raises concerns about the tension that exists between personal freedom and protection of the public's health. How can the public health and healthcare systems contribute to reaching a balance on this contentious issue?
10. Identify three resources, other than the CDC, that you would use in your work to stay abreast of an evolving health situation impacting the population for which you serve.

REFERENCES

American Hospital Association (AHA). (2020). *Population health management.* https://www.aha.org/center/population-health/population-health-management

Boston University School of Public Health (BUSPH). (2016). *Standardized rates of disease.* http://sphweb.bumc.bu.edu/otlt/MPH-Modules/EP/EP713_StandardizedRates/EP713_StandardizedRates2.html

CDC. (2012). *Principles of epidemiology in public health practice: Introduction to applied epidemiology and biostatistics* (3rd ed.) U.S. Department of Health and Human Services.

CDC. (2014). *The public health system and the 10 essential public health services – Powerpoint.* https://www.cdc.gov/publichealthgateway/publichealthservices/essentialhealthservices.html

CDC. (2016). *Lesson 6: Investigating an outbreak – section 2 – steps of an outbreak investigation.* https://www.cdc.gov/csels/dsepd/ss1978/lesson6/section2.html

CDC. (2017). *Quarantine and isolation.* https://www.cdc.gov/quarantine/index.html

CDC. (2020a). *10 Essential Public Health Services Futures Initiative Task Force.* 10 Essential Public Health Services. https://phnci.org/uploads/resource-files/EPHS-English.pdf

CDC. (2020b). *Coronavirus disease 2019 (COVID-19).* https://www.cdc.gov/coronavirus/2019-ncov/faq.html#Coronavirus-Disease-2019-Basics

CDC. (2020c). *Case investigation and contact tracing: Part of a multipronged approach to fight the COVID-19 pandemic.* https://www.cdc.gov/coronavirus/2019-ncov/php/principles-contact-tracing.html

CDC. (2020d). *COVID-19—investigating a COVID-19 case.* https://www.cdc.gov/coronavirus/2019-ncov/php/contact-tracing/contact-tracing-plan/investigating-covid-19-case.html

Framingham Heart Study. (2020). About. https://framinghamheartstudy.org/fhs-about/

Friis, R. H., & Sellers, T. A. (2014). *Epidemiology for public health practice* (5th ed.) Jones & Bartlett Learning.

Health and Medicine Division. (2020). *Roundtable on population health improvement.* Retrieved February 13, 2020, from http://nationalacademies.org/HMD/Activities/PublicHealth/PopulationHealthImprovementRT.aspx

Institute of Medicine (IOM). (1988). *The future of public health.* National Academies Press.

Jernigan, D. B. (2020). Update: Public health response to the coronavirus disease 2019 outbreak — United States, February 24, 2020. *Morbidity and Mortality Weekly Report, 69*, 216–219. http://doi.org/10.15585/mmwr.mm6908e1

Kindig, D. A. (2012). *Is population medicine population health?* https://www.improvingpopulationhealth.org/blog/2012/06/is-population-medicine-population-health.html

Last, J. M. (Ed.). (2001). *Dictionary of epidemiology* (4th ed.). Oxford University Press.

Oleske, D. M. (Ed.). (2001). *Epidemiology and the delivery of health care services* (2nd ed.). Kluwer Academic/Plenum Publishers.

Patel, A., & Jernigan, D. B. (2020). Initial public health response and interim clinical guidance for the 2019 novel coronavirus outbreak — United States, December 31, 2019–February 4, 2020. *Morbidity and Mortality Weekly Report, 69*, 140–146. http://doi.org/10.15585/mmwr.mm6905e1

Porta, M. (Ed.). (2014). *A dictionary of epidemiology* (6th ed.). Oxford University Press.

Public Health Agency of Canada. (2013). *What is the population health approach?* https://www.canada.ca/en/public-health/services/health-promotion/population-health/population-health-approach/what-population-health-approach.html#history

Public Health England. (2020). *Covid-19: Epidemiology, virology, and clinical features.* https://www.gov.uk/government/publications/wuhan-novel-coronavirus-background-information/wuhan-novel-coronavirus-epidemiology-virology-and-clinical-features

Szumilas, M. (2010). Explaining odds ratios. *Journal of the Canadian Academy of Child and Adolescent Psychiatry, 19*(3), 227–229.

Tulen, A. D., Vennema, H., van Pelt, W., Franz, E., & Hofhuis, A. (2019). A case-control study into risk factors for acute hepatitis E in the Netherlands, 2015–2017. *Journal of Infection, 78*(5), P373–P381. https://doi.org/10.1016/j.jinf.2019.02.001

Turnock, B. J. (2001). *Public health: What it is and how it works.* Aspen Publishers, Inc.

Tyler, C. W., & Last, J. M. (1992). Epidemiology. In J. M. Last & R. B. Wallace (Eds.), *Maxcy-Rosenau-Last: Public health and preventive medicine* (14th ed., pp. 11–39). Appleton & Lange.

Winslow, C. E. A. (1920). The un-tilled fields of public health. *Science, 51*(1306), 23–33. https://doi.org/10.1126/science.51.1306.23

World Health Organization (WHO). (1946). *Constitution.* https://www.who.int/about/who-we-are/constitution

CHAPTER 3

Assessing Population Health: Community Health Needs Assessments

Anne M. Hewitt and Don Dykstra

KEY TERMS

Community Benefit
Community Health Improvement Matrix
Community Health Improvement Plan (CHIP)
Community Health Needs Assessment (CHNA)
Community Health Assessment Toolkit

County Health Rankings and Roadmaps
Mobilizing for Action Through Planning and Partnership Model (MAPP)
Patient Protection and Affordable Care Act (PPACA)
PolicyMap
Social Determinants of Health

LEARNING OBJECTIVES

1. Explain the community benefit mandate and the emphasis on community engagement.
2. Assess the Patient Protection and Affordable Care Act (PPACA) of 2010's impact on the role of population health management (PHM) in the community.
3. Identify diverse interactive databases and mapping technologies appropriate for community health needs assessments (CHNAs).
4. Describe the CHNA process.
5. Compare CHNA models on their ease of use and potential outcomes.

> Podcasts that exemplify the content of this chapter are available at Springer Publishing Connect™
>
> Podcast 3.1. Why Does a Hospital Need to Demonstrate Community Benefit?
> Podcast 3.2. Who Needs a Community Health Needs Assessment?

Access the podcast online at http://connect.springerpub.com/content/book/978-0-8261-4427-0/part/part01/chapter/ch03

INTRODUCTION

Populations consist of people who live, work, and play in local communities (Carlson, 2020). Community healthscapes impact the health status and quality of life outcomes of every population-of-interest. For many communities, hospitals and health systems are the major or largest employers and serve as an anchor for local economies (Zuckerman, 2013). Each of these roles emphasizes the deep relationship between communities and the health sector. A primary goal, for population health managers, centers on ensuring the optimum health of their community. This chapter covers the hospitals and health system's efforts and activities to ensure community quality of life via CHNAs and community health improvement plans (CHIPs).

Initial Population Health and Community Alignments: Community Benefit

Maintaining a community's quality of life is an integrated priority in addition to PHM's twin goals of increasing health access and lowering cost. The Internal Revenue Service (IRS) established a community benefit standard in 1969 (James, 2016). **Community benefit** focuses on ensuring that nonprofit hospitals/healthcare systems serve the needs of their community to be eligible for tax exempt status and to operate as a 301c organization (Community Benefit Connect [CBC], 2020). Hospitals and health systems who meet the standards and criteria can be best described as a "public trust" initiative.

"Community benefits are clinical or nonclinical programs or activities providing treatment and/or promoting health and healing that are responsive to identified community needs, not provided for marketing purposes" (James, 2016). Common examples are health fairs with disease screening, mobile health vans, and community gardens all sponsored by the health system or hospital.

DID YOU KNOW?

What Is a Community Benefit?

Community benefit goes far beyond the brick walls of the local community hospital. This video provides multiple examples of hospital efforts to demonstrate community benefit.
https://www.youtube.com/watch?v=cRXDVTq69XY
Catholic Health Association (n.d.-b)

The Catholic Health Association (CHA) remains one of the premier leaders in defining, implementing, and assessing community benefit. Since 2008, tax-exempt hospitals have been required to report their community benefit and other information related to tax exemption on the IRS Form 990 Schedule H, and over the years, additional requirements have been added (CHA, n.d.-a).

TABLE 3.1 Community Benefit Objectives and Criteria

Community Benefit Objectives	Community Benefit Criteria
• Address community need • Improve access to health services • Enhance population health • Advance knowledge • Demonstrate charitable purpose	• Have a board made up of community members • Qualified physicians in the area must have medical privileges at the hospital • Have an emergency department • Admit all types of patients without discrimination and • Funding must be directed to benefit the patients served by the hospital

DID YOU KNOW?

IRS Form 990 Schedule H

Today, Schedule H serves as the primary reporting mechanism for community benefits. Click this link to view the form: www.irs.gov/pub/irs-pdf/f990sh.pdf.

As the primary goal of hospital/health system and community relationships is to improve the health of all residents, PH managers have a responsibility and accountability to meet and achieve all community health objectives. The community benefit standards are specific and detailed for all nonprofit hospitals, which must meet established criteria. Table 3.1 displays both community benefit objectives and criteria (IRS, 2020).

DID YOU KNOW?

The Importance of Hospitals' Benefit to the Community

A recent free eBook is available with the latest information and review of the impact of community benefit. The eBook titled *Hospitals' Benefit to the Community: Research, Policy and Evaluation*, a collection of recently published, peer-reviewed papers, is now available as a free eBook from *Frontiers in Public Health*. The link is here: https://www.frontiersin.org/research-topics/9723/hospitals-benefit-to-the-community-research-policy-and-evaluation.

As the healthcare sector transitions and enters nontraditional entrepreneurial types of partnerships and business relationships, various community stakeholders have questioned if local hospitals provide an appropriate amount of community benefit to their constituents in need (Ofri, 2020). Do hospitals consistently and systematically address the most appropriate healthcare needs of their communities? Are there any missed opportunities for alignment?

Health Policy Implications for Community and Population Health Alignment

The U.S. health sector is one of the most regulated industries in the world, and health policy greatly impacts the parameters of health sector/community relationships. In 2010, the **Patient Protection and Affordable Care Act (PPACA)** (HealthCare.gov., 2010) became one of the most far-reaching policy mandates since the beginnings of Medicare and Medicaid in the 1960s (Goldstein et al., 2016).

> **? DID YOU KNOW?**
>
> **The PPACA—Past and Present**
>
> The PPACA can be considered one of the major catalysts for population health. This legislation's impact list includes many major innovations, some of which have flourished such as the Accountable Care Organization model for value-based care. Other ideas have yet to be fully accepted or integrated into the healthcare sector. The impact list can be categorized into three major areas: health promotion, delivery of care, and value-based initiatives.
>
> Health Promotion Policy
> - National Prevention, Health Promotion, and Public Health Council
> - Prevention and Health Fund
> - **Community Health Needs Assessment Mandate**
>
> Access and Delivery of Care Initiatives
> - Health insurance marketplace (public exchange)
> - Coverage of preventive health services
> - Coverage for annual Medicare wellness visit
> - Expanded Medicaid options for states
>
> Value-Based Models
> - Accountable care organizations
> - Medicare Shared Savings Programs
>
> The PPACA's primary goal targeted universal health coverage for Americans. A review of the Act's impact 10 years later suggests a significant reduction in the number of uninsured people and an increase in access to healthcare services, especially for low-income and people of color (Blumenthal et al., 2020).

The PPACA has transformed the delivery of healthcare, and a prime example is the support for innovation and program waivers. The ACA established the Center for Medicare and Medicaid Innovation (CMMI) within the Centers for Medicare and Medicaid Services (CMS) (CMS, 2020). Soon states began integrating population health approaches, such as disease management programs, in high-cost populations such as Medicaid and Medicare recipients. State health departments also began implementing chronic disease self-management programs (SMPs) as an effective PHM strategy.

> **? DID YOU KNOW?**
>
> **State Health Promotion Example**
>
> One public example of a population health initiative is the adoption of general health promotion initiatives tailored to seniors. New Jersey's Department of Human Services, Division of Aging Services publishes a monthly e-newsletter available to the public—"HealthEASE." Provided in the following is a sample list of health promotion–inspired SMPs, which were transferred to virtual formats due to the COVID pandemic.
>
> **HealthEASE**
>
> A Matter of Balance–
> Move Today–

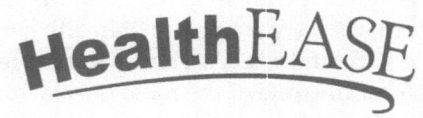

Project Healthy Bones–
Stress Busters for Family Caregivers–
Tai Ji Quan: Moving for Better Balance–
Take Control of Your Health–
The various CMMI demonstration programs and other delivery models align with PHM goals that emphasize access, quality initiatives, and value-based initiatives (Shepard et al., 2021).

Community Health Needs Assessments: Population Health Alignment

The PPACA also introduced the requirement for CHNAs, which focuses on accessing and meeting each community's needs to maintain nonprofit status. This expansive policy, under the IRS jurisdiction, also establishes protocols detailing a hospital's financial assistance and emergency medical policy, limitations of charges and billing, and collection procedures.

Over the years, community benefit criteria had established the necessity of addressing community need but lacked a systematic process, plan, and assessment framework. Local health departments regularly complete mandated community health assessments (CHAs) of their constituents based on geographic location, as directed by state and federal guidelines, but this was not the case with community hospitals. Note the terms CHNA and CHAs are often used interchangeably (Public Health Accreditation Board [PHAB], 2011).

The PPACA of 2010 required hospitals to conduct, every 3 years, CHNAs in partnership with other stakeholder community agencies, such as the local health departments. The purpose was twofold—(1) to assess the current population's health status (CHNA) and (2) to develop an appropriate community implementation plan, commonly known as a CHIP (IRS, 2020). Figure 3.1 presents the specific CHNA requirements in outline form.

Completion of a CHNA is a complex and detailed process, involves many hours of data collection, analysis, and interpretation, and begins usually more than a year in advance. After the CHNA is completed, the CHIP development process requires input and collaboration with diverse and representative community stakeholders. The PPACA stipulates a financial penalty tax of $50,000 per hospital for noncompliance, and the IRS can revoke hospital tax-exempt status.

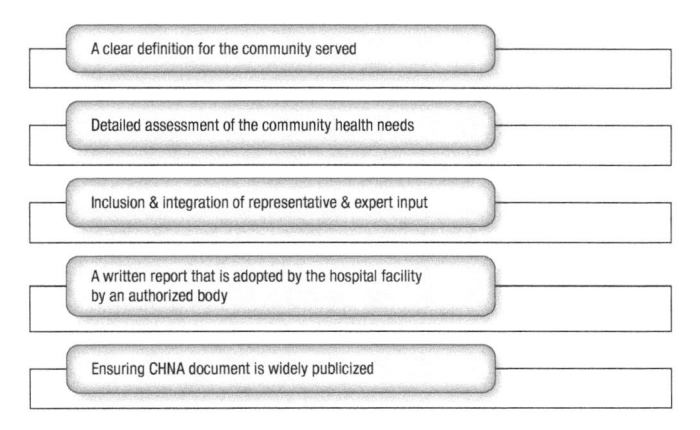

- A clear definition for the community served
- Detailed assessment of the community health needs
- Inclusion & integration of representative & expert input
- A written report that is adopted by the hospital facility by an authorized body
- Ensuring CHNA document is widely publicized

FIGURE 3.1 Outline of Core CHNA Requirements

CHNA, community health needs assessment.

Step-by-Step Community Alignment

Given the CHNA mandate to work with all community stakeholders, population health managers should strongly align with their local public health department or office. Assessment is one of public health's three core functions, and local public health departments have completed CHAs regularly for many years. The professional organization National Association of County and City Health Officials (NACCHO) provides supporting models and materials applicable for completing a CHA process (NACCHO, n.d.-a). Public health professionals often follow the **Mobilizing for Action through Planning and Partnerships (MAPP) model**, which is a recently revised multiphase model based on a community-driven strategic planning process (NACCHO, n.d.-c). In Exhibit 3.1, the original six MAPP phases are presented. As a strategic planning processes, there are multiple activities and deliverables associated with each of these six outlined stages of the community framework.

To support local community hospitals, the American Hospital Association (AHA) sponsored the Association for Community Health Improvement's (ACHI's) **Community Health Assessment Toolkit** (ACHI, 2020).

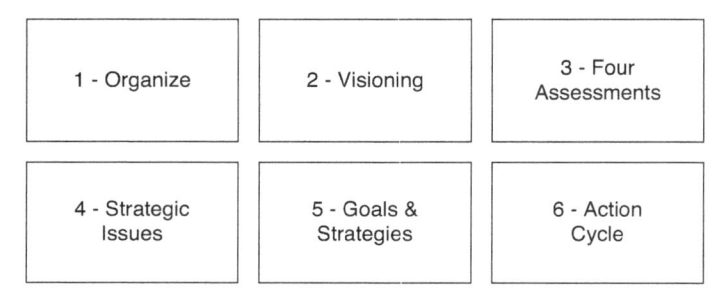

1 - Organize	2 - Visioning	3 - Four Assessments
4 - Strategic Issues	5 - Goals & Strategies	6 - Action Cycle

EXHIBIT 3.1 Mobilizing for Action Through Planning and Partnership Model
Source: Adapted from National Association of County and City Health Officials. (2020). *Mobilizing for action through planning and partnerships (MAPP)*. https://www.naccho.org/programs/public-health-infrastructure/performance-improvement/community-health-assessment/mapp

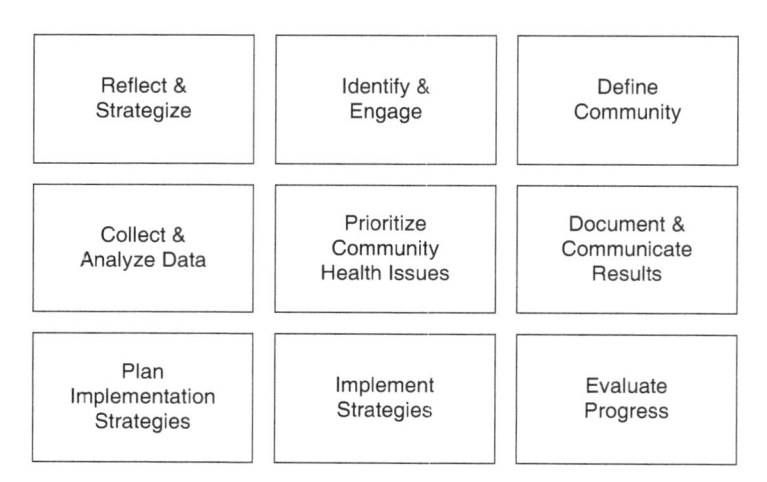

Reflect & Strategize	Identify & Engage	Define Community
Collect & Analyze Data	Prioritize Community Health Issues	Document & Communicate Results
Plan Implementation Strategies	Implement Strategies	Evaluate Progress

EXHIBIT 3.2 Nine Phases of Community Health Assessment Toolkit
Source: Adapted from AHA Community Health Improvement—Community Health Improvement. (2020). *Community health assessment toolkit*. https://www.healthycommunities.org/resources/community-health-assessment-toolkit

This detailed Toolkit provides a nine-step process to successfully complete a CHNA. Each of the nine phases reflects a community oriented, transparent process to improve community health outcomes (see Exhibit 3.2).

> **① DID YOU KNOW?**
>
> **Models of Community Health Needs Assessment**
>
> Take the time to read in-depth about each of the two models that are briefly discussed—MAPP and the CHNA Toolkit (NACCHO, n.d.-b); https://www.naccho.org/programs/public-health-infrastructure/performance-improvement/community-health-assessment/mapp; (ACHI, 2020) https://www.healthycommunities.org/resources/community-health-assessment-toolkit.
>
> Since the passage of the PPACA, both local public health departments and community hospitals have aligned to coproduce CHNAs that are valuable and useful to each partner. In fact, these relationships have led to better data collection and sharing processes (Stoto et al., 2019).

Although differences exist between these two CHA models, each approach produces clearly identified goals to be used for developing a CHIP. As a community is made of many members with diverse agendas, these recognized priorities provide a framework for action and the potential for creating community coalitions focused on similar health priorities. There is no other way to get a complete and comprehensive picture of the health status of the community. As healthcare needs continue to increase, reducing delivery redundancies and addressing the community's health needs is the only way to improve the health of any population.

Community Health Needs Assessments Tools and Applications

Frequently, hospital and health system personnel rely on electronic medical records, also known as electronic health records, and clinical, usage, or claims data for planning purposes. Primary sources, such as the AHA, Medicare, and the Dartmouth Atlas of Health Care (Dartmouth Atlas Project, 2020), provide detailed hospital specific information. Other types of data available include the International Classification of Diseases (ICD) data and specific disease registry information, such as the Surveillance, Epidemiology and End Results Program (SEER) sponsored by the National Cancer Institute (SEER, 2020). As technology capabilities enable greater access to diverse health indicators resulting in new data, industry information and marketing statistics will become available. For instance, access to over-the-counter medications information can serve as complementary data source for a community (Das et al., 2005).

Population and public health researchers, planning, and policy experts regularly access national databases for basic population health information including standard federal and state data on vital statistics (morbidity, mortality, births, deaths, etc.) and the American Community Survey based on U.S. Census data. CDC Wonder, an interactive web-based tool, sponsored by the CDC provides public use data and information (CDC WONDER, 2020). Another valuable CDC resource, the Behavioral Risk Factor Surveillance Survey (BRFSS) analyzes population's health risk behaviors, health conditions and status, and use of preventive services with an emphasis on documenting actual behaviors (Centers for Disease and Health Prevention, 2020).

Each state annually has the option to add specific questions-of-interest targeting emerging health issues. This information helps enhance and provide a more detailed snapshot of a population's health status.

County Health Rankings and Roadmap *and PolicyMap*

Two important community databases and CHNA tools are the RWJ Foundation's sponsored **County Health Rankings and Roadmap** (CHRR) (CHRR, 2020a), and **PolicyMap** (PolicyMap, 2020). Both interactive digital platforms provide supplemental data that permit population health planners to access and manipulate easily. Often state and local public health agencies lack comprehensive, representative, or up-to-date health statistics at a county level or municipal level. Using a four-category system (clinical care, health behaviors, social and economic factors, and physical environment), CHRR ranks the health of nearly every county in the nation and demonstrates ways location affects how well and long we live. Key findings, summarized each year, provide useful comparison metrics that encourage benchmarking analysis to state standards and other top performing county peers (CHRR, 2020b) (https://www.countyhealthrankings.org/reports/2019-county-health-rankings-key-findings-report).

While the CHRR provides user-friendly integration of available county health data, PolicyMap, an online mapping tool, offers a vast assortment of data from multiple databases to describe a population at a defined and specific geographic location (PolicyMap, 2020). PolicyMap, an example of a geographical information system (GIS), is an interactive, visual resource that aligns multiple determinants of health metrics with pinpointed locations. Another PolicyMap benefit is the opportunity to layer personalized data or other relevant information onto a three-layer map. With this level of analysis, health planners and programmers have access to valuable visual evidence to target the most vulnerable communities.

? DID YOU KNOW?

What Happens When a Community Is Ignored?

Understanding a community and the population requires trust, patience, and listening. You only need to listen to the first 3½ minutes of this humorous TEDx video (Ernesto Sirolli: Want to help someone? Shut up and listen!) to understand the importance of valuing the community's voice: https://www.youtube.com/watch?v=chXsLtHqfdM.

The Impact of Recent Community Health Needs Assessment Findings

The first CHNA results became available in 2013, and policy-makers were interested in whether hospitals would adopt the process and integrate outcomes into their strategic plans and programs. An initial study reported substantial variation among hospitals in respect to meeting implementation progress as outlined by the federal CHNA requirements (Cramer et al., 2017). Early research identified the top rural health community needs in two categories: (a) community concerns—alcohol/substance abuse, cancer, and obesity and (b) healthy community issues—access to healthcare, good jobs and a healthy economy, and healthy behaviors and lifestyle (Barnett, 2012).

Later research on a rural area, the Appalachian Ohio region, suggested that hospitals formalize their processes, focus on developing an evidence base, cultivate local partnerships, and reflect on the role of the hospital in public health (Franz, Skinner, & Kelleher, 2017).

Other reports focused on single issues such as a study noting that in U.S. cities with the highest violent crime rates, 74% of CHNAs mentioned violence-related terms, but only 32% designated violence prevention as a priority need (Fischer, 2018). Another targeted CHNA review of Florida hospitals that provided pediatric services revealed that the top four mentioned community health priorities were access to care, nutrition/exercise/obesity, mental health, and health education (Gruber et al., 2019). Researchers also report hospitals predominantly identified health needs related to access to care, insurance coverage, and costs, but dental care, behavioral health, substance abuse, social factors, and healthcare and prescription drugs were infrequently targeted for strategic action (Powell et al., 2018). Results from a significant national analysis using a random sample of 496 U.S. nonprofit hospitals found mental health, access to care, obesity, substance abuse, diabetes, cancer, and the social determinants of health were the most identified needs. However, the rate at which hospitals chose to address each of these needs in their implementation strategies varied considerably, ranging from 56% (cancer) to 85% (obesity) (Franz, Cronin, & Singh, 2021). In addition to chronic care diseases, social determinants of health began to appear as a category of need.

DID YOU KNOW?

Social Determinants of Health

There are many types of determinants of health including physical, genetics, personal (genetics, gender), and external influencers such as education, social status (income), relationships (social support networks), health services (access and availability of care), and even the physical environment (Caron, 2017). Today, social and economic factors are believed to contribute up to 40% of an individual's health status (CHRR, 2020a).

Social determinants of health are defined as "conditions in which people are born, grow, live, work, and age, these circumstances are shaped by the distribution of money, power, and resources at the global, national, and local levels" (World Health Organization [WHO], 2008). Although these were acknowledged several years ago, today's data show their extremely significant impact on health status and quality of life. The WHO definition further describes SDOH as "circumstances are shaped by the distribution of money, power, and resources at the global, national, and local levels."

The PPACA's increased emphasis on mandating healthcare system alignment with community health needs resulted in a greater recognition of SDOH's role in the health of every American. Community and location (place-based) issues gained prominence as risk factors for positive health outcomes.

Concerned with the importance of social determinants of health as reported in CHA and CHNAs, NACCHO released a 2014 report assessing SDOH activities described in local health department CHIPS and nonprofit hospitals strategic implementation plans (NACCHO, 2014). After an extensive review and analysis, the findings suggested that assessing the alignment between SDOH identification (CHNA, CHA) and the resulting strategy or activity (CHIP) required a bivariate analysis on two levels—the level of prevention and the amount or intensity of intervention. The **Community Health Improvement Matrix** presents a visual depiction of an SDOH goal achievement (see Table 3.2).

TABLE 3.2 Community Health Improvement Matrix—Asthma Reduction Example

	Objective: Decrease Asthma in Children					
P R E V E N T I O N	TERTIARY	Pediatric Clinic		School-Asthma Trained Nurses		
	SECONDARY	Peer Support Groups		School Screenings		
	PRIMARY	Action Plan/ Prescription Access Programs	Family Support Groups	Home Weatherization Program		
	PRIMORDAL	Safe Play Areas	Clean and Safe Homes	Home Visits	Clear Air Regulations/ No Smoking Zones	Environmental and Pollution Policy
		Individual	Interpersonal	Organizational	Community	Public Policy
	INTERVENTION LEVEL					

Source: Adapted from National Association of County and City Health Officials. (2014). *Addressing the social determinants of health through the community health improvement matrix. Research brief.* https://www.health.state.mn.us/communities/practice/resources/equitylibrary/docs/AddressingtheSocialDeterminantsofHealthCommHealthMatrix.pdf

Frameworks for assessing population health outcomes highlight the importance and role of CHA as an expected competency for both PH managers and their organizations. In July 2020, the AHA and other health-related professional organizations requested the Secretary of Treasury provide an extension of the next CHNA due date because of the extraordinary burden placed on hospitals due to the COVID-19 challenge (Heath, 2020). The next series of CHAs and CHNA reports will undoubtedly show greater community health needs especially for vulnerable American subpopulations.

SUMMARY

Hospitals continue to maintain their role and position as a community's primary hub and safety net for the populations served. National policies, including the recent PPACA of 2010, hold hospitals accountable for positive population health outcomes. Data informed decision-making based on analysis of multiple health databases and interactive GIS platforms require competencies in both CHNAs and development of community health implementation plans. Future community collaborations will need to focus on the social determinants of health to attain an equitable level of health for all Americans.

DISCUSSION QUESTIONS

1. What is the primary role of the hospital/healthcare system in the community?
2. List and explain at least three major PHM innovations from the PPACA of 2010?
3. Compare the community benefit and CHNAs commonalities and differences.
4. Identify the CHI Toolbox model and describe which of the various 9 steps might pose the largest management challenge.
5. Describe primary benefits for both the CHRR and PolicyMap.
6. Which datasets and which metrics would you select to create a community dashboard?

Toolkit Competency Application—Mini-Case Study: Designing a CHNA Process

ABC Health System: Community Health Needs Assessment

Compliance with IRS guidelines for CHNAs requires the input of the community in the creation of the CHNA. Organizations can employ a broad array of methods to collect, analyze, and ultimately build actionable reasoned insights from community input data derived relative to health issues faced by the population.

The ABC Health System (ABC-HS) consists of six acute care hospitals. The ABC-HS, through its hospitals, ambulatory sites, physician practices, and other partner organizations serves about a million area residents annually, with many in multiple care settings. The health system's geographic footprint ranges from urban to rural setting and from the most to the least

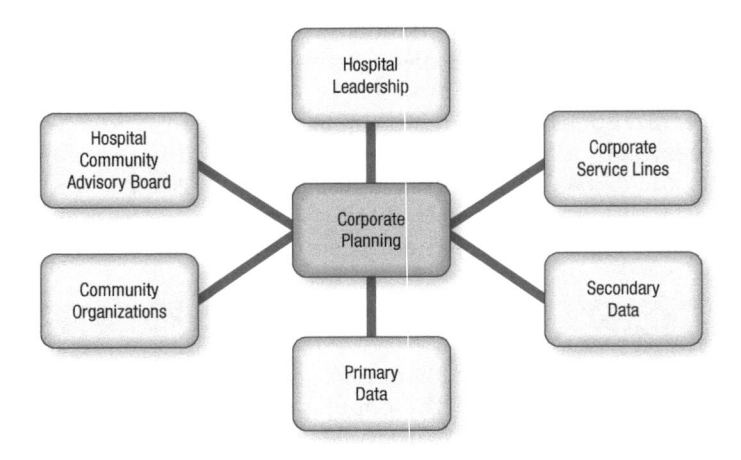

FIGURE 3.2 Necessary Stakeholders and Components for a CHNA

densely populated portions of the state. Building a network of care that provides access to health care services for such a diverse population is informed by the CHNA process, which the ABC-HS developed beginning in 2010 and continues to refine and enhance with each iteration of its CHNA.

Part of any successful CHNA is a clear definition of the contribution that each participant, group, or data set brings to the process. Figure 3.2 depicts the stakeholders and components necessary for a CHNA.

Corporate Planning

In the model employed by the System, corporate planning functions act as the responsible party for completion of the CHNA in accordance with Federal guidelines and timeframes. Planning also serves to identify constituencies and data sources that will inform the process as well as providing substantial support to each constituency as they review secondary data, process findings from primary research and distill qualitative and quantitative elements down to substantive and reasonable targets for community health improvement efforts based on identified needs or disparities in the populations served by the System. Ultimately, planning produces a publicly available report of the CHNA that is approved and adopted by hospital Community Advisory Boards (CABs).

Hospital Community Advisory Board

The System's hospitals all operate a CAB. One of the many functions of this board is to provide leadership of the CHNA process for each hospital and to adopt the CHNA for that cycle. As part of the "kickoff" of the CHNA process, corporate planning provides the CAB an in-depth review and assessment of health factors and behaviors in their community. In most instances, this review serves to inform the CAB with baseline knowledge and often generates questions or inquiries from CAB members about sub-populations the hospital serves. As the CHNA moves through the remaining process steps, the CAB is periodically informed of progress and preliminary findings. Ultimately a numerically prioritized list of health indicators, having been informed by community input, vetted through hospital leadership and relevant service line leads, is presented to the CAB for their final prioritization and adoption.

Data Sources: Secondary Data Options

The basis for any successful CHNA is in the data. Since the inception of the CHNA process, secondary data sources have evolved from extremely limited county or national indicators to extremely granular census tract or block group data sets that allow for identification of disparities and health needs at a hyper-local level.

The first CHNA's were largely informed by aggregated data from state health departments or national estimates from the Centers for Disease Control or the U.S. Department of Health and Human Services. These initial data sets, while informative to hospitals and community organizations seeking to identify opportunities for health improvement, were woefully inadequate at the local level and ultimately became relegated to informing the CHNA process at a remarkably high level.

To make CHNA's more actionable at a local level, forward thinking organizations began mining their own de-identified organizational data. What better way could there be to identify specific clinical and geographic opportunities for health improvement than to look inward to the very individuals the System treated daily. The aggregation of this type of data allowed for much more targeted analyses and sharing of more actionable insights with the community and local public health departments.

Today, there have been tremendous strides made by large data collectives (national, commercial, and local) that allow the System to provide a wide-ranging secondary data analysis of health factors and behaviors in the communities the System serves. This analysis and findings are shared with constituencies in the next process step.

Primary Data and the Role of Community Organizations

Given the limitations of secondary data analyses and driven by blind spots created by a relevant lack of granularity and/or general absence of available data, it is critical that some level of primary research be used to inform the CHNA process. The ABD-HS engages community partners in this process, rather than develop widely distributed public survey instruments. Time and iteration have shown that identifying a core group of community representatives (public health officials, clinical partners, clergy, grass-roots community organizations, etc.) to respond to survey instruments reveals similar substantive community health concerns as would a public survey data collection methodology. Participating organizations and groups are recommended or selected by CAB (CAB members, hospital administrative and clinical leads, and other community organizations with strong ties to populations served by the hospital. The results of this primary data are integrated into findings from secondary data sources, which are weighted by frequency and ultimately form the prioritized list of health factors and behaviors presented to the CAB.

Hospital Leadership and Corporate Service Lines

Administrative and clinical leads at the hospitals play a crucial role in informing the CHNA process. Ultimately, the individual hospitals will carry the responsibility of developing an annual CHIP that is based on the health priorities adopted in the CHNA. Ensuring that hospital leadership and service line leads are informed of health disparities in their communities, can provide insight and direction on how the hospital is currently/not currently addressing a particular health factor or behavior. Corporate service line leads can best deploy resources across a large population and geographic region where similar disparities exist. Their engagement and participation will ultimately create a CHNA that is actionable, measurable, and successful in its goal of improving the health of the communities served by the System.

CASE STUDY SUMMARY

The key organizational element that must be present for a CHNA to be useful, transformative, and to provide a sustainable process is a commitment to substantive and ongoing communication between the community and hospital about how partnerships and resources can best be identified and utilized to alter the direction of identified health disparities.

CASE STUDY QUESTIONS

1. Assess the alignment of ABC-HS's CHNA process with the nine phases of the Community Health Assessment Toolkit.
2. Identify the strengths and weaknesses of the ABC-HS's approach as represented in the Figure 3.2.
3. Describe the multiple roles of the Community Advisory Board in this model.
4. What data sources would you recommend for ABC-HS to help address their healthscape needs for both rural and urban areas?

REFERENCES

Association for Community Health Improvement—Community Health Improvement. (2020). *Community health assessment toolkit*. https://www.healthycommunities.org/resources/community-health-assessment-toolkit

Barnett, K. (2012, February). *Best practices for community health needs assessment and implementation strategy development: A review of scientific methods, current practices, and future potential report of Proceedings from a Public Forum and Interviews of Experts Public Forum convened by the Centers for Disease Control and Prevention Atlanta, Georgia (July 11–13, 2011)*. Public Health Institute. http://www.phi.org/wp-content/uploads/migration/uploads/application/files/dz9vh55o3bb2x56lcrzyel83fwfu3mvu24oqqvn5z6qaeiw2u4.pdf

Blumenthal, D., Collins, S., & Fowler, E. (2020, February 26). The affordable care act at 10 years: What is the effect on health care coverage and access? *The Commonwealth Fund*. https://www.commonwealthfund.org/publications/journal-article/2020/feb/aca-at-10-years-effect-health-care-coverage-access

Carlson, L. M. (2020). Health is where we live, work and play—And in our ZIP codes: Tackling social determinants of health. *The Nation's Health, 50*(1), 3. http://www.thenationshealth.org/content/50/1/3.1

Caron, R. (2017). *Population health: Principles and applications for management*. Health Administration Press. Association of University Programs in Health Administration, Washington, DC.

Catholic Health Association. (n.d.-a). *About community benefit*. https://www.chausa.org/communitybenefit/resources/defining-community-benefit

Catholic Health Association. (n.d.-b). *What is a community benefit?* Video. https://www.youtube.com/watch?v=cRXDVTq69XY

CDC WONDER. (2020). *CDC wide-ranging online data for epidemiologic research.* https://wonder.cdc.gov/

Centers for Disease and Health Prevention. (2020). *Behavioral risk factor surveillance survey (BRFSS).* https://www.cdc.gov/brfss/index.html

Centers for Medicare and Medicaid Services. (2020, November 25). *About the CMS Innovation Center.* Center for Medicare and Medicaid Services. CMS.gov. https://innovation.cms.gov/about

Community Benefit Connect. (2020). *What is community benefit?* Community Benefit Connect. www.communitybenefitconnect.org/about-us/about_what-is/

County Health Rankings and Roadmaps. (2020a). *County health rankings model.* https://www.countyhealthrankings.org/explore-health-rankings/measures-data-sources

County Health Rankings and Roadmaps. (2020b). *2020 county health rankings: State reports.* https://www.countyhealthrankings.org/

Cramer, G. R., Singh, S. R., Flaherty, S., & Young, G. J. (2017). The progress of US hospitals in addressing community health needs. *American Journal of Public Health, 107*(2), 255–261. https://doi.org/10.2105/AJPH.2016.303570

Dartmouth Atlas Project. (2020). *Dartmouth Atlas of Health Care.* https://www.dartmouthatlas.org/

Das, D., Metzger, K., Heffernan, R., Balter, S., Weiss, D., & Mostashari, F. (2005, August 26). Monitoring over-the counter medication sales for early detection of disease outbreaks-New York City. *MMWR Supplement.* https://www.cdc.gov/mmwr/preview/mmwrhtml/su5401a9.htm

Fischer, K. R., Schwimmer, H., Purtle, J., Roman, D., Cosgrove, S, Current, J. J., & Greene, M. B. (2018). A content analysis of hospitals' community health needs assessments in the most violent U.S. cities. *Journal of Community Health, 243*(2), 259–262. https://doi.org/10.1007/s10900-017-0413-9

Franz, B., Cronin, C. E., & Singh, S. (2021). Are nonprofit hospitals addressing the most critical community health needs that they identify in their community health needs assessments? *Journal of Public Health Management and Practice, 27*(1), 80–87. https://doi.org/10.1097/PHH.0000000000001034

Franz, B., Skinner, D., & Kelleher, K. (2017). The impact of the Affordable Care Act on hospital-led community health evaluation in the U.S. Appalachian Ohio. *Journal of Evaluation in Clinical Practice, 23*(4), 882–887. https://www.aacom.org/docs/default-source/hpf-2018/2018-05_seminar/franz_et_al-2017-journal_of_evaluation_in_clinical_practice.pdf?sfvrsn=99eb2097_2

Goldstein, F., Shephard, V., & Duda, S. (2016). Policy implications for population health: Health promotion and wellness. In D. B. Nash, R. J. Fabius, J. L. Clarke, A. Skoufalos, & M. R. Horowitz (Eds.), *Population health: Creating a culture of wellness* (2nd ed., pp. 43–58). Jones & Bartlett Publishing.

Gruber, J. B., Wang, W., Quittner, A., Salyakina, D., & McCafferty-Fernandez, J. (2019). Utilizing Community Health Needs Assessments (CHNAs) in nonprofit hospitals to guide population-centered outcomes research for pediatric patients: New recommendations for CHNA reporting. *Population Health Management, 22*(1), 25–31. https://doi.org/10.1089/pop.2018.0049

HealthCare.gov. (2010). *Patient protection and affordable care act (PPAC).* https://www.healthcare.gov/glossary/patient-protection-and-affordable-care-act/

Heath, S. (2020, July 10). AHA calls for community health needs assessment extension. *Patient Care Access News.* https://patientengagementhit.com/news/aha-calls-for-community-health-needs-assessment-extension

Internal Revenue Service. (2020). *Community health needs assessment for Charitable Hospital Organizations - Section 501(r)(3).* https://www.irs.gov/charities-non-profits/community-health-needs-assessment-for-charitable-hospital-organizations-section-501r3

James, J. (2016). Health policy brief: Nonprofit hospitals community benefits requirements. *Health Affairs.* https://www.healthaffairs.org/do/10.1377/hpb20160225.954803/full/

National Association of County and City Health Officials. (2014). *Addressing the social determinants of health through the community health improvement matrix. Research brief.* https://www.health.state.mn.us/communities/practice/resources/equitylibrary/docs/AddressingtheSocialDeterminantsofHealthCommHealthMatrix.pdf

National Association of County and City Health Officials. (n.d.-a). *Community health assessment and improvement planning.* https://www.naccho.org/programs/public-health-infrastructure/performance-improvement/community-health-assessment

National Association of County and City Health Officials. (n.d.-b). *Mobilizing for action through planning and partnerships (MAPP).* https://www.naccho.org/programs/public-health-infrastructure/performance-improvement/community-health-assessment/mapp

National Association of County and City Health Officials. (n.d.-c). *Mobilizing for action through planning and partnerships (MAPP). Evolution blueprint executive summary.* https://www.naccho.org/uploads/downloadable-resources/MAPP-Evolution-Blueprint-Executive-Summary-V3-FINAL.pdf

Ofri, D. (2020, February 20). Why are nonprofit hospitals so highly profitable? *Opinion. New York Times.* https://www.nytimes.com/2020/02/20/opinion/nonprofit-hospitals.html

PolicyMap. (2020). *2020 PolicyMap: Online GIS maps.* https://www.policymap.com/maps

Powell, R. E., Doty, A. M. B., Rising, K. L., Karp, D. N., Baehr, A., & Carr, B. G. (2018). A content analysis of nonprofit hospital community health needs assessments and community benefit implementation strategies in Philadelphia. *Journal of Public Health Management and Practice, 24*(4), 326–334. https://doi.org/10.1097/PHH.0000000000000062

Public Health Accreditation Board. (2011). *Public health accreditation board: Standards & measures.* https://phsharing.org/resources/public-health-accreditation-board-standards-measures/

Shepard, V., Park, M., & Lee, B. (2021). Policy and advocacy. In D. Nash, A. Skoufalos, R. Fabius, & W. Oglesby (Eds.), *Population health: Creating a culture of wellness* (3rd ed., pp. 251–273). Jones & Bartlett Publishing.

Stoto, M. A., Davis, M. V., & Atkins, A. (2019). Making better use of population health data for community health needs assessments. *eGEMS, 7*(1), 44. https://doi.org/10.5334/egems.305

Surveillance, Epidemiology and End Results Program. (2020). *About SEER.* National Cancer Institute. https://seer.cancer.gov/

World Health Organization. (2008). *Social determinants of health key concepts.* http://www.who.int/social_determinants/thecommission/finalreport/key_concepts/en/

Zuckerman, D. (2013). *Hospitals building healthier communities: Embracing the anchor mission.* Contributions by H. J. Sparks, S. Dubbs, & T. Howard. *The Democracy Collaborative at University of Maryland.* https://community-wealth.org/content/hospitals-building-healthier-communities-embracing-anchor-mission

CHAPTER 4

Social Determinants of Health: Health Promotion for Diverse Populations

Rhonda BeLue, Teaniese Davis, and Michaila Dix

KEY TERMS

Biopsychosocial Model
Community Health Workers
Diversity and Inclusion
Electronic Health Record
Health Disparities
Health Equity and Equality
Health in All Policies

PRAPARE
Social Determinants of Health
Social Justice
Social Vulnerability Index
Structural Racism
Upstream, Midstream, Downstream

LEARNING OBJECTIVES

1. Define and discuss **social determinants of health (SDOH)** and their relationship to quality of life.
2. Describe measures of SDOH.
3. Explain the relationship between SDOH and health disparities.
4. Analyze current population health problems and develop responses to SDOH challenges.
5. Demonstrate the use of SDOH data strategies and applications.

> 🔊 Podcasts that exemplify the content of this chapter are available at Springer Publishing Connect™
>
> Podcast 4.1. The Impact of Social Determinants of Health-on-Health Outcomes

Access the podcast online at http://connect.springerpub.com/content/book/978-0-8261-4427-0/part/part01/chapter/ch04

INTRODUCTION

This chapter focuses on the role of SDOH and their effect on health and well-being of diverse communities. **SDOH are defined by the Centers for Disease Control (CDC) as the places where people live, learn, work, and play** (CDC, 2020a).

The social determinants of health are the social and cultural things that determine how healthy you are. They are things that are outside of your genes. They are things that are outside of what you do as an individual...social determinants of health as those things that actually have a lot of influence on how healthy you are, that are outside of your individual personhood. They are really the context in which individual behaviors arise. It's an important thing for people to realize that when we're dealing with health issues, the medical care system will not be able to make everybody well.

—Camara Jones, MD, PhD (2010)

Awareness of the effects of social and environmental factors on health has been documented and in existence since the mid-1800s (Irwin & Scali, 2007), where early scientists conducting sanitary campaigns noticed that social and living conditions severely affected people's health. For example, individuals who were exposed to low-quality housing were more likely to fall ill. These types of public health observations continued for more than 100 years until the rise of community-based approaches to health in the 1960s to 70s, including the global emergence of the use of community health workers (CHWs; APHA n.d.-a; Perry, 2013). CHWs are frontline public health workers who serve as liaisons between the community and needed health and social services. These individuals have a trusted relationship with the population they serve and easily facilitate access to community-centered and culturally grounded care. CHWs were charged with extending the availability of primary care as well as facilitating social transformation including cultural, environmental, and social factors known to be associated with health. Until population health strategies became integrated into the health delivery system, the medical model focused on disease treatment and contributing SDOH factors were not widely recognized. Today, addressing SDOH remains an important and ongoing issue for population health managers and public health practitioners.

Healthy People 2020 (HP, 2020) categorizes SDOH factors into the following five domains:

- Economic stability
- Education access to quality educational programs
- Health and healthcare access to appropriate and timely healthcare services
- Neighborhood and built environment, and safe environments
- Social and community context

These basic categories help population health managers align the various external factors that can affect quality of life and ultimately positive health outcomes. Exhibit 4.1 offers a visual representation depicts over 15 different subcategories that can ultimately impact populations-of-interest (US DHHS, n.d.).

Multiple federal organizations have plans and initiatives to address SDOH to improve the nation's health, including the U.S. CDC's emphasis on

SDOH				
Economic Factors	Access to Education	Healthcare Access	Built Environment Neighborhood Safety	Social/ Community Context
Employment Housing instability Poverty	Quality schooling Access to early childhood education	Access to healthcare Access to preventive care and screenings	Quality housing Transportation Public safety Access to healthy foods	Civic engagement Structural racism/ discrimination Social Cohesion

Health Disparities
1. Differences in SDOH lead to disparities in health outcomes. 2. SDOH disparities exist among racial/ethnic group resulting in health disparities. 3. SDOH are an upstream issue that requires systematic policy and practices changes to resolve.

Health Outcomes
Morbidity, Mortality. Life expectancy, Mental health status, physical and role functioning, mobility, well-being

EXHIBIT 4.1 Social Determinants of Health (SDOH), Disparities, and Outcomes

Souce: Adapted from https://www.kff.org/disparities-policy/issue-brief/beyond-health-care-the-role-of-social-determinants-in-promoting-health-and-health-equity/

https://www.healthypeople.gov/2020/topics-objectives/topic/social-determinants-of-health

SDOH research (CDC, 2020a), the Office of Disease Prevention and Health Promotion's (ODPHP) strategy to adopt health impact assessments (ODPHP, 2020), and the American Public Health Association's (APHA) focus on health equity (APHA, n.d.-b).

The Impact of Social Determinants of Health for Population Health

Up to 80% of health outcomes are determined by SDOH, such as safe housing or access to healthy foods (Manatt et al., 2019). The literature shows that healthcare only accounts for approximately 10% of positive outcomes in overall morbidity and mortality in the United States (Braveman & Gottlieb, 2014). Initiatives addressing SDOH can reduce the cost of care substantially. Significant evidence already exists to warrant healthcare system involvement in addressing SDOH and to facilitate the integration of health and social services to improve health outcomes for diverse communities (NASM, 2019; Solomon & Kanter, 2018). Addressing SDOH is critical to eliminating health disparities, as individuals, communities, and families who experience poor social conditions are more likely to experience poor health.

SDOH are considered upstream challenges. According to the "upstream/ downstream" parable, *SDOH are an upstream issue* (Manchanda, 2019: Merck, 2018).

DID YOU KNOW?

The Upstream/Downstream Parable

A group of friends was fishing in a river and noticed a person in the river struggling against the current. They saved the first person and then the next. The group of friends decided to go upstream and figure out why, how, and which people were falling into the river and needed to be rescued. When they arrived upstream, they found a scenic bridge with a desirable view. However, to enjoy the view, you had to risk falling in the river. The group of friends worked with the community to build a barrier so that no one would fall in the river again. Addressing SDOH is like putting up this barrier. How do you address upstream issues to avoid downstream problems, in the case of the parable, potential drowning, and obtain the required resources to save the person in the river?

- **Upstream Issues.** Addressing SDOH. In the case of the parable, this would include installing the barrier. In general, this would refer to improving education systems, housing, and economic opportunities.
- **Midstream.** In the case of the parable, this would refer to educating individuals to improve their swimming ability or how to negotiate the bridge without falling. In general, this would include factors related to individual-level behavior change such as promoting healthy eating, healthy family relationships, and exercise.
- **Downstream.** In the case of the parable, this would include costs of treating near-drowning and expenses related to the rescue. In general, this would include treatment of chronic and relapsing conditions such as diabetes and related complications including dialysis or treatment for diabetic retinopathy.

As prominent population health professional David Nash, MD, MHA, promotes, "Shut off the faucet and stop mopping the floor" (Nash, 2018), meaning that if we do not address these upstream issues, we will continue to invest more resources in downstream resources which tax our healthcare system.

DID YOU KNOW?

How Do Social Determinants Affect Health?
- Think about persons living with diabetes. How would SDOH play a role in diabetes management?
- Think about your community. What do you notice about SDOH in your community?

The Impact of Social Determinants of Health on Health Status and Vulnerable Populations

How do SDOH affect health? SDOH can affect health outcomes in several significant ways. The biopsychosocial model (Borrell-Carrió et al., 2014; Wade & Halligan, 2017) was one of the first theoretical models to posit that biology alone does not influence health and that health is also a function of SDOH and psychological well-being (see Figure 4.1).

Social Determinants of Health and Vulnerable Populations

Vulnerable populations, often racial/ethnic groups in the United States, are disproportionately affected by morbidity and mortality compared with other groups. For example, African Americans have a higher rates of heart disease, diabetes, asthma, and obesity. This excess burden of poor health has been associated with stress, socioeconomic challenges, limited access to healthcare, structural/social injustices, and underemployment (Noonan et al., 2016). Unfortunately, the constellation of conditions is also thought to increase

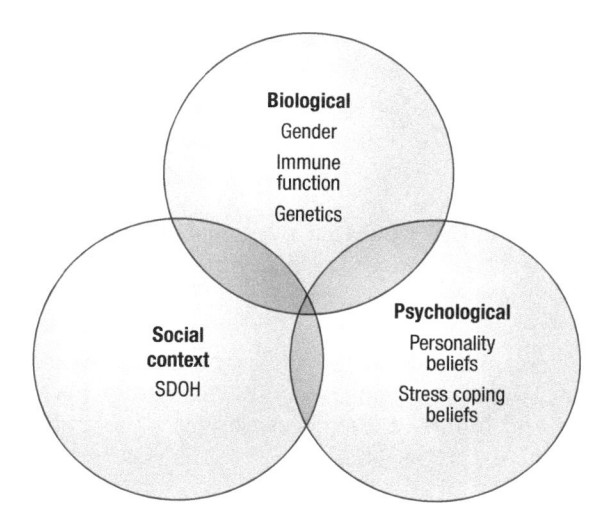

FIGURE 4.1 The Biopsychosocial Model

morbidity and mortality of COVID-19 among African Americans (Ray, 2020). Healthcare organizations can play a role in addressing these health equity issues in their organizations and in the community only if population health managers fully understand the impact of SDOH issues.

As population health managers are responsible for developing, supporting, and sustaining health promotion and disease prevention programs and ensuring safe and quality healthcare, their role far exceeds being culturally competent. Health equality needs to be health equity, and potential negative SDOH should be viewed as risk factors to be addressed with every population health initiative. The following definitions serve as clear illustrations of the potential to positively impact the quality of health for all populations.

- Diversity and Inclusion
  - **Diversity** "encompasses acceptance and respect. It means understanding that everyone is unique and recognizing our individual differences. These can be along the dimensions of race, ethnicity, gender, sexual orientation, socio-economic status, age, physical abilities, religious beliefs, political beliefs, or other ideologies" (QCC CUNY, n.d.).
  - **Inclusion** is "a state of being valued, respected and supported. It's about focusing on the needs of every individual and ensuring the right conditions are in place for each person to achieve his or her full potential" (HUD, n.d.).
- Health Equality and Health Equity
  - **Health equality** is "ensuring that every individual has an equal opportunity to make the most of their lives and talents. Further, it is the belief that no one should have poorer life chances because of the way they were born, where they come from, what they believe, or whether they have a disability" (The Equality and Human Rights Commission, 2018).
  - **Health equity** is "defined as the absence of unfair and avoidable or remediable differences in health among population groups defined socially, economically, demographically or geographically" (WHO, n.d.).

- Health Disparity
  - **Health disparities** are "preventable differences in the burden of disease, injury, violence, or opportunities to achieve optimal health that are experienced by socially disadvantaged populations" (CDC, 2008).
- Social Justice
  - **Social justice** is "the view that everyone deserves equal economic, political and social rights and opportunities" (The San Diego Foundation, 2016).
- Structural Racism
  - **Structural racism** is defined as "the macrolevel systems, social forces, institutions, ideologies, and processes that interact with one another to generate and reinforce inequities among racial and ethnic groups" (Powell, 2008).

SDOH such as exposures to neighborhood socioeconomic degradation, the immigration process (Tuggle et al., 2018), racism, and sexism can cause biological inflammation and dysregulation through the body's reaction to psychological stress caused by poor social circumstances (Davis, 2020). This process can be referred to as allostasis and contributes to one's allostatic load or the cumulative wear and tear on the body and brain (McEwen, 2005). Increased allostatic load is associated with a plethora of health conditions including cardiovascular disease, periodontal disease, and birth outcomes (e.g., low birthweight, etc.).

Second, social determinants can affect health by limiting healthy behaviors and activities such as living in a food desert with limited access to food or a food swamp with access to primarily unhealthy foods (e.g., fast foods), opportunities to exercise (e.g., high crime or no green space), and gaps in access to necessary healthcare that limit access to health facilities and jobs with health insurance benefits. These examples represent only a small sampling of the SDOH impact on vulnerable populations.

The role of a population health manager is to integrate SDOH into daily healthcare practice to reduce and prevent health equities (Braveman et al., 2011). While health disparities contribute to higher healthcare costs and poor patient outcomes, it is also a moral imperative to eliminate health disparities, as they are a result of historical and systematic disenfranchisement based on race/ethnicity, gender, social status, and identity (Jones, 2010).

> **DID YOU KNOW?**
>
> **Social Determinants of Health and Social Needs Are Not the Same!**
>
> A caveat: SDOH and social needs are not the same. While healthcare systems are incorporating vehicles to identify and address individual patients' social needs, addressing SDOH in your healthcare organizations catchment area requires systematic policy change, advocacy, and multistakeholder initiatives to develop sustainable upstream interventions and policy changes (e.g., policies that improve economic stability of the region) to effect downstream outcomes (e.g., patients are unemployed and cannot afford cost of medical care; BMJ, 2018). As a population health manager, it is within your purview to address patient social needs

and SDOH in your healthcare organizations community as they are intrinsically related.
1. Can you describe the relationship between SDOH, psychological response, biological response, and health outcomes?
2. What is the relationship between SDOH and social needs?

Measuring and Monitoring Social Determinants of Health to Improve Population Health Outcomes

Now that we have established that addressing SDOH is critical to the amelioration of health disparities and assisting individuals and communities in improving population health outcomes, the next step is addressing the impact on reimbursement payment systems and the financial bottom line of healthcare systems and organizations. SDOH metrics are increasingly being used in risk adjustment formulae and algorithms, and other emerging alternative care delivery payment structures.

Successful value-based reimbursement initiatives require healthcare systems to provide high-quality care at lower costs (LaPoint, 2019), and both healthcare systems and providers are reimbursed based on patient outcomes as opposed to fee-for-service (FFS) models that reimburse regardless of the patient outcome. For example, in the FFS framework, providers are reimbursed for conducting a hemoglobin A1c test to assess glycemic control among people living with diabetes, whereas a value-based reimbursement framework provides reimbursement partially on whether the patient's hemoglobin A1c indicates proper diabetes management. Risk factors associated with SDOH contribute to a much larger percentage of health than receipt of medical care.

To address the impact of SDOH, the identification and the monitoring of appropriate SDOH via appropriate measures and metrics are required. In this section, you will find examples of ways in which population health managers measure how SDOH protocols can integrate seamlessly into provider's healthcare practices. While SDOH measurement is not universal nor standardized, significant efforts are being made to integrate SDOH measurement into diverse healthcare settings.

Applications and Tools for Addressing Social Determinants of Heath

Four strategies appropriate for population health managers to implement are the enhanced use of electronic medical records, specific software SDOH data collection tools (PRAPARE), ICD-10 SDOH Z-codes, and the use of other external data, such as the Area Resource Files (ARF), the Vulnerable Populations Footprint Tool, and the Social Vulnerability Index.

Electronic Health Records

The Affordable Care Act (ACA) encouraged the development of electronic health records (EHRs) to decrease healthcare costs and improve health outcomes by centralizing and improving the quality of patient information (Tobin-Tyler & Ahmad, 2020). The federal government has invested billions of dollars into EHR development including increasing the number of EHRs available to providers, and training of health information technology professionals for implementation (Schilling, n.d.). In 2012, the ACA implemented a disincentive program that financially penalized healthcare facilities for patients readmitted into the hospital within 30 days for the same encounter, which is an indicator of poor quality of care. If readmission is due to financial issues (e.g., inability to pay for medication, or housing insecurity), having a record of the related SDOH in an EHR will enable the healthcare organization to address the issues and avoid poor outcomes. As the key tool and repository for patient information, and now accessible across platforms and different healthcare providers, SDOH indicators need to be fully integrated.

Incorporating SDOH metrics into the electronic medical record has promise and challenges for population health managers. First, there is no national standard on which measures of SDOH and how to specify them in EHRs. Second, once incorporated into the EHR, how to assure and document that action is taken (Cantor & Thorpe, 2018; Gold et al., 2017). Gottlieb and colleagues (2015, 2016) suggest that EHR data can be aggregated and used for population-level efforts; however, standardization of SDOH data collection and suggested action would be required. The next action step would be the development of referral tools (e.g., referral to community-based resources) within the EHR to serve as a mechanism for action after identification.

PRAPARE

One example of a systematic SDOH data collection and action tool is the Protocol for Responding to and Assessing Patient Assets, Risks and Experiences (PRAPARE). PRAPARE was developed by the National Association of Community Health Centers (NACHE) in 2019. PRAPARE measures are standardized, align with the Healthy People 2020 SDOH goal, and include EHR templates (see Figure 4.2).

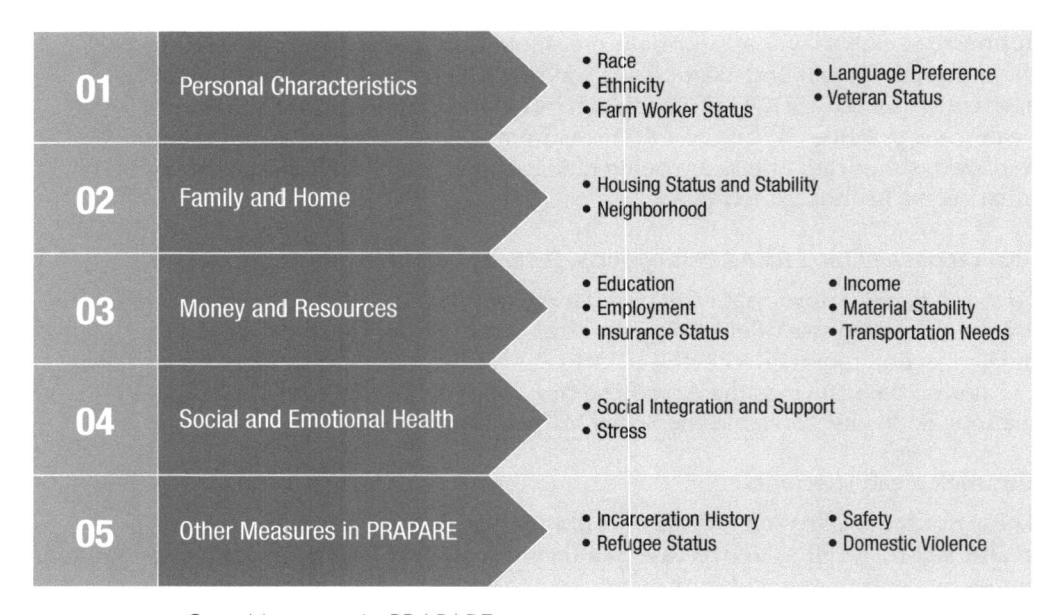

01	Personal Characteristics	• Race • Ethnicity • Farm Worker Status • Language Preference • Veteran Status
02	Family and Home	• Housing Status and Stability • Neighborhood
03	Money and Resources	• Education • Employment • Insurance Status • Income • Material Stability • Transportation Needs
04	Social and Emotional Health	• Social Integration and Support • Stress
05	Other Measures in PRAPARE	• Incarceration History • Refugee Status • Safety • Domestic Violence

FIGURE 4.2 Core Measures in PRAPARE

Adapted from National Association of Community Health Centers PRAPARE TOOL (NACHC, 2019).

The PRAPARE Protocol Document is available in Appendix A.

ICD-10 SDOH Z-codes

In early 2018, ICD-10 Cooperating Parties created diagnostic SDOH Z-codes to facilitate the diagnosis of social factors (Gottlieb et al., 2016; Missouri Hospital Association, 2018). While Z-codes measure SDOH, they can indicate medical necessity. The capturing of SDOH in the ICD-10 system, while still universally implemented, has the potential to assist in the identification of high-risk patients (HITEQ, 2017). For example, Z59.4 indicates lack of adequate food, and Z59.0 indicates homelessness. Z-codes are available to providers as primary or other diagnoses just as other ICD codes are used.

External Data That Address Social Determinants of Health

As a healthcare manager, it is critical to be aware of existing data sources that can assist you in benchmarking your community and catchment area in terms of SDOH measurement. These data sources can also inform your community health needs assessment (Carlton & Singh, 2018). National data sets such as the *ARF* can assist managers in identifying the availability of healthcare resources (e.g., number of hospital beds and number of pediatricians) and by state and county (HRSA, n.d.).

The CDC (2020b) provides a list of national data sources that measure SDOH at the census tract, city, county, and state levels; notably, *the Vulnerable Populations Footprint Tool* creates identifies through geographic mapping of poverty and education levels.

The *Social Vulnerability Index* uses U.S. census variables at tract level to identify factors that are indicative of a community's resilience or ability to recover after disaster. Social vulnerability is an important concept to understand for a population health manager as natural disasters such as hurricanes and tornadoes, and pandemics such as COVID-19 can exacerbate poor health outcomes already experienced by vulnerable communities (Nayak et al., 2020). Unfortunately, constellation of conditions is also thought to increase morbidity and mortality of COVID-19 (Ray, 2020). This disproportionate burden of COVID-19 morbidity and mortality may further exacerbate physical and mental health, as well as socioeconomic disparities in vulnerable families and communities through further loss of income, additional stress, and continued poor access to healthcare. However, the CDC recommended that all vaccine distribution policies reflect consideration of the Social Vulnerability Index and other mapping tools to alleviate disparities (CDC, 2020c).

The integration of SDOH data requires population health managers to recognize important ethical considerations. Once measurement of SDOH needs is identified, there is a moral imperative to act and address these needs. Sometimes resources and infrastructure to address SDOH is lacking or unavailable. The ability to respond should be addressed when implementing SDOH measurement. A second responsibility is for managers to ensure SDOH data and measures are used in an unbiased way to design and deliver the best possible care for patients with SDOH needs and not result in poor care or discrimination. Third, when SDOH data are collected and action is taken to refer patients to community partners for services or to identify service needs, efforts must be taken to protect the patient confidentiality (eHealth Initiative, 2019). Adopting appropriate strategies to address these concerns requires population health management skills and personal commitment.

> **? DID YOU KNOW?**
>
> **Social Determinants of Health and Population Health Manager Accountability**
>
> Assume you are a population health manager. What would you tell your colleagues about why it is important to measure SDOH? What would you say to prepare your colleagues for the challenge? Could you explain the three action steps necessary to ensure that SDOH information is integrated?

Social Determinants of Health in Practice for Population Health Managers

The mandates for integrating SDOH into population health require organizations to move from theory to action (Dean et al., 2013). Given the advent of population health management and value-based care, providers are being held accountable for patient outcomes and controlling costs (NEJM, 2017). As we have reviewed in the previous section, patient outcomes are intrinsically related to SDOH. Due to rising healthcare cost with quality-of-care lagging behind these costs, the Institute for Healthcare Improvement developed the Triple Aim framework to (1) improve quality of care, (2) reduce cost, and (3) improve population health (Dean, 2020).

Data technologies and improved access to SDOH indicators now provide health promotion and population health managers with the tools to effectively address these upstream risk factors of at-risk populations. Developing appropriate interventions and acting on SDOH requires a multisectoral approach with collaborations between healthcare, public health, and non–health sector entities.

Health in All Policies/Non–Health Sector Approach

The World Health Organization and the APHA both support a Health in All Policies Approach (HiAP) to addressing SDOH (APHA 2020; Follow & Hinton, 2018). HiAP is a collaborative approach that brings together policy-makers and practitioners from all sectors related to SDOH under the assumption that all multisectoral policies affect health outcomes. Action on SDOH requires coordination from organizations and partners that fall outside of the traditional healthcare such as housing, transportation, the education system, criminal justice, grocery/food resources and farming, and other social services. While access to transportation and adequate housing effect health, policies and practices to improve access to healthy food and housing must come from organizations that address these issues (APHA 2020; Follow & Hinton, 2018).

Healthcare Systems Approaches

What are healthcare systems doing to address SDOH? SDOH have become a significant focus in the U.S. healthcare system to improve patient outcomes and reduce costs. The ACA has helped to advance the role of healthcare systems in addressing SDOH. As of 2010, not-for-profit hospitals are required to conduct a community health needs assessment and implementation plan to help identify and act on SDOH in their catchment areas to maintain their tax-exempt status. For example, Centers for Medicaid and Medicare Services

(CMS) now facilitate reimbursement and incentives for healthcare systems to respond to enrollees' social needs. (DeSalvo & Leavitt, 2019). In some states, Medicaid managed care organizations (MCOs) are required to develop community partnerships with organizations that provide SDOH-related services such as housing support. Other states include SDOH-related services such as access to food banks and emergency housing in Medicaid benefits packages by also partnering with social services organizations.

Despite the moral imperative and the potential for improved patient outcomes and cost savings, return on investment (ROI) for healthcare systems investment in SDOH has proven to be complex and not without challenges (Gilfillan, 2020). Patient needs are complex, and there is no standard intervention that addresses the diversity of patient SDOH needs; however, significant investments in SDOH by healthcare systems are ongoing.

Population Health Management

Given that healthcare only accounts for less than a quarter of healthcare outcomes, SDOH challenges can contribute to increased healthcare costs. Population health managers should demonstrate leadership by aligning with their community and their catchment area and create best practices that integrate strategic tools and collaborative relationships. Use the following checklist (Table 4.1) as a tool to ensure competency development in this crucial area.

SUMMARY

SDOH have been found to be one of the most significant drivers of population health outcomes. Assessing, monitoring, and addressing SDOH presents challenges and opportunities for population health managers. Recently, strong evidence has supported the necessity of eliminating health disparities and inequities in healthcare outcomes. Social justice issue's recognition and the framing of racial structuralism have resulted in new strategic initiatives and tools to mitigate the impact of SDOH for all vulnerable populations and

TABLE 4.1 Manager-in-Training: SDOH Leadership Competencies

√	SDOH Leadership Competency
	Become familiar with the social and healthcare landscape of your community. Get to know diverse healthcare providers in your area (e.g., FQHCs and other community centers).
	Review your organization's Community Health Needs Assessment and health status reports from your local public health department.
	Volunteer and make a commitment to serving at a community organization that addresses SDOH.
	Provide training to management team and clinical providers regarding the effects of SDOH on patients.
	Establish and integrate diversity and inclusion protocols to avoid any social or cultural biases that could impact vulnerable population health outcomes.
	Learn how to build meaningful community partnerships with organizations that serve diverse communities to address health disparities, social inequities and social justice Building strong community relationships is critical to improving population health and addressing SDOH.
	Adopt a four-tiered approach to healthcare organizations can use to measure and prioritize health equity issues including (a) access to care, (b) care transitions such as referrals from primary to specialty care, (c) quality of care, and (d) social, economic, and environmental impact such as community economic conditions (Sivashanker et al., 2020).

facility high-quality healthcare. New macrostrategies include use of Health in All Policies approaches, while technology advancements include EHR adaptations and mapping software (PRAPARE), and various assessment tools such as the Social Vulnerability Index. Developing skills and competencies related to building community partnerships and collaborations with help ensure population health managers address all the social health determinants that impact their populations-of-interest.

FQHC, federally qualified health center; SDOH, social determinants of health.

DISCUSSION QUESTIONS

1. Why is it important for healthcare systems and provides to measure SDOH? What could be potential consequences?
2. The director of an ED at a hospital in a large city has noticed an increase in ED encounters among individuals who are housing insecure.
    a. How would you confirm the ED director's observations?
    b. What is the relationship between housing insecurity and ED visits?
    c. Suggest community partnerships that would be necessary in addressing this issue.
3. You are the CEO of a behavioral health facility. Your organization maintains a database of SDOH among individuals with severe mental health issues.
    a. Why would addressing SDOH be important in providing high-quality mental healthcare?
    b. Describe potential ethical issues you would have to consider in connecting clients to SDOH-related services.
4. The director the OB/GYN maternity unit in your hospital informed you that a significant number of pregnant women receiving services have nutritional deficiencies and are often food insecure. Please identify potential solutions you can implement in your facility to address this issue.
5. As a healthcare manager, you will lead diverse groups of employees. Describe how you would assess SDOH needs among your workforce and what types of employee-based programs you would consider assisting your employees.
6. Identify one collaborative initiative in your local community developed to address SDOH.
    a. Describe the activities.
    b. Who are the stakeholders?
    c. Is a healthcare facility involved?
        i. If yes, how?
        ii. If not, how could or should a healthcare facility be involved?

For example: Generate Health, a not-for-profit in St. Louis, Missouri, conducts advocacy work to reduce health disparities in the St. Louis region by addressing SDOH. One of their main SDOH activities is the *Social Determinants Tour,* which invites various health profession students to view two disparate neighborhoods and engage in learning how history, policy, and other economic factors have created health disparities (Generatehealth, n.d.).

Toolkit Competency Application

Addressing Social Determinants of Health and Health Disparities
Directions: Population Health often focuses on the most vulnerable populations especially those with chronic disease conditions. The following mini case study provides one example of how a national program addressed risk factors related to diabetes.

In the United States, 34.2 million people have diabetes, of whom 90% to 95% have type 2 diabetes. The prevalence of diabetes will rise considering 88 million adults have prediabetes and 80% of people are unaware they have prediabetes. Prediabetes is defined as having blood sugar levels that are elevated but not yet high enough to be categorized as having diabetes. The total cost of medical care and lost work is $327 billion for people with diagnosed diabetes. Healthcare costs are twice as high for people with diabetes compared with people without diabetes. Lifestyle changes such as healthy eating and physical activity to lose weight are the best methods of preventing prediabetes from developing into diabetes. Engaging in these lifestyle changes can reduce the risk of diabetes by over half among people with prediabetes (CDC, 2020a). Without making the appropriate lifestyle changes, within 5 years, 15% to 30% of people with prediabetes will develop type 2 diabetes (New York State Department of Health, 2020).

The National Diabetes Prevention Program (NDPP) is offered to patients who are prediabetic, HbA1c between 5.7 and 6.4. The NDPP is a year-long evidence-based lifestyle change program (LCP) to prevent or delay type 2 diabetes. NDPP is offered at public and private organizations in communities across the United States (CDC, 2019b). The NDPP can reduce the risk of developing type 2 diabetes by 58% among adults and 71% among people aged >60 years (CDC, 2018).

The NDPP has recognized some racial and ethnic minority groups enroll in the LCP at lower rates than other groups. Therefore, the CDC has funded 10 national organizations in the United States to offer NDPP in underserved areas, defined as regions with fewer resources do address health disparities (CDC, 2019b). Increasing availability and access to NDPP is the start of addressing the concerns regarding "place" in health disparities, helping people who live in areas of high diabetes prevalence with low access. Figure 4.3 maps the location of NDPP programs to diabetes disease prevalence in the United States. The CDC also used the Area Deprivation Index (ADI) to map NDPP availability to socioeconomic disadvantage status in the United States (see Figure 4.4). In both maps, the prevalence of diabetes and socioeconomic disadvantage are more concentrated in the southeast and middle states; however, the availability of programs are not concentrated in the same areas (CDC, n.d.-a).

Program availability is a start to addressing high incidence of prediabetes and diabetes. There are other barriers to care recognized by NDPP program providers. In an integrated healthcare system in the southeastern United States, the NDPP program is offered freely to patients with prediabetes or at an increased risk of diabetes as indicated by the prediabetes risk score, which includes metrics related to family history of diabetes, diagnosis of high blood pressure, level of physical activity, and BMI. Despite being free to

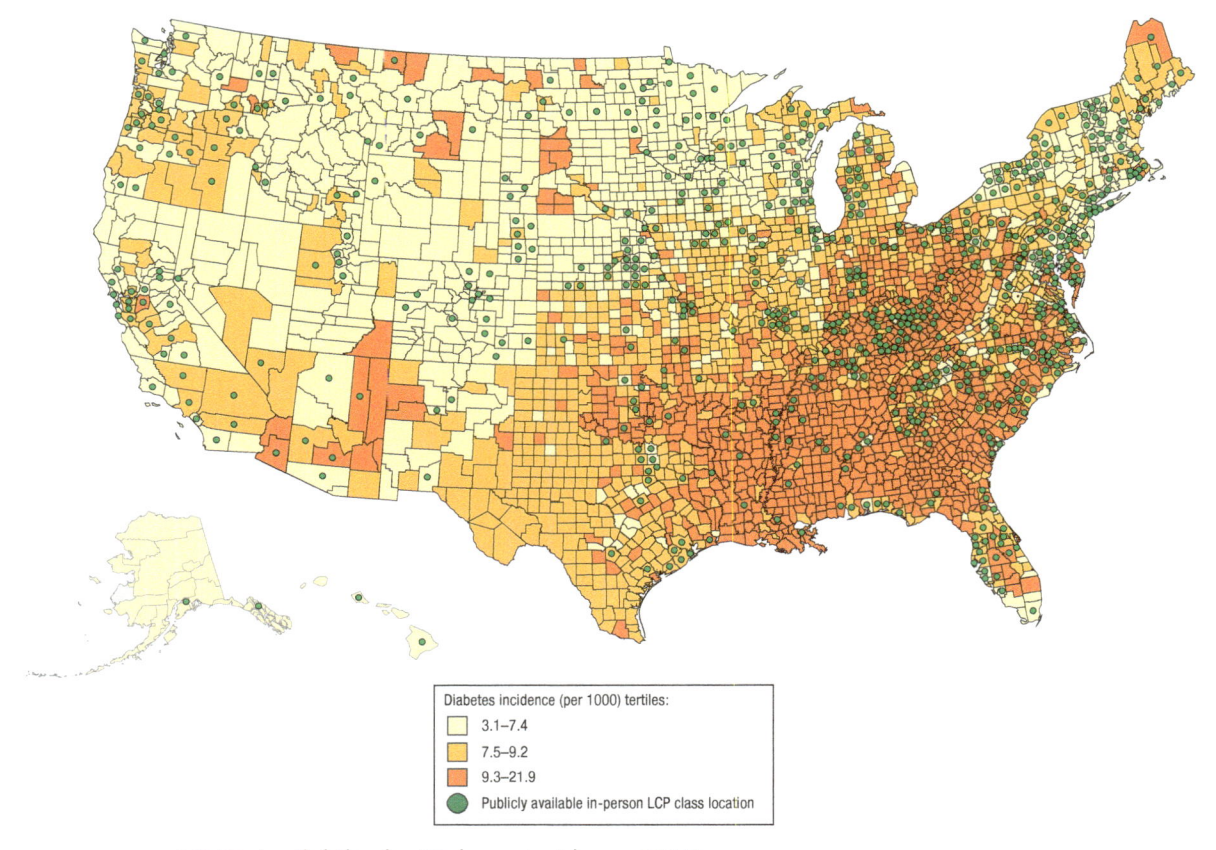

FIGURE 4.3 NDPP Availability by Diabetes Incidence 2017
Source: Centers for Disease Control and Prevention (2017). National Diabetes Prevention Program (LCP) in United States Counties as of March 2017: Counties with at least one CDC-recognized publicly available in-person LCP class location as of March 2017, by county-level diabetes incidence. https://cdc.gov/diabetes/programs/national-dpp-maps/index.html

the patient, there are still barriers in initiating participation and remaining in the program upon joining. Members have discussed challenges related to competing priorities, length of time traveling to a clinic to participate in the program, consistent access to transportation, childcare, and elderly care. While NDPP is offered both online and in-person, this organization offered in-person only prior to the COVID-19 pandemic changing healthcare delivery in the United States.

Program retention for this program met the CDC's guidelines for minimum 60% participation over the course of 12 months. However, there are strategies to improve program retention despite the barriers. Among groups that are vulnerable, research indicates more frequent contact and individualized contact can support higher program retention, therefore keeping people engaged in the program who most need it. A person's decision to participate in a study, or in this case a year-long program, comes with a litany of conflicting motivating factors (Emerson, 1976; Lawler, 2001), some of which the individual is unaware, including fear of failure (Fisher et al., 2012) Therefore, there are individual-level (intrinsic fears or motivating factors), interpersonal-level (commitment to provide childcare or elder care or other

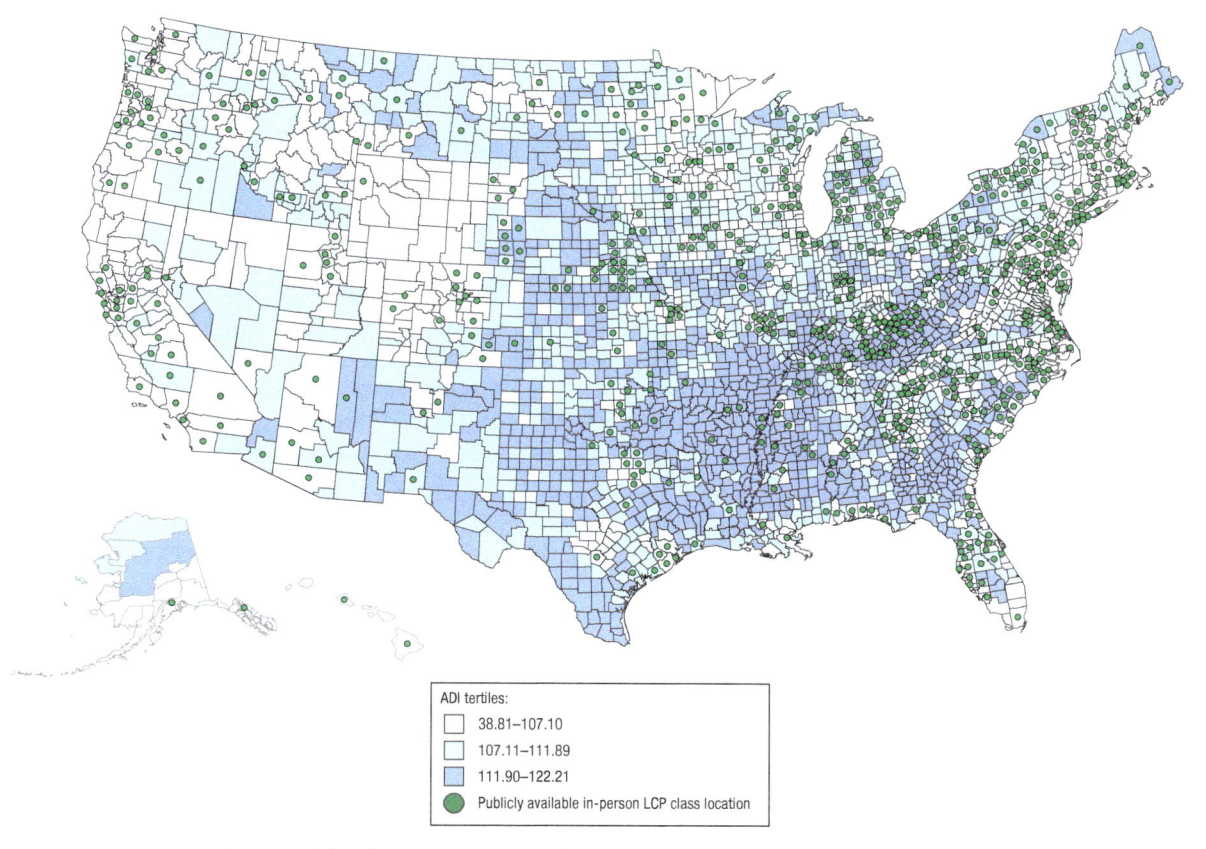

FIGURE 4.4 NDPP Availability for Socioeconomic Disadvantage Status 2017
Source: Centers for Disease Control and Prevention (2017). National Diabetes Prevention Program (LCP) in United States Counties as of March 2017: Counties with at least one CDC-recognized publicly available in-person LCP class location as of March 2017, by socioeconomic disadvantage status of counties.

ADI tertiles:
- 38.81–107.10
- 107.11–111.89
- 111.90–122.21
- Publicly available in-person LCP class location

family and work priorities), and community-level (ability to access) barriers to program engagement. These barriers may be more prevalent among communities at greatest need. In this southeastern area where this NDPP program is located, NDPP has the same concerns that are seen nationally, areas with the highest ADI did not have NDPP program.

CASE STUDY QUESTIONS

1. Review the mini case study. Briefly outline (bullet points) the major community intervention of the NDPP including population eligibility, time frame, and outcomes.
2. Assume you are a population health manager and plan to offer an LCP with elevated risk of diabetes. What strategies will you use to engage subgroups with barriers preventing their participation in your program?
3. This chapter introduces four SDOH databases and tools that can assist in identifying and categorizing populations by specific social determinant

risk factors. Discuss which of these tools or strategies would you adopt for developing a local NDPP program.

- PRAPARE
- Area Resource File (https://data.hrsa.gov/topics/health-workforce/ahrf)
- Vulnerable Populations Footprint Tool (https://www.communitycommons.org/entities/60847319-e438-44be-a5c3-5b8d298845e1)
- Social Vulnerability Index Fund (https://svi.cdc.gov/factsheet.html)

4. Assume you are a population health manager, and your Chief Population Health Officer has shared this article with you and asks you to prepare a one/two pages summary. How would you summarize the population health managerial best practices outlined? What take-aways should be included for in improving a Community Health Action Team (CHAT)?

The Commonwealth Fund is a nonprofit organization that focuses on improving the healthcare system in the United States. The Commonwealth Fund focuses on healthcare **practice and policy**, which makes it unique among the other approaches and tools previously discussed. They recognize not only the importance of SDOH and how to document the impact but also what is necessary to make quality changes. In a recent article, *Improving Population Health Through Communitywide Partnerships*, the authors give best practice examples of CHATs (https://www.commonwealthfund.org/publications/newsletter-article/improving-population-health-through-communitywide-partnerships).

CASE STUDY REFERENCES

Centers for Disease Control and Prevention (CDC). (2018). *About the National DPP*. https://www.cdc.gov/diabetes/prevention/about.htm

Centers for Disease Control and Prevention (CDC). (2019a). *Addressing health disparities in diabetes*. https://www.cdc.gov/diabetes/disparities.html?CDC_AA_refVal=https%3A%2F%2Fwww.cdc.gov%2Fdiabetes%2Fprograms%2Fvulnerable.html

Centers for Disease Control and Prevention (CDC). (2019b, August). *National diabetes prevention program*. https://www.cdc.gov/diabetes/prevention/index.html

Centers for Disease Control and Prevention (CDC). (2020). *A snapshot: Diabetes in the United States*. https://www.cdc.gov/diabetes/library/socialmedia/infographics/diabetes.htm

Centers for Disease Control and Prevention (CDC). (n.d.-a). *National diabetes prevention program (lifestyle change program) in United States Counties as of March 2017*. Retrieved May 18, 2021, from https://www.cdc.gov/diabetes/programs/national-dpp-maps/index.html

Centers for Disease Control and Prevention (CDC). (n.d.-b). *The growing threat of pre-diabetes*, (Infograph). Retrieved May 18, 2021, from https://www.cdc.gov/diabetes/prevention/pdf/NDPP_Infographic.pdf

Emerson, R. M. (1976). Social exchange theory. *Annual Review of Sociology, 2*, 335–363. https://doi.org/10.1146/annurev.so.02.080176.002003

Fisher, L., Hessler, D., Naranjo, D., & Polonsky, W. (2012). AASAP: A program to increase recruitment and retention in clinical trials. *Patient Education and Counseling, 86(3)*, 372–377. https://doi.org/10.1016/j.pec.2011.07.002

Lawler, E. J. (2001). An affect theory of social exchange. *American Journal of Sociology, 107*, 321–352. https://doi.org/10.1086/324071

New York State Department of Health (2020). *Prediabetes*. https://www.health.ny.gov/diseases/conditions/diabetes/prediabetes

PRAPARE

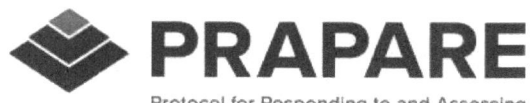

Protocol for Responding to and Assessing Patients' Assets, Risks, and Experiences

PRAPARE®: Protocol for Responding to and Assessing Patient Assets, Risks, and Experiences
Paper Version of PRAPARE® for Implementation as of September 2, 2016

Personal Characteristics

1. Are you Hispanic or Latino?

| Yes | No | I choose not to answer this question |

2. Which race(s) are you? Check all that apply

Asian	Native Hawaiian
Pacific Islander	Black/African American
White	American Indian/Alaskan Native
Other (please write):	
I choose not to answer this question	

3. At any point in the past 2 years, has season or migrant farm work been your or your family's main source of income?

| Yes | No | I choose not to answer this question |

4. Have you been discharged from the armed forces of the United States?

| Yes | No | I choose not to answer this question |

5. What language are you most comfortable speaking?

Family & Home

6. How many family members, including yourself, do you currently live with? _____

| I choose not to answer this question |

7. What is your housing situation today?

| I have housing |
| I do not have housing (staying with others, in a hotel, in a shelter, living outside on the street, on a beach, in a car, or in a park) |
| I choose not to answer this question |

8. Are you worried about losing your housing?

| Yes | No | I choose not to answer this question |

9. What address do you live at?
   Street:_____
   City, State, Zip code: _____

Money & Resources

10. What is the highest level of school that you have finished?

Less than high school degree	High school diploma or GED
More than high school	I choose not to answer this question

11. What is your current work situation?

Unemployed	Part-time or temporary work	Full-time work
Otherwise unemployed but not seeking work (ex: student, retired, disabled, unpaid primary care giver) Please write:		
I choose not to answer this question		

12. What is your main insurance?

None/uninsured	Medicaid
CHIP Medicaid	Medicare
Other public insurance (not CHIP)	Other Public Insurance (CHIP)
Private Insurance	

13. During the past year, what was the total combined income for you and the family members you live with? This information will help us determine if you are eligible for any benefits.

   _____

| I choose not to answer this question |

© 2016. National Association of Community Health Centers, Inc., Association of Asian Pacific Community Health Organizations, and Oregon Primary Care Association. PRAPARE® is proprietary information of NACHC and its partners. All rights reserved. For more information about this tool, please visit our website at www.nachc.org/PRAPARE/ or contact us at prapare@nachc.org.

THE KRESGE FOUNDATION · KAISER PERMANENTE · blue of california foundation · NATIONAL ASSOCIATION OF Community Health Centers · AAPCHO · OPCA Oregon Primary Care Association · Institute for Alternative Futures

APPENDIX A PRAPARE: Protocol for Responding to Assessing Patient Assets, Risks, and Experiences

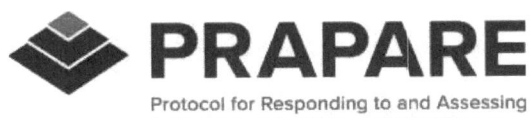

PRAPARE

PRAPARE®: Protocol for Responding to and Assessing Patient Assets, Risks, and Experiences
Paper Version of PRAPARE® for Implementation as of September 2, 2016

14. In the past year, have you or any family members you live with been **unable** to get any of the following when it was **really needed**? Check all that apply.

Yes	No	Food	Yes	No	Clothing
Yes	No	Utilities	Yes	No	Child Care
Yes	No	Medicine or Any Health Care (Medical, Dental, Mental Health, Vision)			
Yes	No	Phone	Yes	No	Other (please write):
		I choose not to answer this question			

15. Has lack of transportation kept you from medical appointments, meetings, work, or from getting things needed for daily living? Check all that apply.

	Yes, it has kept me from medical appointments or
	Yes, it has kept me from non-medical meetings, appointments, work, or from getting things that I need
	No
	I choose not to answer this question

Social and Emotional Health

16. How often do you see or talk to people that you care about and feel close to? (For example: talking to friends on the phone, visiting friends or family, going to church or club meetings)

Less than once a	1 or 2 times a week
3 to 5 times a week	5 or more times a
I choose not to answer this question	

17. Stress is when someone feels tense, nervous, anxious, or can't sleep at night because their mind is troubled. How stressed are you?

Not at all	A little bit
Somewhat	Quite a bit
Very much	I choose not to answer this question

Optional Additional Questions

18. In the past year, have you spent more than 2 nights in a row in a jail, prison, detention center, or juvenile correctional facility?

Yes	No	I choose not to answer this

19. Are you a refugee?

Yes	No	I choose not to answer this

20. Do you feel physically and emotionally safe where you currently live?

Yes	No	Unsure
I choose not to answer this question		

21. In the past year, have you been afraid of your partner or ex-partner?

Yes	No	Unsure
I have not had a partner in the past year		
I choose not to answer this question		

© 2016. National Association of Community Health Centers, Inc., Association of Asian Pacific Community Health Organizations, and Oregon Primary Care Association. PRAPARE® is proprietary information of NACHC and its partners. All rights reserved. For more information about this tool, please visit our website at www.nachc.org/PRAPARE® or contact us at prapare@nachc.org.

APPENDIX A *(Continued)*

The PRAPARE is a SDOH assessment protocol, developed and owned by the National Association of Community Health Centers (NACHC) in partnership with the Association of Asian Pacific Community Health Organization (AAPCHO), the Oregon Primary Care Association (OPCA), and the Institute for Alternative Futures (IAF) (PRAPARE, 2016). For more information, visit www.nachc.org/prapare.

REFERENCES

American Public Health Association. (n.d.-a). *Community health workers*. Retrieved May 18, 2021, from https://www.apha.org/apha-communities/member-sections/community-health-workers

American Public Health Association. (n.d.-b). *Health equity*. Retrieved May 18, 2021, from https://www.apha.org/topics-and issues/health-equity

American Public Health Association (APHA). (2020). *Health in all policies*. APHA. https://www.apha.org/topics-and-issues/health-in-all-policies

BMJ. (2018, July 2). Making a difference by addressing social determinants of health. *BMJ*. https://blogs.bmj.com/case-reports/2018/07/02/making-a-difference-by-addressing-social-determinants-of-health/

Borrell-Carrió, F., Suchman, A. L., & Epstein, R. M. (2014). The biopsychosocial model 25 years later: Principles, practice, and scientific inquiry. *Annals of Family Medicine, 2*, 576–582. https://doi.org/10.1370/afm.245

Braveman, P., & Gottlieb, L. (2014). The social determinants of health: It's time to consider the causes of the causes. *Public Health Reports, 129*(Suppl 2), 19–31. https://doi.org/10.1177/00333549141291S206

Braveman, P. A., Kumanyika, S., Fielding, J., Laveist, T., Borrell, L. N., Manderscheid, R., & Troutman, A. (2011). Health disparities and health equity: The issue is justice. *American Journal of Public Health, 101*(Suppl 1), S149–S155. https://doi.org/10.2105/AJPH.2010.300062

Cantor, M. N., & Thorpe, L. (2018). Integrating data on social determinants of health into electronic health records. *Health Affairs (Millwood), 37*(4), 585–590. https://doi.org/10.1377/hlthaff.2017.1252

Carlton, E. L., & Singh, S. R. (2018). Joint community health needs assessments as a path for coordinating community-wide health improvement efforts between Hospitals and Local Health Departments. *American Journal of Public Health, 108*(5), 676–682. https://doi.org/10.2105/AJPH.2018.304339

Centers for Disease Control and Prevention (CDC). (2008). *Community Health and Program Services (CHAPS): Health disparities among racial/ethnic populations*. U.S. Department of Health and Human Services.

Centers for Disease Control and Prevention (CDC). (2020a, August 19). *Social determinants of health: Know what affects health*. https://www.cdc.gov/socialdeterminants/about.html

Centers for Disease Control and Prevention (CDC). (2020b). *Sources for data on social determinants of health*. https://www.cdc.gov/socialdeterminants/data/index.htm

Centers for Disease Control and Prevention (CDC). (2020c, December 23). Vaccination implementation strategies to consider for populations recommended to receive initial doses of COVID-19 vaccine (persons included in phases 1a–1c). *Vaccinations and Immunizations*. https://www.cdc.gov/vaccines/covid-19/implementation-strategies.html

Davis, B. A. (2020, February 25). *Discrimination: A social determinant of health inequities*. Health Affairs. https://www.healthaffairs.org/do/10.1377/hblog20200220.518458/full/

Dean, C. A. (2020). Social determinants of health associated with Michigan residents 50 years and older health-related quality of life and cardiovascular health. *Gerontology and Geriatric Medicine, 6*, 2333721420979834. https://doi.org/10.1177/2333721420979834

Dean, H. D., Williams, K. M., & Fenton K. A. (2013). From theory to action: Applying social determinants of health to public health practice. *Public Health Reports, 128*(Suppl 3), 1–4. https://doi.org/10.1177/00333549131286S301

DeSalvo, K. & Leavitt, M. O. (2019, July 8). *For An option to address social determinants of health, look to medicaid.* Health Affairs. https://www.apha.org/topics-and-issues/health-in-all-policies

eHealth Initiative. (2019). *Guiding principles for ethical use of social determinants of health data.* An E-health Collaborative Project. https://www.ehidc.org/sites/default/files/resources/files/SDOH%20Ethical%20Guidelines%206.27.19%20FINAL.pdf

The Equality and Human Rights Commission. (2018, August 2). *Understanding equality: What is equality?* https://www.equalityhumanrights.com/en/secondary-education-resources/useful-information/understanding-equality

Follow, A. & Hinton, E. (2018, May 10). *Beyond health care: The role of social determinants in promoting health and health equity.* KFF. https://www.kff.org/disparities-policy/issue-brief/beyond-health-care-the-role-of-social-determinants-in-promoting-health-and-health-equity/

Generate Health. (n.d.). *Generate health equity initiative.* https://generatehealthstl.org/programs/health-equity/

Gilfillan, K. (2020, February 28). *Social determinants of health ROI challenges are not yet outweighing potential benefits to patients.* Healthcare Financial Management Association. https://www.hfma.org/topics/finance-and-business-strategy/article/social-determinants-of-health-roi-challenges-are-not-yet-outweig.html

Gold, R., Cottrell, E., Bunce, A., Middendorf, M., Hollombe, C., Cowburn, S., Mahr, P., & Melgar, G. (2017). Developing Electronic Health Record (EHR) strategies related to health center patients' social determinants of health. *Journal of the American Board of Family Medicine, 30*(4), 428–447. https://doi.org/10.3122/jabfm.2017.04.170046

Gottlieb, L., Tobey, R., Cantor, J., Hessler, D., & Adler, N. E. (2016). Integrating social and medical data to improve population health: Opportunities and barriers. *Health Affairs (Millwood), 35*(11), 2116–2123. https://doi.org/10.1377/hlthaff.2016.0723

Gottlieb, L. M., Tirozzi, K. J., Manchanda, R, Burns, A. R., & Sandel M. T. (2015). Moving electronic medical records upstream: Incorporating social determinants of health. *American Journal of Preventive Medicine, 48*(2), 215–218. https://doi.org/10.1016/j.amepre.2014.07.009

Health Resources and Services Administration (HRSA). (n.d.). *Area resource files.* Retrieved May 18, 2021, from https://data.hrsa.gov/topics/health-workforce/ahrf

HITEQ. (2017, June). *CD-10 Z-Codes for social determinants of health.* HITEQ. http://healthleadsusa.org/wp-content/uploads/2019/03/HITEQ-ICD-10-Z-codes-for-SDoH-June-2017.pdf

Irwin, A., & Scali, E. (2007). Action on the social determinants of health: Historical perspective. *Global Public Health, 2*(3), 235–256. https://doi.org/10.1080/17441690601106304

Jones, C. M. (2010). The moral problem of health disparities. *American Journal of Public Health, 100*(Suppl 1), S47–S51. https://doi.org/10.2105/AJPH.2009.171181

Lapoint, J. (2019). Social determinants of health key to value-based purchasing success. *Value Based Care News.* https://revcycleintelligence.com/news/social-determinants-of-health-key-to-value-based-purchasing-success

Manatt Health & Phelps&Phillips, LLP. (2019, February 1). *Medicaid's role in addressing social determinants of health.* Robert Wood Johnson Foundation. https://www.rwjf.org/en/library/research/2019/02/medicaid-s-role-in-addressing-social-determinants-of-health.html

Manchanda, R. (2019, January 17) *Making sense of the social determinants of health.* http://www.ihi.org/communities/blogs/making-sense-of-the-social-determinants-of-health

McEwen, B. S. (2005). Stressed or stressed out: What is the difference? *Journal of Psychiatry and Neuroscience, 30*(5), 315–318.

Merck, A. (2013, October 08). *The upstream-downstream parable for health equity.* https://salud-america.org/the-upstream-downstream-parable-for-health-equity/

Missouri Hospital Association. (2018). *Policy brief: Decoding social determinants of health.* https://www.mhanet.com/mhaimages/Policy_Briefs/PolicyBrief_SDOH.pdf

Nash, D. B. (2018). Shut off the faucet and stop mopping the floor. *American Health & Drug Benefits, 11*(9), 447–448. https://www.ncbi.nlm.nih.gov/pmc/articles/PMC6322593/

National Academies of Sciences, Engineering, and Medicine; Health and Medicine Division; Board on Health Care Services; Committee on Integrating Social Needs Care into the Delivery of Health Care to Improve the Nation's Health. (2019). *Integrating Social Care into the Delivery of Health Care: Moving Upstream to Improve the Nation's Health*. National Academies Press (US).

National Association of Community Health Centers (NACHC). (2019). *Chapter 1: Understand the PRAPARE Project*. www.nachc.org/wpcontent/uploads/2019/04/NACHC_PRAPARE_Chpt1.pdf

Nayak, A., Islam, S. J., Mehta, A., Ko, Y. A., Patel, S. A., Goyal, A., Sullivan, S., Lewis, T. T., Vaccarino, V., Morris, A. A., & Quyyumi, A. A. (2020). Impact of social vulnerability on COVID-19 incidence and outcomes in the United States. *medRxiv: The Preprint Server for Health Sciences*. https://doi.org/10.1101/2020.04.10.20060962

New England Journal of Medicine (NEJM) Catalyst. (2017, January 1). *What is value-based healthcare?* https://catalyst.nejm.org/doi/full/10.1056/CAT.17.0558

New York State Department of Health. (2020). *Prediabetes*. https://www.health.ny.gov/diseases/conditions/diabetes/prediabetes

Noonan, A. S., Velasco-Mondragon, H. E., & Wagner, F. A. (2016). Improving the health of African Americans in the USA: An overdue opportunity for social justice. *Public Health Review, 37*, 12. https://doi.org/10.1186/s40985-016-0025-4.

Office of Disease Prevention and Health Promotion's (ODPHP). (2020). Social determinants of health. https://www.healthypeople.gov/2020/topics-objectives/topic/social-determinants-of-health

Perry, H. (2013). *A brief history of community health workers*. https://www.mchip.net/sites/default/files/mchipfiles/02_CHW_History.pdf

PRAPARE. (2016). PRAPARE®: Protocol for responding to and assessing patient assets, risks, and experiences. National Association of Community Health Centers. http://www.nachc.org/wp-content/uploads/2018/05/PRAPARE_One_Pager_Sept_2016.pdf

Powell, J. A. (2008). Structural racism: Building upon the insights of John Calmore. *North Carolina Law Review, 86*, 791–816.

Queensborough Community College: The City University of New York (QCC CUNY). (n.d.). *Definition for diversity*. Retrieved May 18, 2021, from https://www.qcc.cuny.edu/diversity/definition.html

Ray, R. (2020, April 09). *Why are blacks dying at higher rates from COVID-19?* The Brookings Institution. https://www.brookings.edu/blog/fixgov/2020/04/09/why-are-blacks-dying-at-higher-rates-from-covid-19/

The San Diego Foundation. (2016, March 24). *What is social justice?* https://www.sdfoundation.org/news-events/sdf-news/what-is-social-justice/

Schilling, B. (n.d.). *The Federal Government has put billions into promoting electronic health record use: How is it going?* The Commonwealth Fund. Retrieved May 18, 2021, from https://www.commonwealthfund.org/publications/newsletter-article/federal-government-has-put-billions-promoting-electronic-health

Sivashanker, K., Duong, K., Resnick, A., Eappen, S. (2020, September 1). *Health care equity: From fragmentation to transformation*. NEJM Catalyst. https://catalyst.nejm.org/doi/full/10.1056/CAT.20.0414

Solomon, L. S., & Kanter, M. H. (2018). Health care steps up to social determinants of health: current context. *The Permanente Journal, 22*, 18–139. https://doi.org/10.7812/TPP/18-139

Tobin-Tyler, E., & Ahmad, B. (2020, May 22). *Marrying value-based payment and the social determinants of health through Medicaid ACOs: Implications for policy and practice*. Millbank Memorial Fund. https://www.milbank.org/publications/marrying-value-based-payment-and-the-social-determinants-of-health-through-medicaid-acos-implications-for-policy-and-practice/

Tuggle, A. C., Cohen, J. H., & Crews, D. E. (2018). Stress, migration, and allostatic load: A model based on Mexican migrants in Columbus, Ohio. *Journal of Physiological Anthropology, 37*(1), 28. https://doi.org/10.1186/s40101-018-0188-4

U.S. Department of Health and Human Services, Office of Disease Prevention and Health Promotion. (n.d.). *Social determinants of health: Interventions and resources*. Healthy

People 2020. Retrieved May 18, 2021, from https://www.healthypeople.gov/2020/topics-objectives/topic/social-determinants-health/interventions-resources

The U.S. Department of Housing and Urban Development (HUD). (n.d.). *Diversity and inclusion definitions*. Retrieved May 18, 2021, from https://www.hud.gov/program_offices/administration/admabout/diversity_inclusion/definitions

Wade, D. T., & Halligan, P. W. (2017). The biopsychosocial model of illness: A model whose time has come. *Clinical Rehabilitation, 31*(8), 995–1004. https://doi.org/10.1177/0269215517709890

World Health Organization. (n.d.). *Social determinants of health: Health equity*. Retrieved May 18, 2021, from https://www.who.int/health-topics/social-determinants-of-health#tab=tab_3

PART II

Population Health Management Strategies and Tools

CHAPTER 5

Health Data Analytics for Population Health Management

Nalin Johri

KEY TERMS

Artificial Intelligence
Electronic Health Record
Fast Healthcare Interoperability Resource (FHIR)
Health Data Analytics
Health Informatics
Health Information Exchanges
Health Information Technology

Interoperability
Machine Learning
Meaningful Use
Patient Registries
Predictive Modeling
Population Health Data
Tableau

LEARNING OBJECTIVES

1. Explain the role of Health Information Technology (HIT) and health data analytics for population health management (PHM).
2. Identify the various federal initiatives, policies, and laws that have influenced the adoption of HIT and population health (PH) data analytics.
3. Describe the utility of an electronic health record (EHR) and other major HIT tools.
4. Explain the concept of interoperability and challenges for real-time use.
5. Assess the impact of artificial intelligence (AI) and predictive modeling for PHM.
6. Provide examples of PH data analytics on improving PH outcomes.

> Podcasts that exemplify the content of this chapter are available at Springer Publishing Connect™
>
> Podcast 5.1. What Happens When Technology Enables the Health Sector to Move Beyond Only Clinical Data?
> Podcast 5.2. Data Analytics as the PHM Challenge

Access the podcast online at http://connect.springerpub.com/content/book/978-0-8261-4427-0/part/part02/chapter/ch05

DID YOU KNOW?

What Is New With Health Data Analytics? (True or False)

1. In 2020, a record was set with $9.4 billion invested in digital health.
2. Digital innovation changed significantly how the healthcare sector responded to COVID-19.
3. PH managers are adopting more noncontact, patient monitoring technology from wearables to video analytics and mobile platforms.
4. Interoperability means the capability of combining systems that provide SDOH data, clinical information, community health status indicators, and claims data.
5. AI is the ability for a computer system to perform a task that an intelligent human could do.

There is no need to double-check the facts in these articles—all these statements are true (1: Landi [2020]; 2: Dyrda [2020]; 3: Lovell [2020]; 4: Leventhal [2020]; and 5: Giannasi [2020]). The role of HIT as an enabler for PHM and the rapid adoption of data analytics will only continue to increase in the coming years.

Key point: Without the capability and accelerated innovation of technology such as the EHR, interoperability capabilities, AI, and data analytics, the adoption rate for PHM strategies would have taken many more years.

INTRODUCTION

The rapid rise of health technology innovation during the past 20 years needs to be considered as a primary factor transforming healthcare delivery. Today's health professions students may not remember a time when the community's main-street doctor, now known as a primary care provider (PCP), relied on stacks of manila folders that contained each patient's personal record. These multiple pages of documentation were often faxed between the PCP, specialist, and local hospital. Now, personal health records are available via patient portals for every patient and their designated provider to view at their own convenience. This capability permits information to be directly exchanged between the patient, various healthcare providers, and organizations. Among the many advances in healthcare technology, personal health records represent one of the significant 21st-century HIT achievements.

Health informatics applications serve as a foundation for PHM. Informatics is the "term used to describe the science of information management in health care" (Mastrian & McGonigle, 2017). A key information technology (IT) component is the DIKW paradigm or universal perspective on understanding the role and flow of data.

$$\text{Data} \longrightarrow \text{Information} \longrightarrow \text{Knowledge} \longrightarrow \text{Wisdom}$$

Population health (PH) managers have plentiful data and information, but the capacity and capability to move to the knowledge level and then wisdom requires the use of data analytics. **Health data analytics** "focuses on the technologies and processes that measure, manage, and analyze healthcare data" (Looker Data Sciences, Inc., 2020).

Health data analytics recognizes the need to go beyond clinical data as clinical data are just a small part of the puzzle of predicting health outcomes. The healthcare industry recognizes that over 80% of outcomes are related to nonclinical factors such as socioeconomic status, lifestyle factors, and other social determinants of health. In order to harness the power of health data analytics, several healthcare organizations are embracing this need to go beyond clinical data and including these additional data (Bresnick, 2019a).

The intersection of PHM and health data analytics creates exciting possibilities and concern at the same time. Over the years, as the concept of PH was operationalized and gained traction, the tendency has been to add more health outcome indicators. The PH manager's role now includes the task of strategically prioritizing and selecting only measures and methods that are pertinent to PHM decision-making. With the help of such innovative analytical tools such as Tableau, artificial intelligence, and machine learning, future PH managers will be prepared to make data informed decisions via health analytics competencies.

DID YOU KNOW?

Health Information Literacy

Information competency is a common goal for all health professionals and a Task Force sponsored by the American Health Information Management Association (AHIMA) and the American Medical Informatics Association (AMIA) identified five competencies:
- Health information literacy and skills
- Health informatics skills using the EHR
- Privacy and confidentiality of health information
- Health Information/data technical security
- Basic computer literacy skills (AHIMA & AMIA, 2008, p. 6)

This chapter introduces health analytics, informatic tools, and strategies that provide useful and necessary applications for successful PHM. Today's PH manager's responsibility and accountability is to know and apply data-driven strategies and approaches and to be able to adequately make comparisons between different systems, platforms, and applications.

Health Information Technology for Population Health Management

Adoption of HIT lagged until the Health Information Technology for Economic and Clinical Health (HITECH) Act of 2009 was passed. HITECH required that healthcare entities install computerized systems and demonstrate their meaningful use (HIPAA Journal, 2020). **Meaningful use** is a term used to describe the requirement for providers to demonstrate performance on defined metrics and measures from their EHR. As part of the American Reinvestment and Recovery Act (ARRA) of 2009, the HITECH Act not only defined meaningful use but also required submission of quality-of-care outcome measures to federal oversight agencies (CMS.gov, 2010). Under the HITECH Act, federal mandates as well as direct financial incentives were used to increase adoption rates of information technology (Brown et al., 2019). The Health Insurance Portability and Accountability Act (HIPAA) and its role in defining privacy and security requirements for healthcare providers and organizations (US DHHS, n.d.) represents a second important federal health policy that impacted the adoption of HIT. The HIPAA Security Rule established standards to protect personal health data and required specific administrative, physical, and technical safeguards to ensure confidentiality, integrity, and security of health information.

Major Health Informatic Tools for Population Health Management

PH managers should be familiar with three major health informatic tools, beginning with the **EHR,** which serves as a universal repository of patient's information. One goal for EHR use is to improve patient safety, which was often impacted by paper records and the inability to assess patient records and conditions in real time. The EHR also enables the transition to value-based care by providing pertinent population data that were used by data analysts to identify high-risk populations (Scherpbier et al., 2021). Today, the EHR forms the information superstructure for PHM..

DID YOU KNOW?

Get Familiar With an Electronic Health Record (EHR) Platform

The following snapshot is one example of an EHR. To learn more about this topic, you can access this Getting Started video from EHRGo (https://www.youtube.com/watch?time_continue=2&v=Y0NJiaTwlpc&feature=emb_logo).

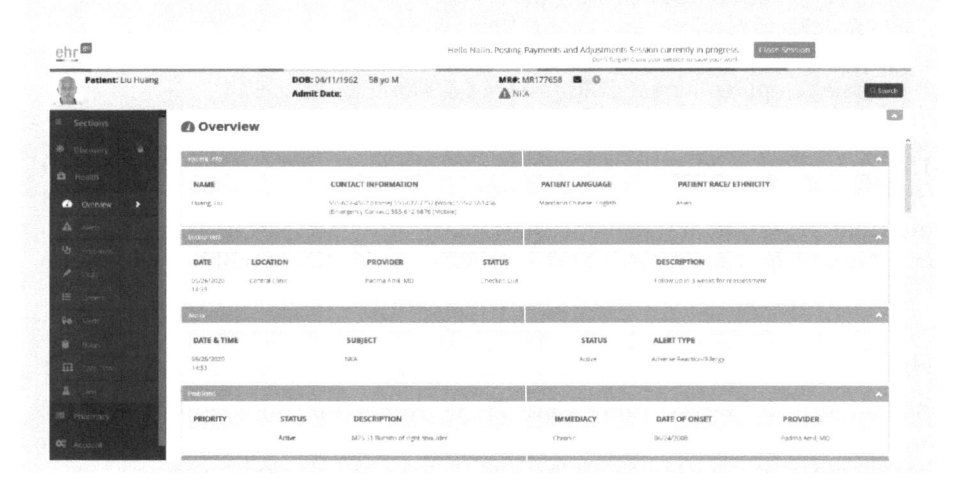

Another example of HIT is the use of complex patient registries. **Patient registries** are patient information repositories that store data related to a health condition or disease. The design is based on technology capabilities of using structured data to provide aggregate information relevant to populations and not just individuals. The data are generally available to qualified health providers and researchers who are interested in a specific disease.

A third PHM tool, a **health information exchange (HIE)** is an example of federal policy that has produced significant benefits by permitting access to patient data and treatment history across heathcare providers and organizations. HIEs can be formed by many diverse organizations (local, state, and regional) and function by providing a database repository of patient data that is easily accessible due to universal standards requirements for all multiple health providers and agencies.

? DID YOU KNOW?

Health Information Exchange

Not all HIEs are sponsored by government agencies, and regional hospitals and heath systems can develop their own HIE. Many state hospital associations were leaders in developing HIEs.

OneHealthNJ is a great example of an HIE. This link includes several video examples: https://www.onehealthnewjersey.com/Home.aspx.

It may seem strange that the Centers for Medicare & Medicaid Services (CMS) would need to provide incentives for hospitals and physician practices to adopt EHRs and other new technologies, but the meaningful use stipulation was the initial catalyst to ensure all health providers and organizations integrated and consistently used health data (CMS, 2010).

Given the rapid rise of easily available data, both ethical and business considerations regarding data transparency became an important managerial responsibility. As with all data collected and used for PH outcomes, the validity of the data is always questioned as to its ability to capture all the important factors that contribute to a single outcome measure. Risk adjustment is a statistical method required for all PHM data to ensure that the outcome truly reflects the health status of a particular individual. The concept of risk, and risk segmentation and stratification are covered in Chapter 6. The process of data analytics produces valuable information that yields meaningful comparative information for informed decision-making.

Health Informatics Strategies for Population Health Management

Technological capabilities have contributed to new PHM strategies including process design and quality improvement initiatives. With the advent of HIT-enabled data analytic tools, opportunities to integrate predictive modeling into population risk segmentation and stratification have become a reality. **Predictive modeling** uses large databases to determine characteristics of vulnerable patients who may be at risk for infection, diseases, or other health needs. Predictive modeling provides PH managers with the option to proactively reach at-risk and rising risk populations without the need to wait for a critical health emergency or seminal event. Predictive modeling also provides managers with business intelligence data that offer a data-supported glimpse of future utilization that is useful for planning (Wills, 2014).

Predictive modeling—an approach that uses mathematical algorithms on existing data to predict the probability of an outcome, future behavior, or consequence (Stiefel, 2016).

Through the use of EHR data on 4 million records, it was found that models were only predicting less than half of the diabetic population. Combining EHRs with claims data and laboratory and medicine data greatly improved the predictive model for diabetic patients (Paruk, 2016).

> **? DID YOU KNOW?**
>
> **Role of Predictive Analytics**
>
> A recent data analytic example highlights the successful role of predictive analytics for a population subgroup—teens (Raths, 2020). Encouraging teenagers to receive important vaccines is a health promotion priority. To achieve this goal, the hospital recognized and followed a data analytics implementation pathway with each level being more sophisticated and complex.
>
> Descriptive ->Diagnostic->Predictive - >Prescriptive
>
> By first combining teen and family profile information with diagnostic information, the analysts were then able to predict those at risk for not being likely to receive an human papillomavirus (HPV) vaccine. Using this methodology, the hospital was able to target families with children not likely to receive HPV vaccines by age 13 with appropriate reminders and support materials. The program outcome showed improvement in the related Healthcare Effectiveness Data and Information Set (HEDIS) score measuring appropriate immunization for teens.

Interoperability

None of the previously described HIT tools or strategies would be available to PH managers without the ability to access various data warehouses synchronously and simultaneously. Today, IT capabilities easily can permit "the secure and seamless exchange of data between two computerized systems" (Wagner, 2018). The **interoperability** of these systems is supported by software known as application programming interface (API; Wagner, 2018). Fast Healthcare Interoperability Resource (FHIR), one of the most popular protocols for joining disparate systems together, refers to standards developed that will enable seamless, on-demand information exchange (Bresnick, 2016). For the myriad databases to be accessed synchronously and simultaneously, they must adhere to established and supported standards and move away from document-based systems.

> **Interoperability**—ability of various systems and organizations to work together to exchange information (Mastrian & McGonigle, 2017).

In 2017, Grady Health System in Atlanta showcased interoperability by exchanging 1.36 million patient records with 1,500 hospitals and 35,000 clinics across the country. Within Grady Health System, interoperability of systems ensured that the infusion pump and EHR communicated to ensure that the right patient got the right medication with the right dose at the right time. Earlier this process was completed manually by nurses programming the infusion pump and transcribing information in the EHR (Wagner, 2018).

FHIR or Fast Healthcare Interoperability Resource is a protocol for ensuring that applications can be seamlessly used across EHRs and HIEs. Northwell Health in New York coordinated with Intersystems to bring out a SMART on FHIR application that allows more efficient collection and storage of patient data across its health system. A key component of this SMART application is the integration of the monitoring of premature baby development. Through this application, the reliance on multiple website and paper documents has been minimized (Jason, 2020a).

Informatics, Big Data, Artificial Intelligence, and Machine Learning

The term "big data" appears as a catch-all phrase to describe data aggregation from diverse sources—clinical, pharmaceutical, claims, social determinants of health, patient profiles, and so forth. Three characteristics distinguish it from traditional data—these data are available in very high volume, these data move at high velocity across healthcare, and these data are highly variable in nature (Catalyst, 2018). Given these characteristics, new possibilities for interpretation continue to emerge and go far beyond traditional quality improvement processes that most hospitals and health providers traditionally rely on for data summaries and reports. AI represents a dominant theme for health IT leaders, as they emerge from the incredible challenges of COVID-19 (Leventhal, 2020). Big data initiatives can be exceptionally challenging as all detailed information reflects multiple populations and infinite personal attributes. While machine learning uses big data sets to "train" the model to accurately pick out patterns in data.

> **Artificial intelligence**—deals with…information tools based on intelligent technologies…that capture the complex process of human thought and intelligence (McGonigle & Mastrian, 2017, p. 65).

AI is a companion to remote patient monitoring and the coordination of the Internet of things equipment for patients who benefit from being taken care at home. AI takes care of the routine tasks such as turning lights on/off, sending patient monitoring results to their provider, and requesting prescriptions as needed.

Machine Learning—uses AI to repeatedly learn from large data sets and improve the identification of patterns in data.

Researchers from MIT's Computer Science and Artificial Intelligence Laboratory used big data to refine the detection of warning signs of acute heart failure based on images of excessive fluid in a patient's lung. Using machine learning with over 300,000 x-ray images and notes from radiologists, the researchers were able to develop a model that accurately found 90% of the most severe cases of acute heart failure (Kent, 2020c).

- Experts suggest that healthcare institutions develop a plan for how data will be used with specific populations and to prepare models and develop interventions in advance.
- AI can also be used to identify an upstream diagnosis on preliminary data, such as developing a tool to detect the severity of excess fluid in the lungs in as an early warning sign for acute health failure (Kent, 2020c).

> **DID YOU KNOW?**
>
> **Data Analytics: Applying Electronic Health Record (EHR) Data for Population Health Management**
>
> Brian Coffey, senior vice president and chief data insight and innovation officer at Southwestern Health Resources (Kent, 2020b), provides insights from mining EHR data. For instance, you could develop a model for complex seniors to be able to predict the risk of fall. What is the risk of fall in 75- to 85-year-old men or women in the population of interest? That is where EHR data becomes powerful, because you can look at the drugs they are taking and whether they have a history of falls, as well as social factors like their living conditions and transportation options. These things can help you understand your population.

With the significant importance of integrating SDOH information, and the added availability of remote monitoring data from wearables and home technology, the future impact of AI will be essential to PHM. New innovations, such as hospitals at home, will grow beyond limited recent use of just targeting healthy individuals for screening, and the management of a few chronic conditions (Kent, 2019).

Health Data Analytics: Sources of Population Health Management Data and Methods

As the definition of what constitutes "population" in healthcare terms expands, so does the range of data that could potentially be relevant for PHM (Univ. of Illinois at Chicago, 2018). In this expanding universe of data, ideal population health outcome measures will more closely resemble the active physical, mental, and social state of the populations they represent for health outcomes overall as well as the distribution of these outcomes across different population groups and geographic regions (Parrish, 2010).

The success of PHM strategies is predicated on access to a range of data on the patient's clinical, financial, and social risks to develop a complete portfolio of data that can then be analyzed for specific risks and appropriate interventions (Nash et al., 2021). Common data categories that should be included are (Bresnick, 2018a) given in Table 5.1.

These varied sources of data and big data are available in fragmented silos that are not interconnected, which limits their access, and use by personnel that need to analyze these disparate sources of data and make decisions (Kent, 2019).

> **DID YOU KNOW?**
>
> **Additional Sources of Population Health Data**
>
> As part of health analytics for PHM, the need to access community-level data on social determinants of health (SDOH) is critical, but hospitals and practices may not have the resources or community connections to immediately make this a reality, and they may start with data within their system. This system-specific data can be enriched by seeking

inputs from patients as well as providers to include some population health perspectives (Sokol, 2019). Currently, there are no established standards for including SDOH data within EHRs creating a barrier for providers to include these data. To address this need, innovative intrastate partnerships are forming to provide stakeholders data on housing, food access, transportation, and other nonmedical factors (Kent, 2020a).

There are several additional sources of population survey data including clearing houses and consolidators of population survey data from a variety of sources.

- Since 2010, the County Health Rankings has been providing data including socio economic, demographic, health, and environmental topics (https://www.county healthrankings.org/ explore-health-rankings/use-data). In its most recent data updation in 2020, over 20 sources of periodic population surveys and registries conducted by a variety of organizations and agencies are used.
- Another source of global and domestic data, sourced from a variety of population surveys and periodically updated, is through the Institute for Health Metrics and evaluation (www.healthdata.org/data-tools). The Institute partners with the University of Washington and provides national and international data on a variety of health subjects and uses models and prediction for the burden of disease estimates including COVID-19 statistics.
- A third source, suited to students and researchers with access to the Inter-University Consortium for Political and Social Research (ICPSR), are the 257-survey series categorized under healthcare facilities (https://www.icpsr.umich.edu/web/pages/ ICPSR/index.html). These surveys provide a variety of socioeconomic, demographic, and health topics and span over 5 million variables. A researched and categorized selection of ICPSR data sets categorized under healthcare facilities is available as a chapter in a recent book on health services research and analytics using Excel (Johri, 2020).
- Another data aggregation platform pushing the boundaries of PHM and SAS is partnering to develop the Healthy Nevada Project that has set an ambitious goal of analyzing citizens' genetic, clinical, environmental, and socioeconomic data in develop a health risk profile of the citizens and predict population health risks based on the totality of these data (SASHealth, n.d.).

TABLE 5.1 Data Categories for Population Health Management Data Analysis

Data Type	Purpose
Patient demographics	Correct identification of individual patients as well as grouping individuals into categories for intervention
Vital signs	To predict risk and potential for chronic conditions
Laboratory results	To predict risk and progress of ongoing interventions
Progress notes	Information from providers is an important source of information on care of patients
Problem lists and diagnoses	Covers what a patient is currently experiencing as well as past conditions that may inform future events
Procedure codes	Utilized for payment and billing purposes as well as use with diagnoses to further analyze conditions
Allergy lists	Includes food sensitivity and adverse drug reactions and interactions
Medication data	To flag potential drug interactions
Admission, discharge, and transfer information	Information to ensure timely and effective follow-up
Skilled nursing, home health, and long-term postacute care	Data to ensure that there are no gaps in information on care received
Social determinants of health	Data that are important for overall wellness of patients

Data Security and Safety

In accessing and using PHM data, which may come from several sources, HIPAA compliance is essential, especially when the data involve protected health information. The Office of the National Coordinator (ONC) in partnership with the Office of Civil Rights (OCR) has developed and updated its Department of Health and Human Services Security Risk Assessment (SRA) tool for use by small and medium healthcare entities to remain HIPAA compliant. This free downloadable SRA tool guides small and medium healthcare entities through assessment of risks in accessing and using electronic protected health information and generates a report that details and rates vulnerabilities and threats (Davis, 2020a).

Multiple data sources, escalating numbers of mergers and acquisitions among healthcare systems, coupled with the rapid scale-up of telehealth in 2020 increased the risk for health data of being breached or hacked. Despite this reality, just 44% of hospitals and healthcare systems reported adhering to the National Institute of Science and Technology's cybersecurity framework standards. Equally worrying is the lack of investment needed to adhere to these standards (Davis, 2020b).

Data Integration

Data integration and interoperability are different processes. Interoperability refers to real-time exchange between systems without middleware, while integration requires a third party or middleware (Robert, 2017). To make advances in value-based care, integration of claims data and clinical data is required. Unfortunately, claims data are proprietary data collected from health plans, and clinical data are proprietary data collected from providers. Health plans typically use claims data to identify populations that account for highest cost of care or care that is delivered inefficiently, while providers tend to focus on clinical data to deliver patient-centered care. These two silos of data need to be integrated and accessed to synergistically apply analytics that can push the boundary on targeted reductions in cost of care and at the same time ensure quality of care (Populytics & Keenan-Nagle Advertising, n.d.). Clearly, competitive and technology barriers need to be transcend these silos to reap analytic advantages (DeloitteHealth, 2017).

Integration ensures that processes are seamlessly included in the same workflow, and the user does not have to switch between applications. In the time of COVID-19, integration of telehealth applications within EHRs ensures that the providers (and patients) are not switching applications such as Facetime, Zoom, or Skype, and there is one single workflow. With an integrated telehealth solution, the front office can check in the patient, and nurse or doctor can also interact with the patient (Jason, 2020b).

The success of PHM strategies, built on sound data analytics tools that use pertinent data, rests on the coherence among these three distinct parts—PHM strategies, analytics, and data—of the PHM analytics puzzle. This coherence is furthered by having a logic model that knits together disparate data elements and applies focused analytics tools to develop targeted PHM strategies for identified populations. A good example of this coherence and logic is provided in the mini case-study at the end of this chapter.

Data Analytics and Population Health Management

The burgeoning list of players providing a variety of population health analytics is a testament to the rapid embrace of PHM and analytics. Filling the demand for PHM, from large healthcare systems to physician practices, the list of providers of population health analytics is rapidly increasing. Becker's Hospital Review has compiled a list of 111 providers as well as their PH analytics niche (Dyrda, 2019). Niche areas include business intelligence, integration with other systems, development of apps, use of mobile phones, risk assessment, transition to value-based care, etc. In a nod to the newer segment of population health management software, the 2020 Best in KLAS report ranked Enli as the top software provider (HealthITAnalytics, 2020).

Selecting Population Health Management Software for Data Analytics

Given the increasing number of PHM solutions-software options, healthcare entities need to begin their decision-making process by identifying measurable goals and aligned activities specific to their population health needs. In the absence of these clearly articulated goals and activities, there is a real danger of overinvesting in technology that may be redundant or worse overinvesting in tools and technology that do not work for their situation (Bresnick, 2018b). Once the goals of PHM are clear, regardless of whether the organization is interested in a standalone PHM software or one that integrates with their EHR, it should include these data-related capabilities (Bresnick, 2018b). See Table 5.2.

Beyond these data-related capabilities, PHM platforms need to include care management, care coordination, and/or patient engagement capabilities (Bresnick, 2018b).

TABLE 5.2 Three Required Data Capabilities for PHM Software

Data Aggregation	Data Analytics	Reporting and Visualization
By pooling or otherwise accessing data (clinical, claims, socioeconomic, etc.) to facilitate the development of individual and community profiles for targeted interventions. Together with pooling data, these data need to be housed somewhere for easy access. Both the pooling and housing require adherence to industry standards to ensure fidelity and security of data and ease of analytics.	To stratify patients by risk as a first step toward developing targeted interventions. Here is where predictive analytics, including artificial intelligence and machine learning tools play a major role in flagging patients who could potentially develop serious events, prior to these events becoming a reality.	Use of dashboards, charts, and figures that highlight important information that is actionable.

PHM, public health management.

❓ DID YOU KNOW?

Population Health Management Data Analyst Career Opportunities—Need a Job?

Recognizing the need to integrate population health and data analytics is evidenced by the growing reflection of these and related terms in position announcements in healthcare. Houser and colleagues in a 2020 study (Houser et al., 2021) curated a sample of 49 position announcements based on their key word search using "population health." In this sample, they found good correspondence between the skill sets in these announcements and the competency domains for accreditation by the Commission on Accreditation for Health Informatics and Information Management Education (American Health Management Information Association (AHIMA), 2020). Based on qualitative analysis of these position announcements, 80% had soft skill requirements, while 25%–36% had skill set requirements that mapped onto the six competency domains for accreditation and included skills related to problem-solving, generating reports, working with spreadsheets, research, data analysis, and visualization.

In a recent survey by Healthcare Information and Management System Society (HIMSS), 90% of respondents were using analytics in clinical area, while 21% reported using it for PHMand just 10% were using analytics for chronic care management (Bresnick, 2019b). A review of articles on PHM published between 2000 and 2015 and found that these articles largely covered the aims of health, cost, and/or quality of care; they very rarely included data management, Triple Aim assessment, risk stratification, evaluation, and feedback (Steenkamer et al., 2017).

The Impact of Health Data Analytics on Population Health Management

With advances in data analytics, population health data are playing a pivotal role in the planning and implementation of health initiatives in communities focused on wellness and prevention (Univ. of Illinois at Chicago, 2018). This has led to some schools emphasizing population health analytics as "applying quantitative methods and technology to reach advanced insight about a group" (Duke University, 2020). However, D. Kindig, an expert in the PHM field, suggested in 2016 that there are far too many measures and indicators for the different facets of population health. He feels that over the years, despite the good intention of simplifying and reducing these population health measures, we are far from achieving this goal (National Academies of Science, Engineering, and Medicine, 2016, p. 1).

A review of articles on PHM published between 2000 and 2015 found that organizations largely covered the aims of health, cost, and/or quality of care; they very rarely included data management, Triple Aim assessment, risk stratification, evaluation, and feedback (Steenkamer et al., 2017). Clearly, opportunities exist for PH managers to imaginatively use and apply the tremendous capabilities of data analytics to the many population health challenges.

Burton suggests that the commonality between PHM and health analytics is the focus on outcomes, which provides value-added through the confluence of three-activity streams (Burton, 2016). See Figure 5.1.

Within this three-stream approach, value-added analytics serves to measure actions that are compliant with best practices and the safety and effectiveness of actions in providing care. In this scenario, analytics adds value by investing more time and resources in understanding the question and

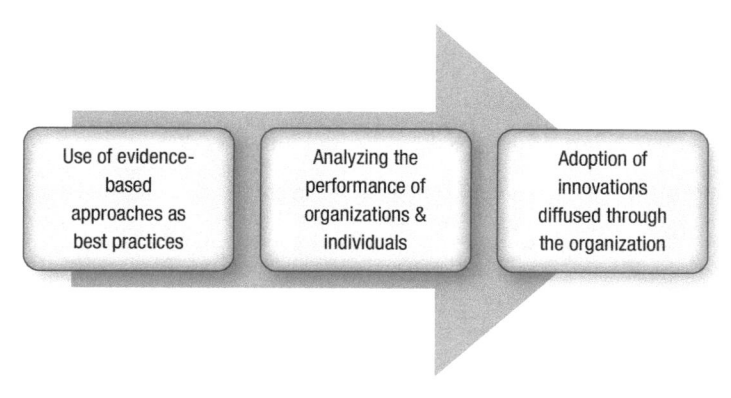

FIGURE 5.1 Data Stream—Health Analytics

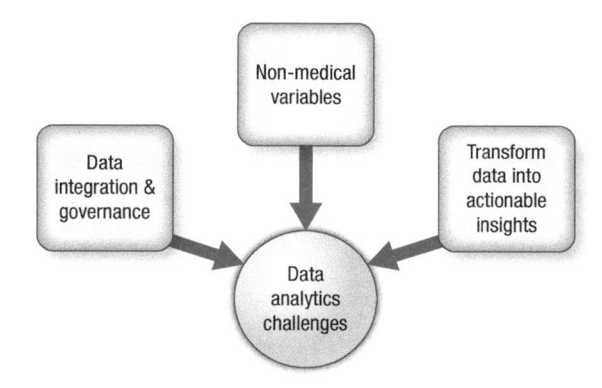

FIGURE 5.2 Current Population Health Analytic Challenges

interpreting data rather than scrambling perpetually to gather data (Burton, 2016). These data can provide actionable insights to reduce variations rather than merely establishing a minimal baseline for organization-wide process improvements that are prioritized for scenarios with the widest variations and most resource use.

Intermingling of Challenges and Opportunities for Population Data Analytics

There are several challenges and opportunities in population health analytics, as indicated in Figure 5.2 (Duke University, 2020).

One of the primary challenges is the growth in volume and types of data that require greater collaboration between healthcare informatics and analytics to ensure that silos of data ownership are overcome. Another area of concern is the impact of nonmedical variables, such as the approach on upstreaming prevention and wellness interventions that require aligning between social, economic, and demographic data with traditional claims and clinical data, and finally, the capacity of PH managers to transform data into actionable insights. Do resources, leadership, and competencies exist to align technology with the health organization's goals and desired population outcomes?

Other drivers of PH analytics focus on operational aspects such as moving from transitional to transformational change. See Table 5.3.

TABLE 5.3 Operational Drivers of PH Analytic

Standardization	Organizational standardization through the use of checklists, for the planning, development, completeness, and aesthetics of dashboards in telling a compelling story (Sisense Inc., n.d.)
EHR data integration	The use of EHR data to flag gaps in care for those who delayed or avoided care, estimated to be 41% of U.S. adults, because of the COVID-19 pandemic and now are at risk of illness or a recurrent disease condition (Czeisler et al., 2020; Sokol, 2020)
Artificial intelligence adoption	The integration of artificial intelligence algorithms into the development of risk scores, and risk stratification, which are key population health activities (Bresnick, 2016; Duke University, 2020)
Budget priorities	The management of health organization's budgets to support the increased demands for PHM analytics (Columbus, 2020)

PH, population health; PHM, public health management.

Population Health Analytics Benefits

PH managers have benefitted from health informatics and data analytics as shown by a variety of positive organizational and patient outcomes.

- Improvement in overall care coordination and transitions of care and even process design
- Increased communication via mobile technology for consumer healthcare
- The introduction and adoption of patient portals for increased patient engagement
- The use of social media and special apps permitting personal management of healthcare and allowing consumers to track their own health status
- The rapid adoption and implementation of telehealth and virtual care (patient monitoring) due to the COVID-19 pandemic

The goal will always be to improve health outcomes for the population of interest.

SUMMARY

Health informatics, IT, and data analytics have converged to dramatically change the healthcare system in the first two decades of this century. Not only have PH outcomes improved, but also HIT technologies have permitted the adoption of new payment models and contributed to advancing new care delivery models that better meet the needs of our consumers and patients. Technology has become an enabler for greater adoption of value-based care. The recent COVID-19 pandemic highlighted the primary and essential role of data analytics for providing quality healthcare and the health sector will continue to aggressively support and fund new technology going forward (Kent, 2020d). A primary goal for all future PH managers is the development of innovative data analytic competencies.

DISCUSSION QUESTIONS

1. Discuss the catalyst for PH management in the context of transformation of data to wisdom.
2. What has been the role of the federal government in encouraging the use of healthcare information technology as it relates to furthering population health data analytics? Should the government have adopted a more hands-on approach? Why or why not?
3. How are EHRs and HIEs related? Look up an existing example of a state-level HIE and discuss.
4. In the context of population health data analytics what is interoperability and how is it overcome?
5. Refer to Kent (2020b) to explain factors behind the success of AI and predictive modeling for PHM.
6. How would you propose to include SDOH in PHM? Be specific in terms of data use, insights, and actions.
7. Explain the confluence of the three data streams (Burton, 2016).
8. What do you consider the three most important challenges and opportunities for population health analytics?

Toolkit Competency Tool

Health Data Analytics and Population Health Management Tableau Application

A great macro example of knitting together disparate data elements is the County Health Rankings Model (see Figure 5.3). In this model developed at the county level, we can see the coming together of data related to health factors that are categorized as health behaviors, clinical care, social and economic factors, and the physical environment. For each of these categorized health factors, there are two or more subcategories that represent the data (from separate data sources) that feed into each of these four categories. A weighted aggregation of these four categories of health factors leads to the health outcomes represented as length of life as well as quality of life that are used for the final ranking of counties in the United States. The simplicity of this logic model belies the complex task of bringing together data from different sources to arrive at the ranking of health outcomes at the county level in the United States. In this model, the population is at the county level. These county-level data can now be used to analyze and assess outcomes and/or risk factors to determine focused and targeted interventions for county-level population.

This is an example of defining a regional or community population as opposed to a discrete or defined population (Lewis, 2014) that the analysis, predictions, and/or intervention would be relevant to. The importance of identifying a population is critical as it identifies the population that the entity will be responsible for (Bresnick, 2016) and provides scope to population health analytics. Healthcare entities may choose a narrower scope by identifying a discrete population of patients enrolled for care at their institution, while other entities or agencies may choose a broader scope of regional or community population, as in the present case.

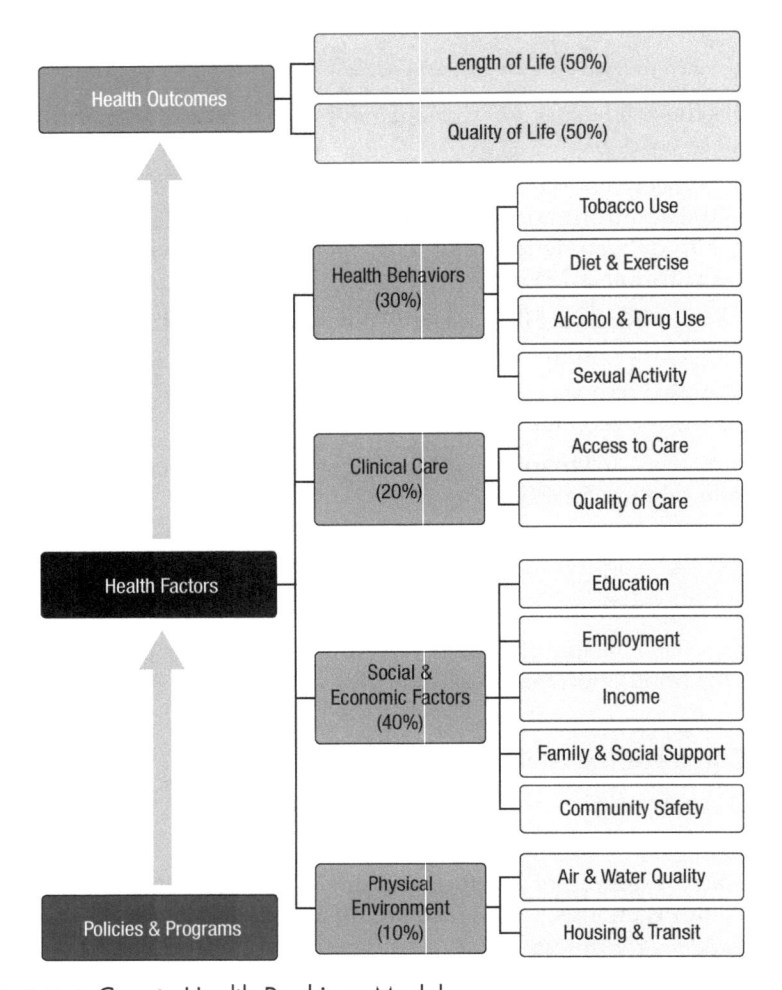

FIGURE 5.3 County Health Rankings Model

The University of Wisconsin Population Health Institute. County Health Rankings & Roadmaps, 2021. www.countyhealthrankings.org

Data from County Health Ranking (https://www.countyhealthrankings.org/explore-health-rankings/use-data) are a good example of curated data from several sources on social and demographic factors (see Figure 5.3). Since these data are at the county and state levels, it provides a wonderful opportunity to analyze these data on community population to assess the implications of these factors on community health outcomes. For example, from the 2017 County Health Rankings data, we can use Tableau to undertake targeted analysis for counties in New Jersey to better understand the relationship between exercise, inactivity, and health status. In Figure 5.4, we have a visualization of counties in New Jersey with average percentage of populations reporting fair/poor health. This shows that three northern counties— Passaic, Essex, and Hudson—and a southern county—Cumberland are on the higher end of the spectrum of counties with populations reporting fair/poor health. In trying to understand this problem further, we can use the same data set to assess, for instance, percentages of population that are physically inactive (Figure 5.5) as well as percentages of population with access to exercise (Figure 5.6). From these two figures, the southern county, Cumberland, has

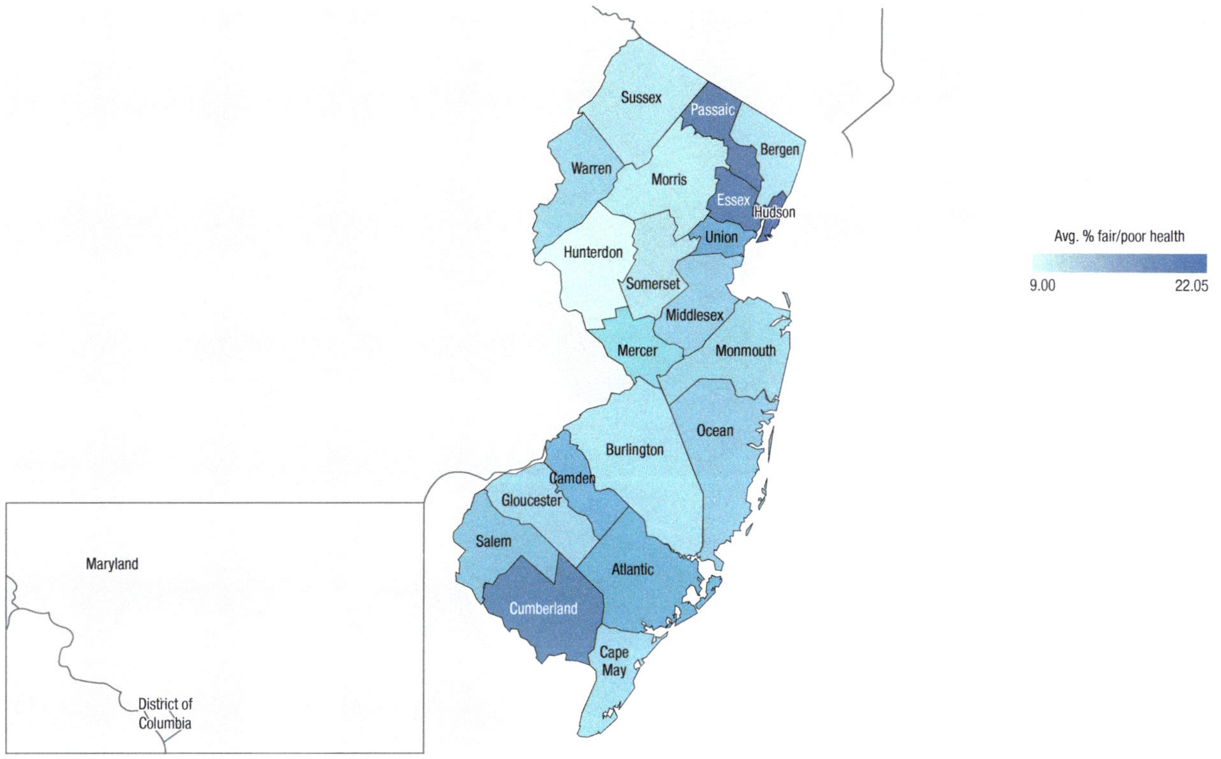

FIGURE 5.4 Average % Reporting Fair/Poor Health in New Jersey Counties, 2017

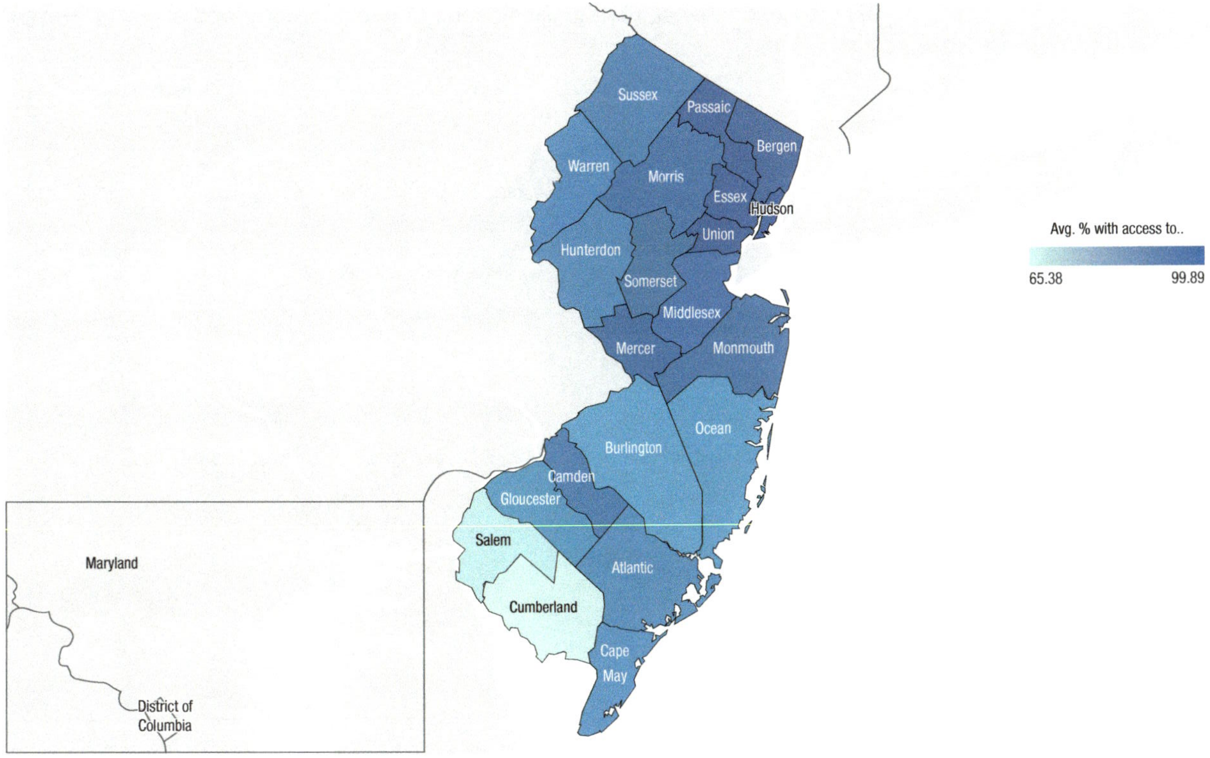

FIGURE 5.5 Average % with Access to Exercise in New Jersey Counties, 2017

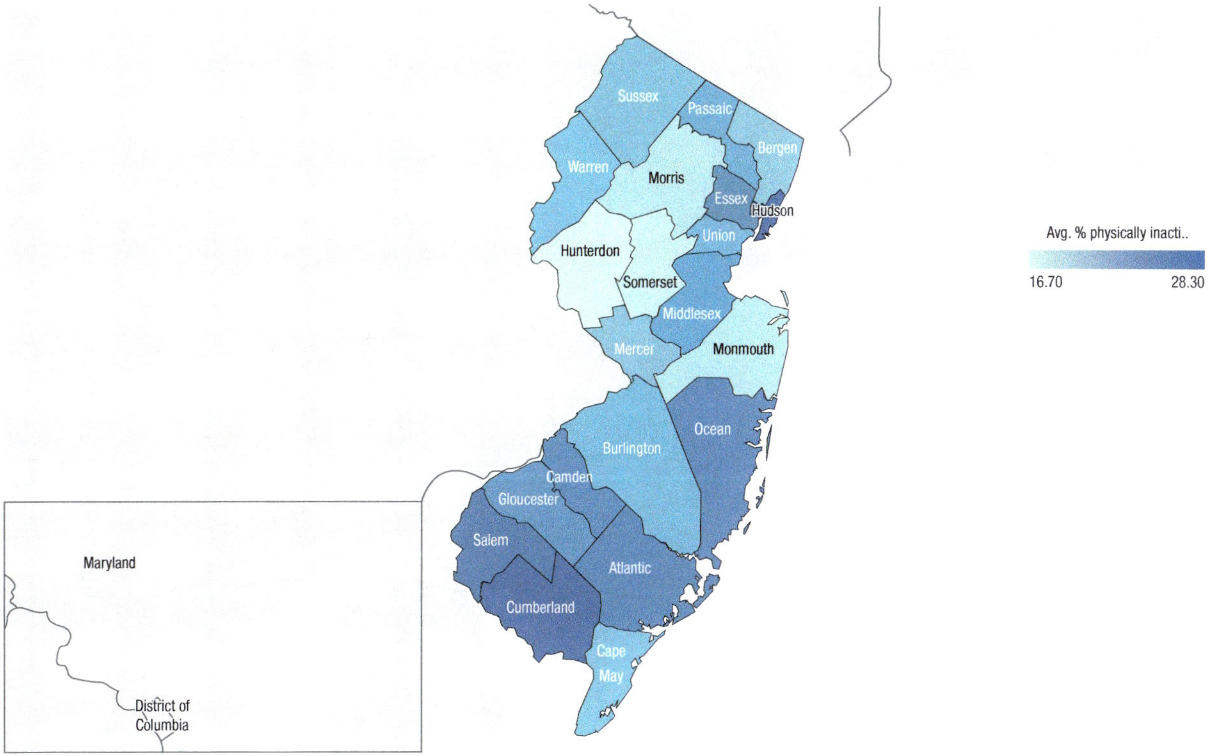

FIGURE 5.6 Average % Physically Inactive in New Jersey Counties, 2017

Exhibit 5.1

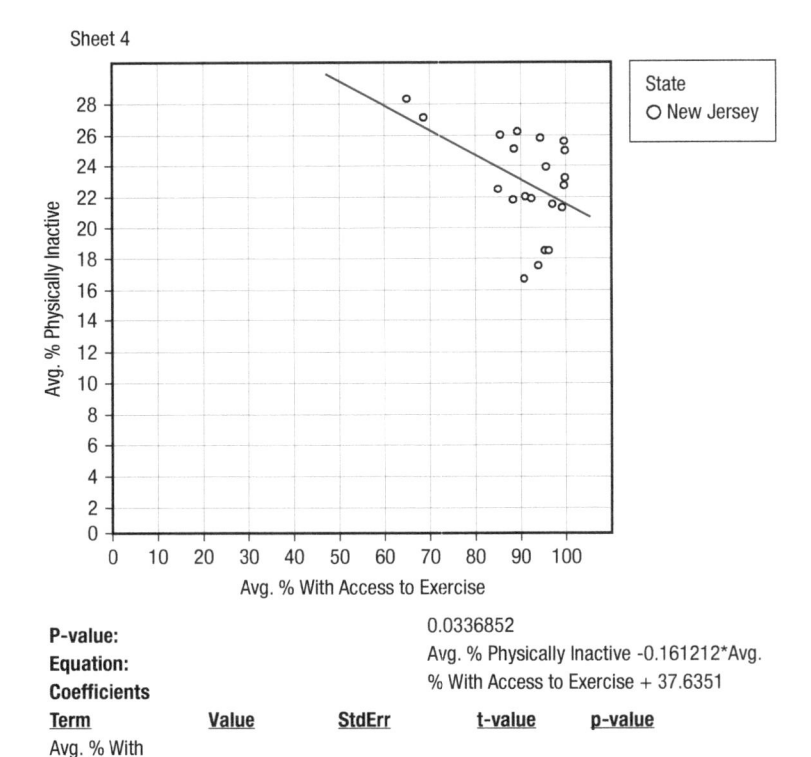

Sheet 4

[Scatter plot showing Avg. % Physically Inactive (y-axis, 0–28) versus Avg. % With Access to Exercise (x-axis, 0–100) for New Jersey counties, with a downward-sloping regression line.]

P-value:	0.0336852			
Equation:	Avg. % Physically Inactive -0.161212*Avg. % With Access to Exercise + 37.6351			
Coefficients				
Term	Value	StdErr	t-value	p-value
Avg. % With Access to Exercise	-0.161212	0.0704208	-2.28926	0.0336852
intercept	37.6351	6.46406	5.82221	<0.0001

EXHIBIT 5.1 Relationship Between Physical Inactivity and Access to Exercise in New Jersey Counties, 2017

the greater average percentages of population that are physically inactive and without access to exercise. The data also show (Exhibit 5.1) that there is a significant ($p < 0.05$) relationship between physical inactivity and access to exercise. Based on this quick analysis, we can see that it is possible that for the southern New Jersey county of Cumberland, interventions related to increasing access to exercise may have a salutary effect on decreasing physical inactivity, and this may be one of the factors in the poor/fair health status of the county residents. However, such interventions may not have as beneficial an effect on the three northern counties, as they are on different parts of the spectrum of physical inactivity and access to exercise. The need for a county-specific approach to such interventions and analysis is underscored here as you explore more fully other determinants of fair/poor health.

CASE STUDY QUESTIONS

1. Consider data sources in Figure 5.3 to identify data that you could potentially use in developing a population health model related to fair/poor health status at county level.

2. Based on Figures 5.4 through 5.6 and Exhibit 5.1, what relationships are you able to develop based on the data visualizations. What are other

data/variables that you would like to consider to better explain these relationships.
3. If you were advising a hospital based in Cumberland County, what recommendations would you make to improve the health status of patients drawn from this county.

REFERENCES

American Health Information Management Association (AHIMA), & American Medical Informatics Association (AMIA). (2008, October). *Joint workforce taskforce: Health information management and informatics core competencies for individuals working with electronic health records.* http://library.ahima.org/PdfView?oid=104073

American Health Management Information Association (AHIMA). (2020). *HIM Curricula.* AHIMA. https://ahima.org/him-curricula/

Bresnick, J. (2016, December 16). *Using risk scores, stratification for population health management.* HealthITAnalytics. https://healthitanalytics.com/features/using-risk-scores-stratification-for-population-health-management

Bresnick, J. (2018a, January 2). *Identifying big data sources for population health management.* HealthITAnalytics. https://healthitanalytics.com/news/identifying-big-data-sources-for-population-health-management

Bresnick, J. (2018b, August 28). *How to choose a population health management company.* HealthITAnalytics. https://healthitanalytics.com/features/how-to-choose-a-population-health-management-company

Bresnick, J. (2019a, April 15). *Unleashing the value of health data in the era of artificial intelligence.* HealthITAnalytics. https://healthitanalytics.com/features/unleashing-the-value-of-health-data-in-the-era-of-artificial-intelligence

Bresnick, J. (2019b, April 30). *Data analytics in widespread use, but not for population health.* HealthITAnalytics. https://healthitanalytics.com/news/data-analytics-in-widespread-use-but-not-for-population-health

Brown, G. D., Pasupathy, K. S., & Patrick, T. B. (2019). *Health informatics: A systems perspective* (2nd ed.). Health Administration Press (HAP); Association of University Programs in Health Administration (AUPHA).

Burton, T. D. (2016). *A guide to successful outcomes using population health analytics* (p. 21). Health Catalyst.

Catalyst, N. (2018). Healthcare big data and the promise of value-based care. *NEJM Catalyst.* https://catalyst.nejm.org/doi/full/10.1056/CAT.18.0290

CMS.gov. (2010, July 13). *CMS and ONC final regulations define meaningful use and set standards for electronic health record incentive program.* CMS. https://www.cms.gov/newsroom/fact-sheets/cms-and-onc-final-regulations-define-meaningful-use-and-set-standards-electronic-health-record

Columbus, L. (2020, October). *How COVID-19 is changing analytics spending.* https://www.forbes.com/sites/louiscolumbus/2020/05/10/how-covid-19-is-changing-analytics-spending/?sh=6693bde111cf

Czeisler, M. É., Marynak, K., Clarke, K. E. N., Salah, Z., Shakya, I., Thierry, J. M., Ali, N., McMillan, H., Wiley, J. F., Weaver, M. D., Czeisler, C. A., Rajaratnam, S. M. W., & Howard, M. E. (2020). Delay or avoidance of medical care because of COVID-19–related concerns—United States, June 2020. *MMWR. Morbidity and Mortality Weekly Report, 69*(36), 1250. https://doi.org/10.15585/mmwr.mm6936a4

Davis, J. (2020a, September 15). *HIPAA compliance: ONC updates security risk assessment tool.* HealthITSecurity. https://healthitsecurity.com/news/hipaa-compliance-onc-updates-security-risk-assessment-tool

Davis, J. (2020b, September 23). *Just 44% of healthcare providers meet NIST cybersecurity standards.* HealthITSecurity. https://healthitsecurity.com/news/just-44-of-healthcare-providers-meet-nist-cybersecurity-standards

DeloitteHealth. (2017). *Population health analytics.* Deloitte United States. https://www2.deloitte.com/us/en/pages/life-sciences-and-health-care/articles/population-health-analytics.html

Duke University. (2020, June 20). *Population health and the role of health analytics | Duke Fuqua*. Masters in Health Analytics Online. https://www.fuqua.duke.edu/programs/msqm-health-analytics/articles/population-health-analytics/

Dyrda, L. (2019). *108+ population health management companies to know | 2019*. https://www.beckershospitalreview.com/lists/108-population-health-management-companies-to-know-2019.html

Dyrda, L. (2020, May 5). *5 high-impact areas for digital innovation in response to COVID-19: Insights from Jefferson's Neil Gomes*. https://www.beckershospitalreview.com/digital-transformation/5-high-impact-areas-for-digital-innovation-in-response-to-covid-19-insights-from-jefferson-s-neil-gomes.html

Giannasi, N. (2020, February 27). *How artificial intelligence can make the U.S. Healthcare more efficient*. https://www.beckershospitalreview.com/how-artificial-intelligence-can-make-the-u-s-healthcare-more-efficient.html?tmpl=component&print=1&layout=default

HealthITAnalytics. (2020, February 3). *Best in KLAS ranks top vendors for population health, analytics*. HealthITAnalytics. https://healthitanalytics.com/news/best-in-klas-ranks-top-vendors-for-population-health-analytics

HIPAA Journal. (2020). What is the HITECH act. *HIPAA Journal*. https://www.hipaajournal.com/what-is-the-hitech-act/

Houser, S. H., Flite, C. A., Foster, S. L., Hunt, T. J., Kinnerson, L., Palmer, M. N., Peterson, J., & Damez Pope, R. (2021). Population health: Identifying skill sets and education alignment for HIM professionals. *Perspectives in Health Information Management, 2021* (Winter). https://perspectives.ahima.org/population-health-identifying-skill-sets-and-education-alignment-for-him-professionals/

Jason, C. (2020a, January 30). *NY health system promotes interoperability with SMART on FHIR App*. EHR Intelligence. https://ehrintelligence.com/news/ny-health-system-promotes-interoperability-with-smart-on-fhir-app

Jason, C. (2020b, October 09). *What are the top telehealth, EHR integration in healthcare?* EHR Intelligence. https://ehrintelligence.com/news/what-are-the-top-telehealth-ehr-integrations-in-healthcare

Johri, N. (2020). *Health services research and analytics using excel*. Springer Publishing Company.

Kent, J. (2019, June 21). *Inching toward the data-driven future of population health management*. HealthITAnalytics. https://healthitanalytics.com/news/inching-toward-the-data-driven-future-of-population-health-management

Kent, J. (2020a, May 11). *Sharing SDOH data for improved population health management*. HealthITAnalytics. https://healthitanalytics.com/news/sharing-sdoh-data-for-improved-population-health-management

Kent, J. (2020b, August 13). *Harnessing big data to enhance population health management*. HealthITAnalytics. https://healthitanalytics.com/news/harnessing-big-data-to-enhance-population-health-management

Kent, J. (2020c, October 5). *Machine learning can predict heart failure from a single X-ray*. HealthITAnalytics. https://healthitanalytics.com/news/machine-learning-can-predict-heart-failure-from-a-single-x-ray

Kent, J. (2020d, December 24). *Intersection of big data analytics, COVID-19 top focus of 2020* https://healthitanalytics.com/news/intersection-of-big-data-analytics-covid-19-top-focus-of-2020

Landi, H. (2020, October 7). *2020 breaks record in digital health investment with $9.4B in funding*. Fierce Healthcare. https://www.fiercehealthcare.com/tech/2020-breaks-record-digital-health-investment9funding#:~:text=2020%20breaks%20record%20in%20digital%20health%20investment%20with%20%249.4B%20in%20funding,-by%20Heather%20Landi&text=With%20%249.4%20billion%20invested%20up,for%20digital%20health%20to%20date

Leventhal, R. (2020, September 23). *CIOs put analytics, AI initiatives into sharper focus*. Healthcare Innovation. https://www.hcinnovationgroup.com/analytics-ai/news/21155457/cios-put-analytics-ai-initiatives-into-sharper-focus

Lewis, N. (2014). *Populations, population health, and the evolution of population management: Making sense of the terminology in US Health Care Today*. http://www.ihi.org/communities/blogs/population-health-population-management-terminology-in-us-health-care

Looker Data Sciences, Inc. (2020). *Healthcare analytics*. Looker. https://looker.com/definitions/healthcare-analytics

Lovell, T. (2020, May 29). *COVID-19 has accelerated adoption of non-contact patient monitoring technology, says Frost & Sullivan analysis*. Healthcare IT News. https://www.healthcareitnews.com/news/emea/covid-19-has-accelerated-adoption-non-contact-patient-monitoring-technology-says-frost

Mastrian, K., & McGonigle, D. (2017). Informatics, science, and the foundation of knowledge. In K. Mastrian & D. McGonigle (Eds.), *Informatics for health professionals* (p. 5). Jones and Bartlett Learning.

McGonigle, D., & Mastrian, K. (2017). Introduction to cognitive science and cognitive informatics. In K. Mastrian & D. McGonigle (Eds.), *Informatics for health professionals* (p. 65). Jones and Bartlett Learning.

Nash, D. B., Skoufalos, A., Fabius, R. J., & Oglesby, W. H. (2021). *Population health: Creating a culture of wellness*. Jones and Bartlett Learning.

National Academies of Science, Engineering, and Medicine. (2016). *Metrics that matter for population health action: Workshop Summary*. The National Academies Press. https://www.nap.edu/download/21899

Parrish, R. G. (2010). *Preventing chronic disease: July 2010: 10_0005*. https://www.cdc.gov/pcd/issues/2010/jul/10_0005.htm

Paruk, F. (2016, August 9). *Using claims, lab, and clinical analytics to discover diabetics*. HealthITAnalytics. https://healthitanalytics.com/news/using-claims-lab-and-clinical-analytics-to-discover-diabetics

Populytics, J. N., & Keenan-Nagle Advertising. (n.d.). Population health analytics—increase value, improve care. *Populytics Health Management Solutions*. Retrieved September 26, 2020, from https://www.populytics.com/services/population-health-analytics/

Raths, D. (2020, September 25). *The predictive analytics journey at Texas Children's Hospital*. Healthcare Innovation. https://www.hcinnovationgroup.com/analytics-ai/artifical-intelligence-machine-learning/article/21155910/the-predictive-analytics-journey-at-texas-childrens-hospital

Robert, B. (2017). *Integration vs. interoperability: What's the difference? SIS BLOG*. https://blog.sisfirst.com/integration-v-interoperability-what-is-the-difference

SASHealth. (n.d.). *Population Health Analytics*. Retrieved September 26, 2020, from https://www.sas.com/en_us/industry/health-care/solution/population-health.html

Scherpbier, H., Walsh, K., & Skoufalos, A. (2021). Population health data and analytics. In D. Nash, A. Skoufalos, R. Fabius, & W. Oglesby (Eds.), *Population health: Creating a culture of wellness* (pp. 113–135). Jones and Bartlett Learning.

Sisense Inc. (n.d.). *Dashboard design worksheets & checklists.pdf*. Retrieved September 26, 2020, from https://pages.sisense.com/rs/601-OXE-081/images/Dashboard%20Design%20Worksheets%20%26%20Checklists.pdf

Sokol, E. (2019, September 10). *Data Analytic strategies essential for population health management*. HealthITAnalytics. https://healthitanalytics.com/news/data-analytic-strategies-essential-for-population-health-management

Steenkamer, B. M., Drewes, H. W., Heijink, R., Baan, C. A., & Struijs, J. N. (2017). Defining population health management: A scoping review of the literature. *Population Health Management, 20*(1), 74–85. https://doi.org/10.1089/pop.2015.0149

Stiefel, M. (2016). Decision support. In D. Nash et al. (Eds.), *Population health: Creating a culture of wellness* (pp. 257–276). Jones & Bartlett Learning.

Univ. of Illinois at Chicago. (2018, February 22). *The role of data in population health |UIC Online*. UIC Online Health Informatics. https://healthinformatics.uic.edu/blog/the-role-of-data-in-population-health/

US DHHS. (n.d.) Health Information Privacy. US Department of Health and Human Services. Retrieved May 18, 2021, from https://www.hhs.gov/hipaa/index.html

Wagner, K. (2018, October). *Interoperability success models of digital integration*. Healthcare Executive. https://healthcareexecutive.org/archives/september-october-2018/interoperability-success-models-of-digital-integration

Wills, M. J. (2014). Decisions through data: Analytics in healthcare. *Journal of Healthcare Management, 59*(4), 254–262. https://journals.lww.com/jhmonline/Fulltext/2014/07000/Decisions_Through_Data__Analytics_in_Healthcare.5.aspx

CHAPTER 6

Population Health Decision-Making: Risk Segmentation, Stratification, and Management

Julie L. Mascari and Anne M. Hewitt

KEY TERMS

Health Risk Assessment
Hotspotting
Risk
Risk Factor
Risk Management
Risk Segmentation
Risk Stratification
Spend

LEARNING OBJECTIVES

1. Explain the concepts of risk, risk score, segmentation, and stratification.
2. Identify the basic five risk categories previously used for population segmentation and describe the expanded continuum of care options.
3. Discuss the decision-making process when selecting metrics to segment a population.
4. Assess factors that determine the level and intensity of care coordination and treatment recommended for a particular population.
5. Apply both risk segmentation and stratification strategies to a high-risk population.

> Podcasts that exemplify the content of this chapter are available at Springer Publishing Connect™
>
> Podcast 6.1. Can You Risk Stratify?
> Podcast 6.2. Moving Onto Risk Decision-Making

Access the podcast online at http://connect.springerpub.com/content/book/978-0-8261-4427-0/part/part02/chapter/ch06

INTRODUCTION

One of the most significant difference between population health management (PHM) and previous healthcare approaches is the focus on defining discrete populations for purposes of tailoring interventions and improving health outcomes. Why is it necessary to group or categorize populations for healthcare? A recent well-known story explains the basis for risk segmentation and stratification.

DID YOU KNOW?

Hotspotting

Health professionals and providers may associate the terms "risk segmentation" and "stratification" with the term "**hotspotting**." The idea of "hotspotting" emerged from extensive community experience and effort by the Camden Coalition of Healthcare Providers in New Jersey (Gawande, 2011). Started by a single physician who recognized that one at-risk individual with comorbidities and lacking any coordination of care would be responsible for costing the healthcare system hundreds of thousands of dollars. The ultimate outcome resulted in universal recognition that very few people "Hotspotters" could account for a disproportionate number of medical services and costs (McIntire et al., 2021). Health policy and planners quickly began theorizing that targeting at-risk priority patients with tailored interventions could save any healthcare system millions of dollars.

Today, population health (PH) managers access artificial intelligence, cloud computing, and predictive analytics to replace basic spreadsheets, as they determine which patients are at rising risk for disease or negative health outcomes. But the goal of care coordination and tailored interventions to promote health and prevent disease remains a constant challenge.

This chapter emphasizes the importance of risk segmentation and stratification as PHM techniques. The beginning phase involves successfully identifying the population-of-interest. PH managers combine various data sets to establish the (who). Databases may include the following:

- Managerial epidemiological data
- Public and/or private databases
- Community health needs assessment reports
- Social determinants of health (SDOH) indicators
- Clinical outcomes along with electronic medical record (EMR) data
- Administrative analyses including utilization and hospital admission rates

The next phase involves distinguishing specific risk factors, or the (why). In the third phase, the population groups are placed into risk management categories related to condition or disease (how) that will facilitate design and delivery of care implementation plans (what), which completes the process. This step-by-step method follows the progression identified in the *Population Health Alliance Framework* (PHA, 2018). See Figure 6.1.

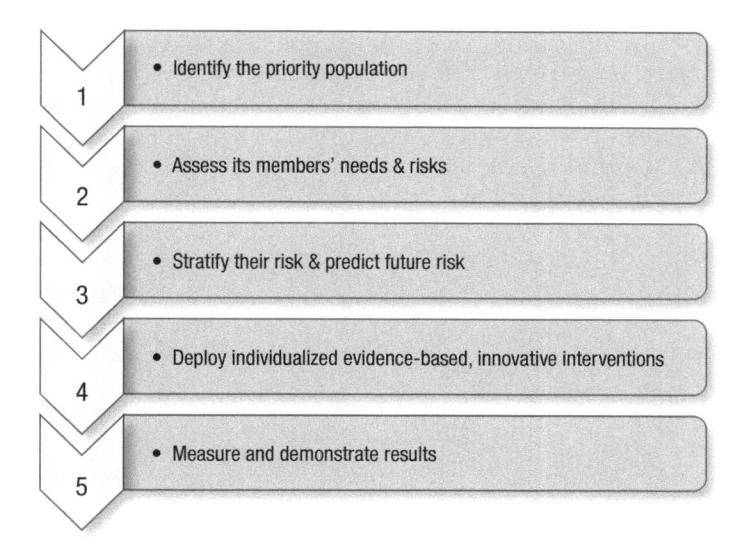

1. Identify the priority population
2. Assess its members' needs & risks
3. Stratify their risk & predict future risk
4. Deploy individualized evidence-based, innovative interventions
5. Measure and demonstrate results

FIGURE 6.1 PHA—Step-by-Step Risk Segmentation and Stratification Process

PHA, Population Health Alliance.
Source: Population Health Alliance (2012).

Understanding Risk Fundamentals in Population Health Management

The first time you visited a primary care physician (PCP), you may have been asked to complete a brief questionnaire about your health conditions and status. Although your own PCP probably did not statistically analyze these data, the information provided a snapshot of your health risks. Formal questionnaires are referred to **health risk assessment**s (HRAs), and the data from thousands of individuals can be aggregated to determine various disease risks across a population. Health risk appraisals help select those patients or consumers who would benefit from participation in a specific type of health promotion program (McAlearney, 2003a). HRAs, usually questionnaires, can be completed in person or digitally and function as screening tools to identify and monitor health status (PDHI, 2020). One of the most common validated HRAs used as a quality-of-life baseline tool is the 36 Item Short Form Health Survey (Rand, n.d.).

❓ DID YOU KNOW?

Health Risk Assessment

The 36 Item Short Form Health Survey (SF-36) evolved from a Medical Outcomes study in the 1990s (McAlearney, 2003b). Today, the 12-Item Short Form Survey is used frequently by health providers as brief health assessment that measures both physical and mental health status.
Click on the link to see the SF-12 questionnaire and review the questions: https://www.hss.edu/physician-files/huang/SF12-RCH.pdf.
Click on this link to complete the online survey and receive a summary document of your health risks (S-12 OrthoToolkit, 2021): https://orthotoolkit.com/sf-12.
What did you discover?

Statistic textbooks often define **risk** as the probability that an *event* will occur (Ranganathan et al., 2015). For PH managers, an event represents different types of risk such as exposure to a contagious disease, an acute episode of care, extreme levels of chronic care, a catastrophic accident, or other types of health needs. Identifying risk factors permits population segmentation for better aligned care coordination.

Risk Factor: If PH managers can correctly identify **a risk factor, which** is an exposure that is associated with a disease or condition, without certainty, that impacts an at-risk population, then the opportunity to reduce or eliminate that risk factor becomes a priority. Researchers have established the link between cigarette smoking and chronic conditions such as cardiopulmonary obstructive pulmonary disease (COPD). Smoking is an example of a risk factor that can be mitigated to produce better health outcomes.

If a population is characterized by a particular risk, such as obesity, the likelihood that this subpopulation will either need or seek care will lead to higher health utilization and ultimately additional costs. A primary PHM issue, always of concern, is the cost or **spend** for individual patients with known risk factors that would identify them for additional interventions. Table 6.1 shows a fictious set of data that analysts would need to analyze for appropriate cost and care utilization trends.

Did you correctly identify those individuals at most risk or rising risk? What criteria and benchmarks did you use?

Health data analytics has provided capabilities to examine multiple and complex population characteristics simultaneously and select only the most relevant metrics for assessing an individual's potential health status. These analyses can be combined to develop a single **risk score.** A risk score may indicate the likelihood of a single event, such as a hospital readmission within the next 6 months. An individual with multiple comorbidities such as hypertension, obesity, and diabetes would generally have a higher risk score than a person with only obesity.

Risk score and risk segmentation—the act of dividing patients into categories of risk based on their clinical and lifestyle characteristics—are often used interchangeably, although the two terms have different connotations.

Risk segmentation uses current and prospective medical costs, health status, attitudes, and level of healthcare engagement *to select individuals* from a population—plan members, patients, or employees. It is the first and primary step in identifying an at-risk population. Common risk segmentation categories are current health status, health service patterns and usage, and medical costs.

The choice and selection of not only the appropriate risk factors, but also pertinent indicators, require data interpretation as well as clinical expertise and the use of predictive modeling. In general, risk segmentation begins by assessing healthcare utilization and/or high costs. The more precise these risk factors in identifying a population of interest, the greater the likelihood of a positive health outcome and lower expenses per patient. Administrative data that represent cost per patient are often referred to as spend.

TABLE 6.1 Fictitious Patient Data Used for Identification and Risk Segmentation

Age	Gender	200x Annualize Medical Expense	200x Annualize Rx Expense	TOTAL MEDICAL COSTS	Primary Chronic Condition	ED	Hospital	PCP Visits
24	M	160,688.73	32,654.45	193,343.18	Chronic skin ulcer	1	2	Y
64	F	114,248.37	111,478.54	225,726.91	Antineoplastics, other episodes	0	0	Y
39	F	87,510.49	83,613.85	171,124.34	Adult rheumatoid arthritis	0	0	Y
19	F	87,149.87	1,196.38	88,346.25	Other urology	0	0	Y
19	F	85,892.92	69,184.16	155,077.08	Immunodeficiencies	0	0	Y
37	M	82,684.98	20,062.54	102,747.52	Chronic skin ulcer	0	1	Y
62	M	78,817.16	8,732.66	87,549.82	Chronic skin ulcer	1	1	Y
23	F	78,744.30	71,469.50	150,213.80	Antineoplastics, Other Episodes	1	0	Y
32	M	75,051.79	1,181.88	76,233.67	Chronic skin ulcer	0	1	Y
63	M	72,847.51	3,985.25	76,832.76	Chronic skin ulcer	2	7	Y
60	M	71,415.32	2,900.82	74,316.14	Atherosclerosis	0	0	Y
39	M	69,325.06	587.65	69,912.71	Chronic skin ulcer	4	0	Y
38	F	68,947.78	65,535.50	134,483.28	Adult rheumatoid arthritis	0	0	Y

PCP, primary care physician.

TABLE 6.2 Sample Population Health Risk Matrix

Patient Segmentation	Patient Stratification Level—Risk Levels		
Risk categories	Low	Medium	High
Risk factor #1	Level a–b	Level c–d	Level e–f
Risk factor #2			

After completing risk segmentation, PH managers engage in a stratification process to assess within a population the levels of risk— low, medium, high, or low, medium, rising risk, high. The goal is to divide the population in tiers and then align the appropriate health responses to prevent negative health outcomes. **Risk stratification** is a systematic process for identifying and predicting *patient's risk levels* relating to healthcare needs, services, and care coordination with the goal of identifying those at highest risk and managing their care to prevent poor health outcomes. Note that risk stratification is completed after risk segmentation.

A risk stratification framework may combine several individual risk scores to create a broader profile of a patient and their complex, ongoing needs. Table 6.2 illustrates a draft risk matrix designed to include all potential risk factors that are categorized according to level of need.

ⓘ DID YOU KNOW?

Practice: Developing a Population Health Risk

Segmentation/Stratification Matrix Health Issue: Recent evidence suggests that many COVID-19-positive patients continue to exhibit debilitating symptoms months after testing positive. This group of individuals have been referred to as long haulers. A regional health system seeks to target this population and develop an evidence-based treatment strategy for managing this condition and preventing future hospital readmissions.

Step 1: After completing a clinical data analysis of recent positive patients and aligning findings with EMR profiles, SDOH risk factors, health service usage, and administrative costs, the following risk factors were selected and placed in the matrix. Although not included specifically in the matrix, many patients identified were found to be female, over one-third of this group represented diverse minorities (Latinx, African Americans), and more than one half were young adults (ages 20–40) with no previous comorbidities.

Step 2: Based on evidence-based conclusions from Step 1, the following levels for risk stratification were selected. See Table 6.3.

TABLE 6.3 Sample (Only)* Population Health Risk Matrix

Patient Segmentation	Patient Stratification Level		
	Low	Medium	High
Fatigue/joint pain and body aches	Continuing	Persistent/affecting daily life	Intense—limiting movement
Continued loss of smell or taste	Somewhat noticeable	Significant/ evidence of loss of appetite	Extreme/ loss of appetite and weight

Patient Segmentation	Patient Stratification Level		
Mental confusion or brain fog	Occasional	Significant/ affecting decision making	Intense—requiring ADL support
Preexisting comorbidities	0–1	2–3	4 or more
Difficulty sleeping	Sporadic	1–2 weekly	Nightly
Coughing or shortness of breath	Chronic, but intermittent	Persistent/affecting daily life escalating	Intense—requiring respiratory assistance
Rapid heart rate	Chronic, responsive to medication	Persistent/affecting daily life	Intense—requiring intervention
Type of healthcare utilization	PCP visits	Use of Urgi Care or ED	Hospital readmission

*Disclaimer: Unvalidated example—not to be used in any type of health practice.
ADL, activities of daily living; PCP, primary care physician.
(Adapted from Bean, 2021; Kastner, 2020)

Today's risk segmentation strategies and applications represent a significant shift away from the dominant view of risk management that has been pervasive in the health insurance industry. We are moving to a proactive stance to support the broad definition of PHM—a variety of approaches developed to foster health and quality of care improvements while managing costs.

Population Health Management Categories and Recent Innovations

When managing a population, healthcare managers need to know the health status of the at-risk population and complete both risk segmentation and stratification before you can create interventions to help keep them healthy. As healthcare providers move toward accepting both medical outcomes and fiscal accountability for their patients and shift to a value over volume approach, it becomes imperative to thoroughly understand the process. Step 3 in the process is risk management of the specific populations once the risk segmentation and stratification are completed.

Risk management is a primary competency for PH managers. The process includes developing and implementing safe and effective patient care practices and pathways, monitoring financial costs, and maintaining safe working environments to ensure optimum health outcomes. Risk management is much more than simply health promotion.

Before the adoption of sophisticated technology options, such as data analytics, predictive modeling, interoperability, and artificial intelligence models, most health providers and insurers generally relied on five major types of risk categories for their insured populations. These categories are presented in Figure 6.2.

> **? DID YOU KNOW?**
>
> **Types of Population Health Management**
>
> Each of the five basic types of PH categories required specific strategies and approaches.
> - Lifestyle management offers a collection of health promotion and disease prevention strategies and approaches to facilitate health behavior change for decreased risk and improved populations' health habits.
> - Demand management emphasizes remote directing consumers within specific populations toward appropriate utilization of medical care services.
> - Disease management is appropriate for populations with a particular disease and includes care coordination (medical and care management) tailored to the specific patients' needs with that condition.
> - Catastrophic care management assembles all the necessary services needed by patients who suffer from serious injuries or catastrophic illnesses identified by either condition or length and intensity of care.
> - Disability management is often offered in connection with employers and designed to align typical healthcare delivery with disability management to improve worker outcome and productivity that may be diminished due to illness or injury (McAlearney, 2003a).

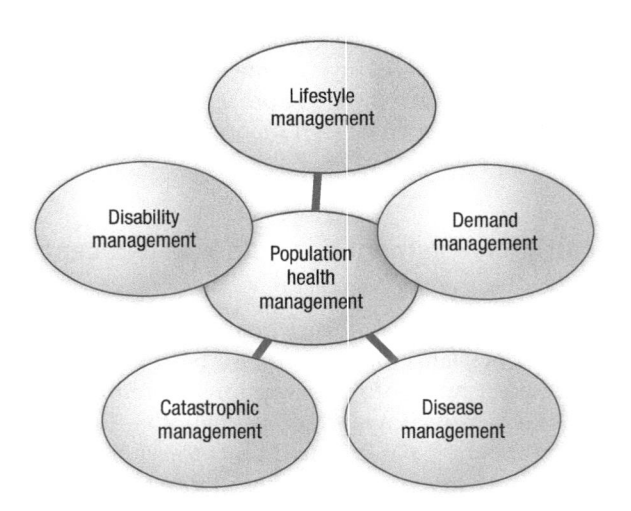

FIGURE 6.2 Initial Population Health Risk Management Categories
Source: Adapted from McAlearney (2003a).

Today, we recognize the necessity for not only risk segmentation but also stratification. For example, many individuals show no immediate risk of disease but would benefit from improving basic lifestyle behaviors, such as increasing exercise. However, others may be overweight in addition to lack of exercise. They both belong in the lifestyle management category but require different health promotion strategies to improve. In disease management, we might first segment patients by the type of disease and then by acuity. Once these steps are accomplished, we move on to deciding the type and frequency of interventions with many new options now available. See Table 6.4 for a visual presentation.

TABLE 6.4 Population Risk Management Category Continuum

Health Promotion and Disease Prevention	Lifestyle Mgt.	Demand Mgt.	Disease Mgt.	Catastrophic Mgt.	Disability Mgt.	Rehabilitation Care Mgt.	Palliative Care Mgt.	Hospice Care Mgt.
Prevention						\multicolumn{3}{c}{Postacute Care}		

As the type of population risk management categories has expanded significantly, so has the health delivery location options and types of interaction such as face-to-face or virtual!

Population Health Management Risk-Based Intervention Strategies

After the initial risk-based segmentation and stratification, selection of intervention strategy requires assessing current health status, patient characteristics and attitudes, level of healthcare engagement to stratify individuals from any population—plan members, patients, or employees. The key to this decision-making process is recognizing the level of need and patient preferences and aligning them with resource capabilities allotted and appropriate for the targeted population. See Figure 6.3.

As shown in Figure 6.3, after the initial risk segmentation and stratification is completed, the population of interest can be further categorized into various levels of engagement capacity, clinical need, appropriate intervention type, and intensity of care level depending on the alignment of risk factors. Note, a distinction should be made between healthcare provider and payer ownership of this process as differences may exist between an insurance model versus an ACO or PCMH with providers focused on specific PH outcomes.

The final PHM step for a priority population is the matching of the type of care (intervention), the choice of health provider, the touchpoint (interaction channel), and the timeline for interaction. Further decisions on the types of interventions available should be based on evidence-based practices as well as health behavior models, patient engagement strategies, and return-on-investment analyses. Table 6.5 presents a sample intervention matrix.

This table also introduces us into PH risk management strategies by showing assigned levels of care. A typical level of care diagram includes four risk levels and identifies types of interventions, health personnel responsible, and

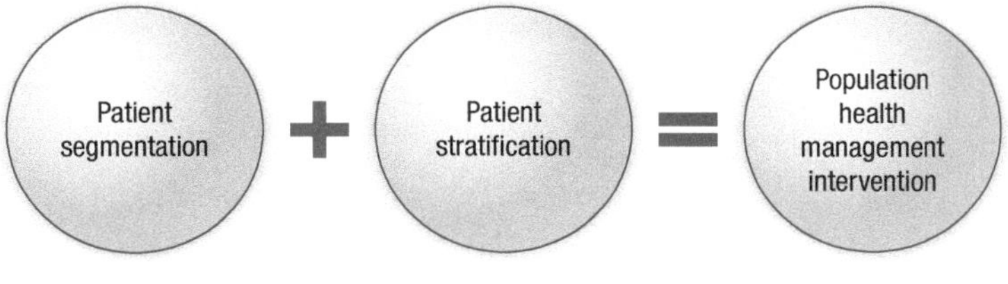

FIGURE 6.3 Relationship Between Risk Segmentation/Stratification and Population Management Intervention

TABLE 6.5 Sample Risk Segmentation/Stratification Management Intervention Matrix

	Low Risk	Moderate Risk	Rising Risk	High Risk
Healthcare provider/ coordinator	Telephonic care manager	Social worker/ other qualified	Qualified care managers	Advanced practitioner care managers
Intervention	Q 6 months telephonic assessment	Q 6-month in-home assessment	Quarterly in-home assessment	Monthly contact

the number of patients covered per provider. A companion table would be needed that outlines the expense per person per month (PPPM). To further illustrate this process, Figure 6.4 shows the relationship between the type of intervention, level of coordination, and potential metrics for assessment.

In addition to the risk segmentation and stratification process described, PH managers would be estimating return on investment (ROI) and completing financial sensitivity analyses for the various healthcare delivery options.

Attaining a positive ROI is a major concern for all constituents of the health sector, but especially for healthcare payers, providers, and PH managers. Over time, as these groups accept more accountability for PH outcomes, ROI can be used as a marker to indicate a population's positive health status leading to greater financial rewards and incentives. In order to achieve that goal, complex risk management skills will be essential for PH managers.

There are multiple and diverse components involved in the implementation phase including aligned incentives, information systems support, communication and coordination, engaged patients, and involved and responsible providers (McAlearney, 2003c). The goal is to improve quality of life for a priority population using a value-added model that should reduce costs.

So, who typically completes the PH segmentation and management processes? For accountable care organizations (ACOs,) the decision makes represent a diverse set of team members. Common ACO team members, necessary for conducting PH segmentation, require a diverse set of health experts including ACO chief medical officers, chief executives, PH directors, health providers, and care management personnel. Others supporting and operations contributors

Intervention specific
- Population-at-risk identified, segmented by intervention type
- #/% of population-at-risk reached
- #/% population-at-risk engaged

Patient specific
- #/% of population-at-risk in maintenance pathway/improvement clinical health status
- #/% of population-at-risk with lowered cost
- #/% of population-at-risk with reduced negative SDOH factors

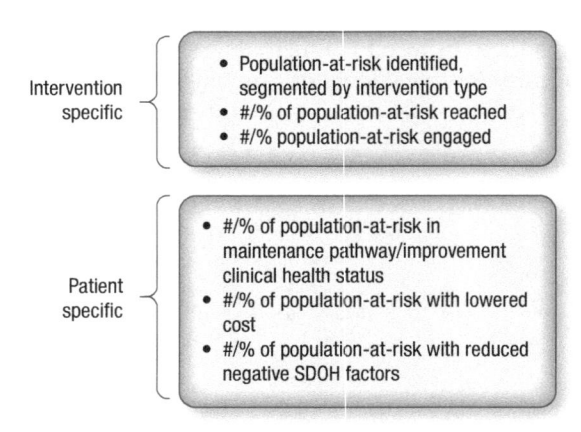

FIGURE 6.4 Sample Risk Matrix—Intervention, Coordination, and Evaluation

would be data analysis staff, and practicing physician and other practitioners as needed (O'Malley et al., 2019). For patient stratification and interventions, subgroups add other frontline clinicians such as PCPs, nurse care managers, social workers, care transition staff, and behavioral health providers. The role of the population manager will be one of convener, integrator, and coordinator.

SUMMARY

PH managers face the most difficult challenge in risk segmenting and stratifying populations correctly. This process currently relies extensively on data analytics, but it is expected that the role of artificial intelligence will increase and be used to inform these decisions. The goal remains to balance the resources and obtain optimum and quality PH outcomes. Once the risk segmentation and stratification components have identified a population at risk, the next step involves in selecting type of intervention, choice of health providers, and appropriate outcome metrics. The entire process should answer the following questions:

- Which metrics will you use to identify your population at risk?
- Once you have identified those at-risk, how will you stratify them by level of risk?
- What types of interventions will you use?
- Who will implement these interventions?
- What outcomes will you expect and how will you measure?

DISCUSSION QUESTIONS

1. True or False
   a. Risk stratification relies on identifying the population's major characteristics, and risk segmentation requires a detailed analytical review of many risk factors. T/F
   b. An individual placed into a demand management risk category probably will not move into the disease management category. T/F
   c. Acuity looks at the level of use of medical services. T/F
   d. Predictive modeling and artificial intelligence often use risk scores to determine care coordination. T/F
   e. "Spend" can refer to an individual or a subpopulation's cost of care. T/F
2. Explain the ways risk segmentation and stratification differ.
3. Review the five basic categories that were previously used for population segmentation. Why have they changed and what additional options that have emerged?
4. What data sources would you seek before developing a risk segmentation and risk stratification for a rising risk population?
5. Define risk, risk score, segmentation, and stratification, and provide examples.
6. What factors determine the level and intensity of care coordination and treatment recommended for a particular population?

Tool Competency Application: Risk Segmentation and Stratification Case Study—Special Needs Plan

Directions: This case study presents *Healthy Populations Inc.'s (HPI)*; (fictitious insurance company) special needs plan (SNP) for an at-risk population. Review the narrative and data carefully and then respond to the questions. Note that Phase 1 of the process has been completed for you. Additional information is provided in Tables 6.6 through 6.11.

Phase 1: Determining, Verifying, and Tracking Eligibility

This phase has been completed for overall and Subpopulations

Following internal protocols and policies, all members of the priority population meet the Centers for Medicare or Medicaid Services (CMS) guidelines for dual eligible Special Needs Plans and are duly enrolled in *HPI* identified plan.

Section B. Overall SNP Population

Phase 2 and 3: Identify Health Concerns of the Overall SNP Population

HPI utilizes multiple reporting tools to gather clinical analytical data on the SNP population. The data include demographic characteristics such as environment, lifestyle, and socioeconomic factors along with cost and utilization patterns for our members. *HPI* is offering a D-SNP in a Midwest state.

Member Composition
Midwest State: HIP's D-SNP population is mostly white, female, between the ages of 60 and 79 years of age, live alone, and have three or more comorbidities. While the majority of our members live alone, 83% report having a caregiver available if needed. 41% of this population speak English, and 56% speak Spanish. 69% of our population is diagnosed with diabetes with chronic complications, 43% with vascular disease, and 40% with congestive heart failure. While diabetes, cardiovascular, and chronic lung diseases are often correlated, our members with these conditions also tend to have comorbidities including morbid obesity (27%) and psychiatric disorders (9%).

- 58% of the population are between the ages of 60 and 79 years of age, 12% are 80 or over, and 30% are under 60 years old.
- 33% are male, and 67% are female.
- 50% are White, 31% are Black, 14% are Hispanic, 4% are Asian or Native American, and 1% have a race classification as other.
- 24% report difficulty with light housework, 43% with kneeling, 59% with walking A quarter of a mile, and 49% with lifting.
- 23% are having problems or worried about purchasing food or medication, and 27% are having problem or worried about paying for rent or utilities.
- 7% are concerned about forgetting to take medication, 9% worry about forgetting appointments, and 6% worry about misplacing important items.
- 7% report feeling down, sad, or blue some of the time and 13% most of the time over the last 2 weeks.
- 8% have zero comorbidities, 23% have one or two comorbidities, and 69% have three or more comorbidities.

- The following are the top five relevant diagnoses:
  1. Diabetes with complications (69%)
  2. Vascular disease (43%)
  3. Congestive heart failure (40%)
  4. Morbid obesity (27%)
  5. Specified heart arrhythmias (19%)

The SDOH help identify issues and opportunities for developing the right plans for health improvement. For example, ethnicity information helps us understand the language and cultural needs of our SNP population.

For the Socioeconomic Factor Report, data are available from several sources. The Social Associations is a measure representing social isolation and community interaction. For example, associations include membership organizations such as civic, religious, recreational, and professional organizations. Food Insecurity is the percentage of the population who did not have access to a reliable source of food during the past year. Income Inequality is the ratio of household income at the 80th percentile to that of the 20th percentile. A higher inequality ratio indicates greater division between the top and bottom ends of the income spectrum.

TABLE 6.6 Prevalence of Chronic Conditions for Special Needs Plan (SNP) Members as of October 2019

	Prevalence of Chronic Conditions for SNP Members							
Population	Diabetes with Complications	Vascular Disease	Congestive Heart Failure	Morbid Obesity	Chronic Obstructive Pulmonary Disease	Major Depressive, Bipolar, and Paranoid Disorders	Drug/ Alcohol Dependence	Rheumatoid Arthritis and Inflammatory Connective Tissues Disease
Midwest State	69%	62%	23%	27%	8%	0%	9%	9%

TABLE 6.7 Lifestyle Factor Report on Special Needs Plan (SNP) Population as of April 2019

	Lifestyle Factors				
Description	Obesity	Tobacco Usage	Physical Inactivity	Physically Unhealthy Days	Mentally Unhealthy Days
National	28%	16%	23%	3.7	3.8
Midwest State	28%	15%	24%	3.7	3.6

TABLE 6.8 Socioeconomic Factor Report on Special Needs Plan (SNP) Population as of April 2019

	Socioeconomic Factors					
Description	Social Association Rate	Food Insecurity	High School Graduate	Median Household Income (K)	Income Inequality	Household With Severe Problems
National	9%	14%	83%	60.4	4.4	19%
Midwest State	8%	16%	89%	57.8	4.6	18%

TABLE 6.9 Environment Factor Report on Special Needs Plan (SNP) Population as of April 2019

	Environment Factors		
Description	Limited Access to Healthy Food	Air Pollution—Particulate Matter	Food Environment Index
National	6%	9.9	7.8
Midwest State	8%	10.2	7.2

TABLE 6.10 Utilization Report on Special Needs Plan (SNP) Population as of April 2019

	Utilization				
Description	Inpatient Admits per 1,000	Average Length of Stay	Admit Costs	ED Visits per 1,000	ED Cost per Visit
National	210	5.6	$12,743	420	$709
Midwest State	215	5.6	$13,117	369	$731

Phase 4: Define Unique Characteristics of the SNP Population

As a result of enrollment qualifications for a D-SNP (low income, disabled, older, and eligible for both Medicare and Medicaid), members have more complex and costly medical needs. Other unique characteristics of this population include having three or more comorbidities, prescribed multiple prescription medications, and tend to be at a higher risk financially and cognitively. Common barriers faced regularly by our members are gaps in care due to poor coordination between Medicare and Medicaid programs and the high rate of prevalence with multiple chronic conditions. Each demographic characteristic causes additional barriers, which are considered when designing our care management programs including providers who are multilinguistic. Care managers who discuss diet restrictions, translators versed in healthcare and multilanguage brochures. Data for SNP-relevant diagnoses are reviewed and analyzed annually to identify initiatives and opportunities for healthcare improvement.

Health disparities mirror differences in socioeconomic status, racial and ethnic background, and education level. Income also contributes to poor and unsafe living conditions within this D-SNP population. Hazards in a member's home may contribute to falls and may result in nutritional deficiencies and even death.

Language barriers may affect educational attainment, income, and access to care. Ethnicity, language, and cultural beliefs may increase the gaps in care faced by our SNP population. These factors are taken into consideration when developing programs. Methods for addressing health literacy and elements of cultural diversity are integrated into the MOC. For example, written materials sent to the member are at a fourth- to sixth-grade reading level based on state requirements. The majority of materials are available in English and Spanish. Most materials are available in English and Spanish. After educational materials are mailed to the member, the care manager or a member of the interdisciplinary care team discusses the information at the next successful contact or next scheduled contact with the member to review, discuss, and answer questions regarding the content. Humana also has bilingual staff and access to a language translation line as needed.

TABLE 6.11 Prevalence of Chronic Conditions for Special Needs Plan (SNP) Members as of October 2019

\multicolumn{10}{c}{Prevalence of Chronic Conditions for SNP Members}
Population	Diabetes with Complications	Vascular Disease	Congestive Heart Failure	Morbid Obesity	Chronic Obstructive Pulmonary Disease	Major Depressive, Bipolar, and Paranoid Disorders	Drug/ Alcohol Dependence	Rheumatoid Arthritis and Inflammatory Connective Tissues Disease
Texas	69%	62%	23%	27%	8%	0%	9%	9%

Additionally, a common barrier faced within our D-SNP membership population is members' ambivalence and readiness for change. Collaborative discussions between a care manager and a member to strengthen a member's motivation and commitment for change is critical for preventative healthcare and avoiding hospitalizations and readmissions.

Table 6.11 is an example of prevalence of chronic conditions based on HPI's Community Scorecard for this population.

Section B: Subpopulation-Most Vulnerable Members

Factor 1: Definition of Most Vulnerable Members

Our D-SNP members are a diverse population with a small percentage bearing the most cost. HPI's most vulnerable population tends to be poor and report poorer health status. The most vulnerable members compared with the general SNP population have more frequent ED visits and/or hospital admissions and presence of complex comorbidities; have experienced a major change in health, functional, or mental status; lack caregiver support; or are members near end of life. Other unique characteristics of the most vulnerable population include having three or more comorbidities, prescribed multiple prescription medications, and tend to have be at a higher risk financially, socially, and cognitively.

HPIs use methods of risk stratification, and evaluating level of acuity is dynamic to best guide the most appropriate level and intensity of intervention. Systematically, the member is stratified according to proprietary algorithms built in the clinical platform based on the results of embedded tools within the HRA. The HRA is the combination of the PRA Screening Instrument, Vulnerable Elder Survey (VES) and PHQ-9, questions related to additional key chronic conditions, Care of Older Adult measures, and preventive screenings.

- The PRA Screening Instrument is a screening tool used to identify members of older populations who are at high risk for using health services heavily in the future.
- The VES-13 is used to assess the risk of health deterioration in older adults by considering a number of factors including age, disabilities functional limitations, and self-reported health status.
- The PHQ-9 is a multipurpose instrument for screening, diagnosing, monitoring, and measuring the severity of depression.

The HRA scoring methodology produces a total risk score, which is used to recommend the appropriate care management for the SNP member. The risk score is calculated using a weighted sum of the risks and needs assigned to individual questions in the HRA by counting the number of medical/social economic/functional/mental health questions. The weight to each question was developed using data collected from earlier surveys with similar questions and the claims history for SNP members to optimize the prediction of the future risk of the members. As an example, based on a tiering of the population in which the top 10% represents the most vulnerable, a total risk score of 35 or greater would place a member in the most vulnerable stratification.

The HRA provides initial stratification for the member of severe, high, medium, and low. Members who refuse care management or unable to be reached are stratified as low. The most vulnerable population are stratified as severe.

Following the stratification level identified by the HRA, the care manager may review recent claims, hospitalizations, or medications or use additional surveys to further evaluate and analyze the system stratification. The care manager may determine whether the member needs higher or lower level of support and reassigns the member to the appropriate risk stratification in the clinical documentation system along with the appropriate reason for reassignment.

In addition, members who are candidates for the stratification of severe are prospectively identified based on their predicted cost and the presence of chronic conditions, rather than reactively targeted because they have already become high-cost users and have high-cost conditions.

HPI provides access to special services and partners with community resources to support the unique needs of our most vulnerable members. The services and resources offered address the medical, socioeconomic, psychological, disease specific conditions, and gaps in coordination between Medicare and Medicaid faced by our SNP population for provision of care to this population. Specially tailored services for the most vulnerable members include but are not limited to a higher frequency of outreach by the care manager. This higher stratification allows for more intensive outreach, where care managers can monitor the progress toward goals, whether interventions have been implemented or whether interventions need to be modified to meet the established goal on a more frequent basis. The model relies on the expertise of the care manager to complete ongoing evaluations of member needs and the flexibility to adjust the member's individualized care plans based on the unique needs of the member. In addition, the most vulnerable members who have a depression severity of moderately severe or higher are also eligible for behavioral health support that is provided by independently licensed behavioral health clinicians who are immediately available to the member as an interdisciplinary care team participant. Other services and programs available include but are not limited to medication therapy, meal-delivery programs, transportation services, financial assistance, end-of-life planning, and social service interventions.

CASE STUDY QUESTIONS

1. Explain the value and benefits in targeting a subpopulation for HPI?
2. Select five major characteristics of the general population that you feel would have the largest impact on positive health status. Provide a rationale.
3. Compare the healthcare barriers of the general SNP population to the priority vulnerable subpopulation.

4. Describe the elements used to configure the risk score for the vulnerable population.
5. Review the weighting for determining the risk score. What range or cut-off would you use to create a "rising risk" category? Provide your rationale and outline potential interventions you would recommend.
6. How does HPI match the interventions and care coordination with the level of risk?

REFERENCES

Bean, M. (2021, January 4). *COVID-19 'long haulers' Identify 205 Virus Symptoms*. https://www.beckershospitalreview.com/patient-safety-outcomes/covid-19-long-haulers-identify-205-virus-symptoms.html?origin=BHRE&utm_source=BHRE&utm_medium=email&utm_content=newsletter&oly_enc_id=1450I5993723C6U

Gawande, A. (2011, January 17). The hot spotters. *The New Yorker, 86*(45), 40–51. https://www.newyorker.com/magazine/2011/01/24/the-hot-spottershttps://www.ncbi.nlm.nih.gov/pmc/articles/PMC4640017/

Kastner, J. (2020, December 16). Young San Diego COVID-19 long-haulers still sick months after testing positive. *ABC News*. https://www.10news.com/news/local-news/san-diego-news/young-san-diego-covid-19-long-haulers-st

McAlearney, A. (2003a). *Population health management: Strategies to improve outcomes*. Health Administration Press/Association of University Programs in Health Administration.

McAlearney, A. (2003b). *Targeting individuals for population health management. Population health management: Strategies to improve outcomes*. Health Administration Press/Association of University Programs in Health Administration.

McAlearney, A. (2003c). Integrating population health management: Concepts and strategies. *Population Health Management: Strategies to Improve Outcomes*. Health Administration Press/Association of University Programs in Health Administration.

McIntire, R., McAna, J. & Oglesby, W. (2021). Epidemiology. In D. Nash, A. Skoufalos, R. Fabius, & W. Oglesby, (Eds.), *Population health: Creating a culture of wellness* (3rd ed., pp. 23–45). Jones and Bartlett Learning.

O'Malley, A., Rich, E., Sarwar, R., Schultz, E., Cannon Warren, W., Shah, T. & Abrams, M. (2019, January 3). *How accountable care organizations use population segmentation to care for high-need, high-cost patients*. The Commonwealth Fund. https://www.commonwealthfund.org/publications/issue-briefs/2019/jan/how-acos-use-segmentation-high-need-high-cost

PDHI. (2020, February). *What is a health risk assessment?* PDHI. https://www.pdhi.com/ncqa/what-is-a-health-risk-assessment/

PHA Population Health Management Framework & Maljanian, R. (2018). *Population health alliance*. https://populationhealthalliance.org/research/understanding-population-health/

Population Health Alliance. (2012). *A population health guide for primary care models*. https://populationhealthalliance.org/population-health-guide-for-primary-care-models/

RAND. (n.d.). *36-item short form survey instrument*. RAND. Retrieved May 18, 2021, from https://www.rand.org/health-care/surveys_tools/mos/36-item-short-form/survey-instrument.html

Ranganathan, P., Aggarwal, R., & Pramesh, C. (2015, October–December). Common pitfalls in statistical analysis: Odds versus risk. *Perspectives in Clinical Research, 6*(4), 222–224. https://doi.org/10.4103/2229-3485.167092

S-12 OrthoToolkit. (2021). *OrthoToolkit*. https://orthotoolkit.com/sf-12/

CHAPTER 7

Population Health Models—Part I

Anastasia Miller

KEY TERMS

Accountable Care Organizations
Comprehensive Primary Care Plus (CPC+)
Horizontal and Vertical Integration
Independent Practice Association (IPA)
Integrated Delivery Networks (IDNs)
Medicare Access and CHIP Reauthorization
Act of 2015 (MACRA)
Multispecialty Group Practice (MSGP)
Patient-Centered Medical Homes (PCMH)
Physician–Hospital Organization (PHO)
Shared Savings Program
Single Specialty Group Practice

LEARNING OBJECTIVES

1. Trace the evolution of population healthcare delivery models.
2. Describe major legislative mandates that impact healthcare reimbursement.
3. Compare and contrast accountable care organizations (ACOs) and Patient Centered Medical Homes (PCMHs).
4. Distinguish between horizontal and vertical integration.
5. Illustrate the realignment of financial incentives for new population health (PH) models.

Podcasts that exemplify the content of this chapter are available at Springer Publishing Connect™

Podcast 7.1. QUICK: Define IDS, ACO, and PCMH
Podcast 7.2. Why Doesn't One Size Fit All for Our Patients?

Access the podcast online at http://connect.springerpub.com/content/book/978-0-8261-4427-0/part/part02/chapter/ch07

INTRODUCTION

For population health management (PHM), there is no one approach, one tool, or one method of managing the health of a given population. Neither is there one answer for which framework would be appropriate to all populations. That is why there are multiple models, each of which have their pros and cons, and more appropriate for certain populations as opposed to others. This chapter covers recognized and validated popular models, most of which did not exist in the 20th century. Recent laws, regulations, and mandates created or enabled these emerging and innovative approaches and strategies. The models that predate the Affordable Care Act were not even officially population health models, they were outgrowths of managed care frameworks (Burns & Pauly, 2002), as minimal financial structures were in place to support a population health approach. These models helped health managers develop innovative financial incentives to properly address population health for the first time in this country.

The Triple Aim: A Foundation for Population Health Management

Although covered extensively in the literature, we need to acknowledge the pivotal roles of the Triple Aim. This conceptual term was coined by researchers at the Institute for Healthcare Improvement (IHI) before the creation of the Patient Protection and Affordable Care Act of 2010 (ACA; Berwick et al., 2008), and it officially became part of the national healthcare strategy when incorporated into the ACA (Whittington et al., 2015). The Triple Aims—simultaneously addressed improving patient experience of care, improving population heath, and reducing the per capita costs of care—continue to serve as major concepts for PHM. The original Triple Aim initiative emphasized the need for an "integrator" who would be responsible for linking "health care organizations (as well as public health and social service organizations) whose missions overlap across the spectrum of delivery" (Berwick et al., 2008). The goal of providing quality care at the lowest possible cost has become the watchword for PHM although the concept presents multiple challenges. Population health agencies and managers seek ways to balance these sometimes-conflicting goals to improve patient outcomes as providing high-quality care is often not done cheaply.

In addition, to the impact of the ACA and the Triple Aim initiative, another legislative mandate, "The Medicare Access and CHIP Reauthorization Act of 2015 (MACRA)," also served as a catalyst for new financial models. MACRA created a national framework for financial rewarding health providers (clinicians) for adopting value over volume models (ACC, 2015).

This chapter introduces the commonly adopted population health models as seen in the United States Health Care System. The optimal choice for any given system will depend on the specific needs of that population, the articulated system goals, and the resources available.

Models of Population Health Management

Integrated Delivery Networks

The need to integrate health systems was originally identified at a World Health Organization conference in 1978 (Thomas et al., 2008). Historically, **integrated delivery networks (IDNs)** were equated with health maintenance systems such as health management organizations (HMOs; Burns &

Pauly, 2002) although there are some key differences. HMOs are organized systems of multiple voluntarily enrolled providers to provide agreed-upon healthcare service for a geographic region.

IDNs can be either single organizations or groups of organizations working together for population health. The goal of an IDN is to integrate the provision of care within a health system. Although different definitions of IDNs exist, one common characteristic is the presence of an organized, coordinated effort by a network of providers, typically under a single unifying name.

> **DID YOU KNOW?**
>
> **A closer look: Veterans Health Administration**
>
> The nation's largest IDN is the Veterans Health Administration (VHA; Mattocks & Yehia, 2017). The VHA has over 9 million enrollees across all 50 states. They are an example of both horizontal integration and vertical integration (Sales, 2008), with integration occurring within as well as between the different levels of care at their 1,074 outpatient clinics and 170 medical centers (Veterans Administration, 2009). To find more information about the VHA, you can visit their website: https://www.va.gov/health/aboutvha.asp.

IDNs also include coordinated economic and clinical agreements across a range of providers necessary to effectively serve a wide range of needs for a specific population or community (Al-Saddique, 2018). Another unifying characteristic of IDN networks is the acknowledged clinical and financial responsibility for their patients who are managed with a holistic approach. Examples of well-known IDNs include Kaiser Permanente (Maeda et al., 2014), the Mayo Clinic (Kumar et al., 2009), and Intermountain Healthcare (James & Savitz, 2011).

Horizontal and Vertical Integration

IDNs exist in a wide range of forms (structures), but there are three levels of integration:

- Linkage
- Coordination
- Full integration (Hebert & Veil, 2004)

IDNs can be at any of these three levels of integration and utilize either of the two major types of integration: **horizontal or vertical** (see Figure 7.1).

Horizontal integration occurs when organizations that provide a similar level of care work together to manage care.

Horizontal integration is between agencies on the **same level** (primary, secondary, or tertiary). Many of today's large health systems began with horizontal integration via mergers or acquisitions of other local hospitals.

The levels of care are primary care (the typical entry point for a patient, including primary care providers [PCPs], pediatricians, and OB-GYNs), secondary care (specialists who focus on specific bodily systems, such as cardiologists),

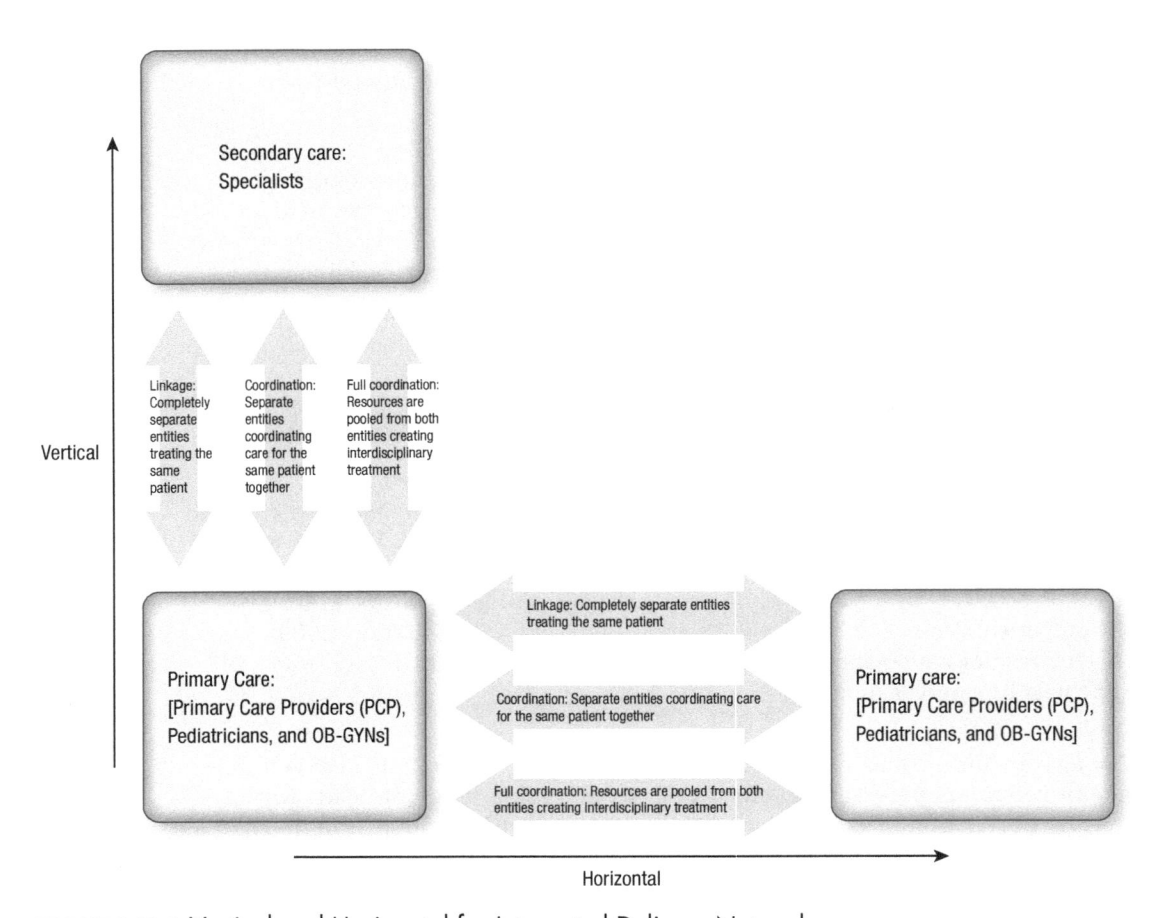

FIGURE 7.1 Vertical and Horizontal for Integrated Delivery Networks

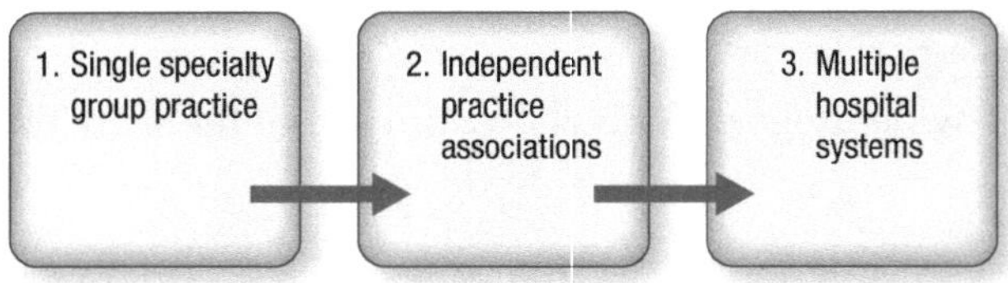

FIGURE 7.2 Horizontal Integration Examples

and tertiary care (specialized care requiring specialized equipment and frequently synonymous with hospitals). When providers or organizations horizontally integrate, they typically join forces under a single brand (see Figure 7.2).

Single specialty group practices are most common type of practice management seen in the United States (Ellis et al., 2018). Practice benefits include shared resources, which yield economies of scale, negotiation leverage and advantages with insurance companies, improved quality of care, and consolidated administrative responsibilities (Casalino et al., 2004). Two major barriers to these types of collaborations have been the physician desire for autonomy and lack of physician leadership (Casalino et al., 2003); however, the economy of scale for information technology has been a major driving force for an increased number of practices. (Payne et al., 2013). These arrangements can cover all three levels of integration.

An **Independent Practice Association (IPA)** is a group of physicians participating as a network to contract with health insurance plans. Under this arrangement, the physicians maintain ownership of their own offices with the IPA serving as an integration network with which to negotiate with insurance companies as well as to jointly create processes to reduce costs and improve quality (Casalino et al., 2013). Under the ACA, this management model can qualify to be an ACO) These arrangements can be at the level of linkage or coordination but fall short of full integration.

Multiple neighboring hospitals can form a tertiary horizontally integrated network. Multihospital systems consist of two or more hospitals sharing common ownership. This includes a wide range of linkage levels, from informal linkages to complete integration. There are multiple advantages for this type of arrangement, including exploiting economies of scale through more efficient management of supplies, simplifying local consumer purchasing options, providing increased financial stability, and expanding the economies of network scope. This partial consolidation arrangement came to prominence after the Medicare and Medicaid Act of 1965 was passed (Dranove & Shanley, 1995). The percentage of hospitals in a multihospital network system went from 32.1% in 1980 to 73.4% in 1997 (Lega, 2005). In the years since, many health entities have also integrated vertically through acquisition of physician practices, ambulatory centers, and postacute care providers, making it hard to sometimes identify the horizontal integration clearly (Heeringa et al., 2020).

All three types of horizonal integration led to improved efficiency and financial savings as well as improving patient outcomes. There are also arguments for the ability to provide patient-centered care more effectively when there is integration (Evans et al., 2013).

Vertical Integration is between agencies on **different levels** (primary to secondary, secondary to tertiary, etc.) and occurs when organizations at different levels of care delivery coordinate the provision of care.

One of the primary rationales behind vertical integration is to pair providers offering complementary services to reduce redundancies and improve quality for the population being served (see Figure 7.3).

The classic example of a **physician–hospital organization (PHO)** is when hospitals purchase physician practices (Heeringa et al., 2020). There is some variation, but PHOs generally have some level of linkage, which results in an

1. Physician–hospital organizations → 2. Multi-specialty group practice → 3. Hospital-sponsored HMOs → 4. Government-facilitated networks

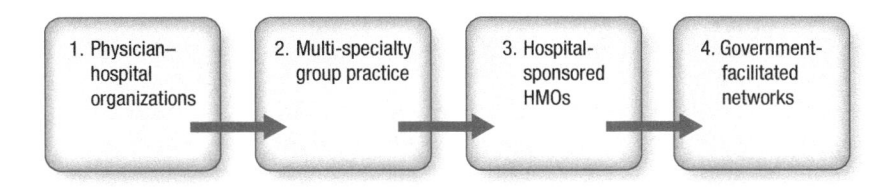

FIGURE 7.3 Vertical Integration Examples

affiliation agreement that allows physicians and the hospital to work cooperatively while being governed independently. PHOs originated as a way for both physicians to gain economies of scale for major capital expenses such as information technology and billing systems, while also spreading malpractice risk across a larger pool of providers and increasing the physician negotiating power with payers (Wise et al., 2012). Hospitals were often partially motivated to take control of the referral pipeline (Burns & Pauly, 2002). Research shows that PHOs are associated with decreased length of stay in uncompetitive rural markets (Burns et al., 2013).

Another vertical example, a **multispecialty group practice (MSGP),** could be technically either horizontally integrated through the coordination of care provided by specialists at the same level or vertically integrated through coordination of both primary and secondary providers. We have placed it under vertical integration to make it distinct from single specialty group practices. MSGPs, which are vertically integrated, allow both primary care and specialist physicians to come together under a shared "common governance, infrastructure, and finances, and refer patients to one another for services offered within the group" (McCarthy, 2015, p. 13). One of the obvious benefits of this type of arrangement is that by offering services across the medical spectrum, these groups can often provide much of the care required by most patients in-house. A classic example of a MSGP is the Mayo Clinic (Heeringa et al., 2020).

Another unique model occurs when hospitals decide to vertically integrate into the insurance market by establishing their own HMOs (Burns & Pauly, 2002). Although some of these arrangements failed with most hospitals abandoning this type of setup, a few remain. Notably Scott &White Healthcare (now Baylor, Scott, & White Health) based in Dallas, Texas, has been very successful (Allison, 2015).

The last example highlights government-facilitated networks. Sometimes the local or regional government is the main driving "integrator" for a region. In this situation, the government takes the active role of organizing providers and agencies to address the needs of the local population (Al-Saddique, 2018). An example of this would be the Community Care of North Carolina initiative (Steiner et al., 2008), which was an outgrowth of a successful regional project and was further adopted with the primary goal of linking patients with a primary care physician (PCP) (Steiner et al., 2008).

Both Horizontal and Vertical Integration: What Do the Data Show?

Between the 1980 and the 1990s, there was a slow but distinct shift away from interest in horizontal integration to vertical integration (Evans et al., 2013), and an increased focus on improving patient care through the continuum of care. Many of the original benefits to justify horizontal integration remained: increased efficiency, reduced costs, and pooled risk, assuming the responsibility for the health status of the local population (Cuellar & Gertler, 2006). The main addition was the goal of economies of scope in addition to economies of scale.

Over the past decade, with the emergence of PHM, there has been a renewed interest in integration, however, in a broader sense. There has been interest in integrating not only both horizontally and vertically, but across sectors such as social services (Evans et al., 2013). The multisector approach is a result of an increased appreciation of the interconnectedness of social determinants of health and health status. This includes a holistic approach to the physical and mental well-being of people as well as considerations for the cultural competencies needed to properly treat communities (Satcher & Rachel, 2017).

The complexity of these IDNs continues to present multiple management challenges, as some horizontal organizations experienced higher costs for multiple reasons (Evans et al., 2013) and vertically integrated organizations faced challenges with higher prices and medical spending along increased utilization (Capps et al., 2018) while showing that a continuum of care can lead to better coordination of care for medically needy patients (Richards et al., 2016).

For population health managers, the question remains—with these expanding networks of organizations, will they be capable of providing the quality of care and at a lowered cost for the targeted populations.

Accountable Care Organizations

Although relatively new, **Accountable Care Organizations (ACOs** are a growing presence in PHM with about 6 million Medicare beneficiaries in an ACOs. As of January 2020, there were 558 ACOs currently providing care to 12.3 million Americans (NAACOS, n.d.). There are ACOs in all 50 states, the District of Columbia, and Puerto Rico (Muhlestein et al., 2017).

ACOs are networks of providers who come together to provide whole-patient centered care to patients, with the primary care physician (PCP) at the center of the network. Two well-known ACOs for their ability to save on cost are Palm Beach ACO and Baylor Scott and White Quality Alliance (Lapointe, 2019b).

In 2012, a voluntary payment model was created by CMS as part of the ACA. Sec. 3022 of ACA amended Section 1899 of Title XVIII (**Shared Savings Program**) specifies that an organization can be ACO if eligibility criteria are met. Organizations that wish to participate must meet seven outlined requirements (see Table 7.1).

TABLE 7.1 Summary of Accountable Care Organization (ACO) Eligibility and Requirements

ACO Eligibility Criteria	ACO Requirements
1) Physicians and other professionals in group practices 2) Physicians and other professionals in networks of practices 3) Partnerships or joint venture arrangements between hospitals and physicians/professionals 4) Hospitals employing physicians/professionals 5) Other forms that the Secretary of Health and Human Services may determine appropriate	1) Have a formal legal structure to receive and distribute shared savings 2) Have a sufficient number of primary care professionals for the number of assigned beneficiaries (a minimum of 5,000) 3) Agree to participate in the program for not less than a 3-year period 4) Have sufficient information regarding participating ACO healthcare professionals 5) Have a leadership and management structure that includes clinical and administrative systems 6) Have defined processes to (a) promote evidenced-based medicine, (b) report the necessary data to evaluate quality and cost measures, and (c) coordinate care 7) Demonstrate it meets patient-centeredness criteria, as determined by the Secretary of Health and Human Services

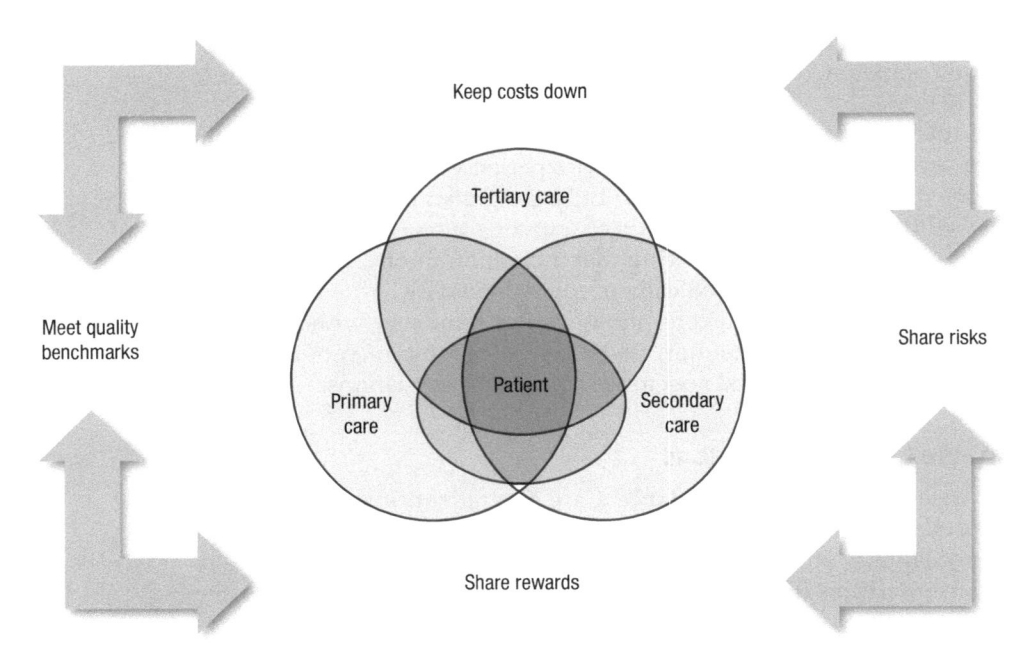

FIGURE 7.4 Patient-Centered Care Coordination

ACOs are networks of providers (both individual providers as well as networks of clinics and hospitals) who come together to provide whole-patient-centered care to patients, with the PCP at the center of the network. In this model, ACOs make providers all jointly accountable for the health of their patients to save money by improving care coordination and sharing information to reduce unnecessary duplication of tests and treatments. The providers can choose the level of financial risk knowing that higher risk can lead to higher rewards. ACOs that can reduce the total costs of their patient populations share in the savings (LaPointe, 2019a) with greater reimbursements going to those who meet quality benchmarks, focus on prevention, and keep chronic care patients out of the hospital. Those practitioners are unable to meet any of the criteria, or benchmarks assume the monetary risk of paying to improve their patient's outcomes (Gold, 2015). See Figure 7.4.

ⓘ DID YOU KNOW?

A Closer Look: Southwestern Health Resources Accountable Care Network, North Texas

The Southwestern Health Resources (SWHR) Accountable Care Network is a physician-led ACO, which is the combination of academic (The University of Texas Southwestern Medical Center) and a large nonprofit entity (Texas Health Resources) aligned with commercial healthcare plans and Medicare to provide quality care. The network serves more than 650,000 patients (with nearly 79,000 Medicare beneficiaries) across 17 counties in North Texas and includes a network of 29 hospital locations and more than 5,000 physicians. It is the fourth largest ACO in the nation.

SWHR operates the nation's highest rated Next Generation ACO for savings 2 years in a row. SWHR saved more than $37 million in 2018 and has saved more than $67 million overall since joining the Next Generation ACO Model in 2017. SWHR has been among the country's top-performing programs since 2015.

"These successful results reaffirm the effectiveness of our clinically integrated network of academic and community physicians and hospitals and doctors," said Andrew Ziskind, MD, senior executive officer of Southwestern Health Resources. "Being ranked No. 1 in the nation for second year in a row further demonstrates the success of the physician-driven strategies, SWHR has designed to build a stronger system of care. While we have achieved significant savings, we also have significantly improved the quality of care delivered to patients." To find more information about the SWHR ACO model, you can visit their website: https://www.southwesternhealth.org/aco-model.

ACOs are sometimes referred to as medical neighborhoods due to the nature of multiple providers working together to take responsibility for their patient's well-being. This phrase helps convey that ACOs are more than a single provider or clinic working together to improve population health outcomes (Southwestern Health Resources Care Network, 2020).

ACOs can be managed by private plans, Medicare, or Medicaid providers. In fact, the plurality ACO contracts are private plans, with the next most being Medicare providers, and relatively few Medicaid providers (Muhlestein et al., 2017). Agencies can form or dissolve ACOs at any time, and this turnover accounts for the difference in numbers of created ACOs and currently practicing ACOs.

There are some criticisms of ACOs. First is that the incentives to coordinate are just leading to an increase to the trend of healthcare mergers and acquisitions, which in turn leads to a reduction in competition and results in higher prices for patients (LaPointe, 2019a). There is, however, evidence that ACOs do result in a reduction of hospitalization and hospital length of stay and in improved quality, although the data on their ability to save costs are conflicted (Blackstone & Fuhr, 2016).

This biggest difference between an ACO and a **patient-centered medical home (PCMH)** is that PCMH is an approach for an individual practice while ACO is for a network of providers

Patient-Centered Medical Homes

Although they are often confused with ACOs, **PCMHs** are distinct in multiple ways. First, PCMHs are medical homes as opposed to medical neighborhoods, even though they are still created with the intention of reducing costs while improving patient outcomes. PCMHs predate the ACA by several decades (Sia et al., 2004) and originated in the 1960s as a concept from the American Academy of Pediatrics (AAP) as "Medical Home for children with special health care needs" and to address fragmented pediatric care (children with special healthcare needs [CSHCN]; O'Dell, 2016; Sia et al., 2004). Later, multiple professional organizations, including the AAP, the American Academy of Family Physicians (AAFP, n.d.), the American College of Physicians (ACP), and the American Osteopathic Association (AOA), came together to define the modern concept of PCMH (Joint Principles of the Patient-Centered

Medical Home, 2007). The Agency for Healthcare Research and Quality (AHRQ) has slightly modified the definitions in creating the five functions and attributes of a PCMH, to be more inclusive of nonphysician medical providers (O'Dell, 2016).

PCMHs are multiple providers under one organizational banner. All 50 states and the District of Columbia have all implemented some type of PCMH (Primary Care Innovations, 2020), and 30 states have implemented at least one Medicaid/CHIP PCMH (Primary Care Innovations, 2020).

Although PCMHs predate the ACA, the status of PCMHs is linked to the ACA. The ACA (Sec. 3021) established the Center for Medicare and Medicaid Innovation within CMS (also known as the Innovation Center or CMMI), which provides an avenue to fund innovative and patient-centered delivery models such as the PCMH. The ACA (Sec. 3502) also specifically authorized the funding of interdisciplinary, community-based primary care teams to provide culturally informed patient-centered care. PCMH models, community based, can and are being implemented by both private insurers and the government (Cunningham, 2015). The most widely adopted PCMH evaluation program in the country is the National Committee for Quality Assurance (NCQA), and as of 2020, they had recognized approximately 13,000 practices with 67,000 clinicians (NCQA, 2020).

Characteristics of Patient-Centered Medical Homes

To qualify as a PCMH, the agency must be more than just an organization. According to the AHRQ, the agency must have a core function of delivering primary care to demonstrate five functions and attributes (AHRQ, 2014). See Table 7.2. These core attributes must be present to be considered a PCMH; however, simply having these attributes alone does not make them a certified PCMH.

Certification Options

The exact number of practicing PCMHs remains unknown as an agency can choose to call itself a PCMH without becoming certified, although obtaining certification can bring an agency better reimbursement rates in some markets. Organizations can either get certified through national accrediting bodies such as the NCQA, the Accreditation Association for Ambulatory Health Care (AAAHC), or the Joint Commission, or they can choose to do it through a state health plan or agency. Interestingly, the AAP, AAFP, ACP, and AOA

TABLE 7.2 Patient-Centered Medical Home Function and Attributes

Function	Attribute Criteria
Patient centered	Requires providing culturally informed care reflecting the patient's values, beliefs, and wishes as well as making the patient an active part of their own care team.
Comprehensive	Ensuring that the majority of all of the patient's care must be met through the PCMH, including the majority of the preventative, acute, and chronic care the patient needs.
Coordinated	Patient's care must be coordinated across the continuum of care, including community-based care if needed.
Accessible	Any patient should be able to access it when urgent needs arise without significant wait times, including 24-hour phone or email support from a care member.
Quality and safety focus	Evidence of continuous performance and quality improvement, use of evidence-based medicine, and other indicators of patient commitment.

may have created the modern-day principles of the PCMH (Joint Principles of the Patient-Centered Medical Home, 2007), but none of these organizations administer certification.

PCMH, patient-centered medical home.

All PCMH recognitions require the agencies to follow specific protocols to ensure patient-centered and coordinated care. The NCQA is the most widely adopted, and the process has three main steps: commit, transform, and succeed (Process—PCMH, 2020). PCMHs must conduct self-assessment, submit performance and quality data online, and finally adopt continuous quality improvement activities for yearly check-ins (Bresnick, 2017a). There are three levels of NCQA PCMH recognition levels ranging from the most basic at level 1 to the most advanced at level 3 (Bresnick, 2017b). See Figure 7.5.

DID YOU KNOW?

A Closer Look: Hackensack Meridian Medical Group:

Primary Care, Jackson, New Jersey

As a participant of the Comprehensive Primary Care Plus (CPC+) program, a NCQA recognized level 3 (the most advanced) PCMH with additional recognition from NCQA as both having a clinician who has received both the DRP—Diabetes Recognition Program and the HSRP—Heart/Stroke Recognition Program, this practice has sufficiently demonstrated that it is able to provide high-quality care to patients in the Jackson, New Jersey, region. To find more information about the Hackensack Meridian Medical Group, you can visit their website: https://www.hackensackmeridianhealth.org/locations/primary-care-jackson-suite-2-1.

Source: NCQA Report Cards. (n.d.). Retrieved September 17, 2020, https://reportcards.ncqa.org/

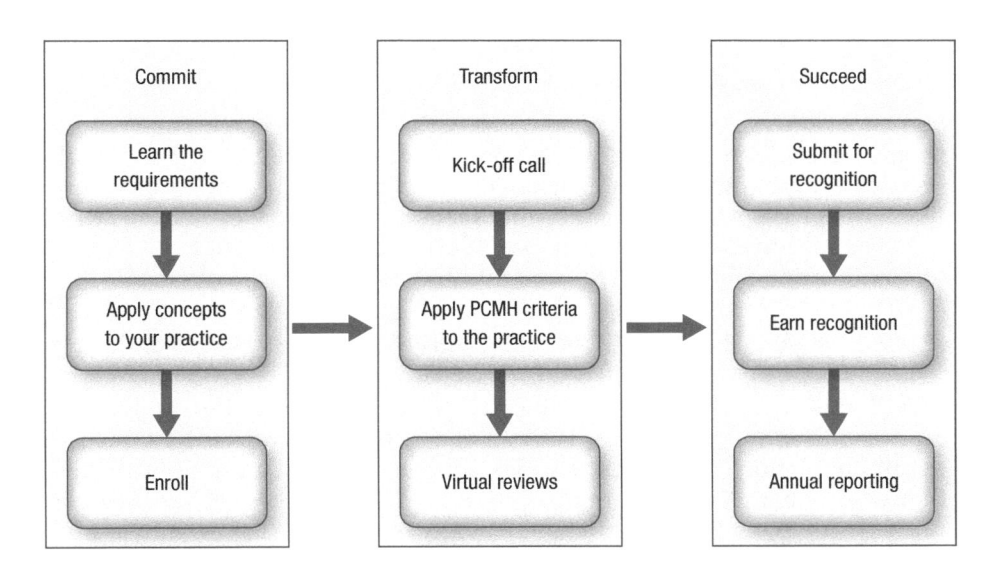

FIGURE 7.5 NCQA Patient-Centered Medical Home Recognition Process

Source: Adapted from Process - PCMH. (2020, August 12). Retrieved August 20, 2020, from https://www.ncqa.org/programs/health-care-providers-practices/patient-centered-medical-home-pcmh/process/

TABLE 7.3 Comparison of PCMH Comprehensive Primary Care Plus Tracks

Comparison of PCMH Models		
	PCMH	**CPC+**
Adhere to medical home model	X	X
Multispecialty practices allowed		X
Rural Health Clinic (RHC) Certified practice allowed	X	
Participant in ACO allowed	X	X
Pediatric practice allowed	X	
Participates in the Medicare Shared Savings Program (MSSP)	X	X
Must adhere to the five functions of a PCMH	X	X

ACO, accountable care organization; CPC+, Comprehensive Primary Care Plus; PCMH, patient-centered medical home.

Source: Adapted from ACP. (2017). Eligibility Assessment for Comprehensive Primary Care Plus (CPC +). https://www.acponline.org/system/files/documents/practice-resources/business-resources/payment/models/other-care/acp_cpc_plus_eligibility_assessment_revised_v3.pdf

Comprehensive Primary Care Plus (CPC+) is a national private–public partnership, which currently supports 2,804 primary care practices and 52 aligned payers in 18 regions through a unique multipayer payment system. It includes two primary care practice tracks with incrementally advanced care delivery requirements and payment options (Track 1 is for agencies building capabilities to become a PCMH, while Track 2 is for those already functioning as such). Agencies in both tracks make changes to care delivery based on the CPC functions:

- Access and Continuity
- Care Management
- Comprehensiveness and Coordination
- Patient and Caregiver Engagement
- Planned Care and Population Health (U.S. HHS, 2019)

Similar to the ACP's recommendations, CPC+ includes three payment elements. There is the standard payment under the Medicare FFS as usual, risk-adjusted monthly care management fees, and performance-based incentives. The performance-based incentives include both prospective and retrospective incentives. They are still essentially PCMHs, but held at to slightly different and higher standards (see Table 7.3).

SUMMARY

This chapter described and explained the most common population health models currently available for PH managers. There is no one right answer for all populations or regions, and multiple models can be used in conjunction with one another to better improve patient outcomes and reduce per capita costs. What is promising is the alignment of financial incentives and improving patient care. For example, before providers were finally able to get reimbursement for telemedicine services through both public and private insurance, there was little motivation for the average provider to offer these services (Neufeld et al., 2016). The Quality Payment Program is an example of a shift from the single largest payer in the U.S. health system

(Gordon & Siegel, 2020) to formalize pay-for-performance instead of pay-for-service (Rathbun et al., 2018). By making providers financially tied to the outcomes of their patients, significant savings occur (Haas et al., 2019) and improved outcomes such as reduction in ED visits and improved chronic disease management (Kaufman et al., 2019). This is a rapidly evolving field, and while there is no way to predict exactly what PHM models will look like in the future, we can be sure that it will involve leveraging information technology, utilizing evidence-based data, and coordinating care for the holistic patient care.

DISCUSSION QUESTIONS

1. Managed care was a precursor to population health in many ways. What are some of the key differences between traditional managed care models and these population health models?
2. Create a diagram showing the various types of IDNs.
3. Under what circumstances might it make more sense for an agency to not get certified as a PCMH?
4. Provide an example of an ACO setup with horizontal integration and a separate example of an ACO with vertical integration
5. Explore the properties of PCMHs in your state at https://www.pcpcc.org/initiatives/state. Are they mostly private or publicly funded? Do any have proven outcomes? How does your state compare to neighboring states?
6. Describe the similarities and differences between ACOs and PCMHs.

Toolkit Competency Application

Recognition Options for Patient-Centered Medical Homes

As a director of strategic planning for your community hospital, you were instrumental in the acquisition of both primary care and specialty practices joining your health system. The CEO has just requested that you assess two potential credentialing/ recognition opportunities and report back with a **brief two-page summary recommendation**. The CEO and other executives know the basic structure of the CPC+ and the AHQR models and their primary interest. It is up to you to identify the potential top five challenges for implementation. In addition to Table 7.3 that provides a comparison between the two models, basic implementation toolkits are available for your review. See Resources #1 and #2. Given the short time frame for completion, the executive summary will highlight the most common barriers and challenges to implementation.

RESOURCES

CMS Comprehensive Primary Care Plus CPC+: https://innovation.cms.gov/files/x/cpcplus-rfa.pdf (open resource)
Getting Started Toolkit: Get Started With NCQA PCMH Recognition: https://www.ncqa.org/programs/health-care-providers-practices/patient-centered-medical-home-pcmh/getting-started-toolkit/3 (available for free download)

REFERENCES

ACC. (2015, April 28). *Medicare Access and CHIP Reauthorization Act of 2015: What you need to know*. American College of Cardiology. https://www.acc.org/latest-in-cardiology/articles/2015/04/28/15/59/medicare-access-and-chip-reauthorization-act-of-2015-what-you-need-to-know

ACP. (2017). *Eligibility assessment for Comprehensive Primary Care Plus (CPC+)*. American College of Physicians. https://www.acponline.org/system/files/documents/practice-resources/business-resources/payment/models/other-care/acp_cpc_plus_eligibility_assessment_revised_v3.pdf

Agency for Healthcare Research and Quality. (2014). AHRQ updates on primary care research: The AHRQ patient-centered medical home resource center. *The Annals of Family Medicine, 12*(6), 586–586. https://doi.org/10.1370/afm.1728

Allison, J. (2015). Interview with Joel T. Allison, FACHE, CEO of Baylor Scott & White Health. *Journal of Healthcare Management, 60*(2), 81–85.

Al-Saddique, A. (2018). Integrated delivery systems (IDSs) as a means of reducing costs and improving healthcare delivery. *Journal of Healthcare Communications, 3*(1), 19. https://doi.org/10.4172/2472-1654.100129

American Academy of Family Physicians. (n.d.). *Joint Principles of the Patient-Centered Medical Home*. https://www.aafp.org/dam/AAFP/documents/practice_management/pcmh/initiatives/PCMHJoint.pdf

Berwick, D. M., Nolan, T. W., & Whittington, J. (2008). The triple aim: Care, health, and cost. *Health Affairs, 27*(3), 759–769. http://dx.doi.org/10.1377/hlthaff.27.3.759

Blackstone, E. A., & Fuhr, J. P. (2016). The economics of Medicare accountable care organizations. *American Health & Drug Benefits, 9*(1), 11–19.

Bresnick, J. (2017a, April 7). *NCQA revamps patient-centered medical home to ease adoption*. Health IT Analytics. https://healthitanalytics.com/news/ncqa-revamps-patient-centered-medical-home-to-ease-adoption

Bresnick, J. (2017b, July 17). *How does an ACO differ from the patient-centered medical home?* Health IT Analytics. https://healthitanalytics.com/news/how-does-an-aco-differ-from-the-patient-centered-medical-home

Burns, L. R., Goldsmith, J. C., & Sen, A. (2013). Horizontal and vertical integration of physicians: A tale of two tails. *Advances in Health Care Management Annual Review of Health Care Management: Revisiting The Evolution of Health Systems Organization, 15*, 39–117. https://doi.org/10.1108/s1474-8231(2013)0000015009

Burns, L. R., & Pauly, M. V. (2002). Integrated delivery networks: A detour on the road to integrated health care? *Health Affairs, 21*(4), 128–143. https://doi.org/10.1377/hlthaff.21.4.128

Capps, C., Dranove, D., & Ody, C. (2018). The effect of hospital acquisitions of physician practices on prices and spending. *Journal of Health Economics, 59*, 139–152. https://doi.org/10.1016/j.jhealeco.2018.04.001

Casalino, L. P., Devers, K. J., Lake, T. K., Reed, M., & Stoddard, J. J. (2003). Benefits of and barriers to large medical group practice in the United States. *Archives of Internal Medicine, 163*(16), 1958–1964. https://doi.org/10.1001/archinte.163.16.1958

Casalino, L. P., Pham, H., & Bazzoli, G. (2004). Growth of single-specialty medical groups. *Health Affairs, 23*(2), 82–90. https://doi.org/10.1377/hlthaff.23.2.82

Casalino, L. P., Wu, F. M., Ryan, A. M., Copeland, K., Rittenhouse, D. R., Ramsay, P. P., & Shortell, S. M. (2013). Independent practice associations and physician-hospital organizations can improve care management for smaller practices. *Health Affairs, 32*(8), 1376–1382.

Cuellar, A. E., & Gertler, P. J. (2006). Strategic integration of hospitals and physicians. *Journal of Health Economics, 25*(1), 1–28. https://doi.org/10.1016/j.jhealeco.2005.04.009

Cunningham, P. J. (2015). Many Medicaid beneficiaries receive care consistent with attributes of patient-centered medical homes. *Health Affairs, 34*(7), 1105–1112. https://doi.org/10.1377/hlthaff.2015.0141

Dranove, D., & Shanley, M. (1995). Cost reductions or reputation enhancement as motives for mergers: The logic of multihospital systems. *Strategic Management Journal, 16*(1), 55–74. https://doi.org/10.1002/smj.4250160107

Ellis, S. D., Karim, S. A., Vukas, R. R., Marx, D., & Uddin, J. (2018). Four needles in a haystack: A systematic review assessing quality of health care in specialty practice by practice type. *INQUIRY: The Journal of Health Care Organization, Provision, and Financing, 55*, 1–13. https://doi.org/10.1177/0046958018787041

Evans, J. M., Baker, G. R., Berta, W. B., & Barnsley, J. (2013). The evolution of integrated healthcare strategies. In *Academy of management proceedings* (Vol. 2013, No. 1, p. 13931). Academy of Management. https://doi.org/10.5465/ambpp.2013.159

Gold, J. (2015, September 14). *Accountable care organizations, explained.* https://khn.org/news/aco-accountable-care-organization-faq/

Gordon, D., & Siegel, D. (2020). Machine learning and the future of medicare fraud detection. *Journal of the American Academy of Dermatology, August*, e133. https://doi.org/10.1016/j.jaad.2020.03.059

Haas, D. A., Zhang, X., Kaplan, R. S., & Song, Z. (2019). Evaluation of economic and clinical outcomes under Centers for Medicare & Medicaid Services mandatory bundled payments for joint replacements. *JAMA Internal Medicine, 179*(7), 924–931. https://doi.org/10.1001/jamainternmed.2019.0480

Hebert, R. R., & Veil, A. A. (2004). Monitoring the degree of implementation of an integrated delivery system. *International Journal of Integrated Care, 4*, e05. https://doi.org/10.5334/ijic.106

Heeringa, J., Mutti, A., Furukawa, M. F., Lechner, A., Maurer, K. A., & Rich, E. (2020). Horizontal and vertical integration of health care providers: A framework for understanding various provider organizational structures. *International Journal of Integrated Care, 20*(1), 2. https://doi.org/10.5334/ijic.4635.

James, B. C., & Savitz, L. A. (2011). How Intermountain trimmed health care costs through robust quality improvement efforts. *Health Affairs, 30*(6), 1185–1191. https://doi.org/10.1377/hlthaff.2011.0358

Joint Principles of the Patient-Centered Medical Home. (2007). *American Academy of Family Physicians.* https://www.aafp.org/dam/AAFP/documents/practice_management/pcmh/initiatives/PCMHJoint.pdf

Kaufman, B. G., Spivack, B. S., Stearns, S. C., Song, P. H., & O'Brien, E. C. (2019). Impact of accountable care organizations on utilization, care, and outcomes: A systematic review. *Medical Care Research and Review, 76*(3), 255–290. https://doi.org/10.1177/1077558717745916

Kumar, V., Duncan, A. K., & Breslin, M. A. (2009). Innovating health care delivery: The design of health services. *Journal of Business Strategy, 30*(2/3), 13–20.

LaPointe, J. (2019a, December 18). *Understanding the fundamentals of accountable care organizations.* Revcycle Intelligence. https://revcycleintelligence.com/features/understanding-the-fundamentals-of-accountable-care-organizations

LaPointe, J. (2019b). *Top 10 accountable care organizations by shared savings in 2019.* Revcycle Intelligence. https://revcycleintelligence.com/news/top-10-accountable-care-organizations-by-shared-savings-in-2019

Lega, F. (2005). Strategies for multi-hospital networks: A framework. *Health Services Management Research, 18*(2), 86–99. https://doi.org/10.1258/0951484053723135

Maeda, J. L. K., Lee, K. M., & Horberg, M. (2014). Comparative health systems research among Kaiser Permanente and other integrated delivery systems: A systematic literature review. *The Permanente Journal, 18*(3), 66–77. https://doi.org/10.7812/TPP/13-159

Mattocks, K. M., & Yehia, B. (2017). Evaluating the veterans choice program: Lessons for developing a high-performing integrated network. *Medical Care, 55*, 1–3. https://doi.org/10.1097/MLR.0000000000000743

McCarthy, D. (2015) Integrated healthcare delivery models in an era of reform. In J. M. Shiver, & J. Cantiello, (Eds.), *Managing integrated health systems* (pp. 1–24). Jones and Bartlett.

Muhlestein, D., Saunders, R. S., & McClellan, M. B. (2017, June 28). Growth of ACOs and alternative payment models in 2017. *Health Affairs.* https://www.healthaffairs.org/do/10.1377/hblog20170628.060719/full/

NAACOS. (n.d.). *Home.* Retrieved August 22, 2020, from https://www.naacos.com/

NCQA Patient-Centered Medical Home (PCMH). (2020, August 12). *National Committee for Quality Assurance.* https://www.ncqa.org/programs/health-care-providers-practices/patient-centered-medical-home-pcmh/

Neufeld, J. D., Doarn, C. R., & Aly, R. (2016). State policies influence medicare telemedicine utilization. *Telemedicine and e-Health, 22*(1), 70–74. https://doi.org/10.1089/tmj.2015.0044

Newsroom. (2020, January 27). *Southwestern health resources accountable care network listed No. 1 in U.S. for Medicare savings for second straight year.* UT Southwestern. https://www.utsouthwestern.edu/newsroom/articles/year-2020/swhr-aco-medicare-savings.html

O'Dell, M. L. (2016). What is a patient-centered medical home? *Missouri Medicine, 113*(4), 301–304.

Payne, T. H., Bates, D. W., Berner, E. S., Bernstam, E. V., Covvey, H. D., Frisse, M. E., Graf, T., Greenses, R. A.., Hoffer, E. P., Kuperman, G., Lehmann, H. P., Liang, L., Middleton, B., Omenn, G. S., & Ozbolt, J. (2013). Healthcare information technology and economics. *Journal of the American Medical Informatics Association, 20*(2), 212–217. https://doi.org/10.1136/amiajnl-2012-000821

Primary Care Innovations and PCMH Map by State. (2020, August 20). *Patient centered primary care collaborative.* https://www.pcpcc.org/initiatives/state

Process - PCMH. (2020, August 12). *National Committee for Quality Assurance.* https://www.ncqa.org/programs/health-care-providers-practices/patient-centered-medical-home-pcmh/process/

Rathbun, J., Johnson, B., Woo, K., & Copeland, T. P. (2018). Quality Payment Program year 2. *Journal of Vascular Surgery, 67*(3), 984. https://doi.org/10.1016/j.jvs.2017.12.015

Richards, M. R., Nikpay, S. S., & Graves, J. A. (2016). The growing integration of physician practices. *Medical Care, 54*(7), 714–718. https://doi.org/10.1097/MLR.0000000000000546

Sales, A. E. (2008). The Veterans Health Administration in the context of health insurance reform. *Medical Care, 46*(10), 1020–1022. https://doi.org/10.1097/MLR.0b013e318184aa75

Satcher, D., & Rachel, S. A. (2017). Promoting mental health equity: The role of integrated care. *Journal of Clinical Psychology in Medical Settings, 24*(3–4), 182–186. https://doi.org/10.1007/s10880-016-9465-8

Sia, C., Tonniges, T. F., Osterhus, E., & Taba, S. (2004). History of the medical home concept. *Pediatrics, 113*(Supplement 4), 1473–1478.

Steiner, B. D., Denham, A. C., Ashkin, E., Newton, W. P., Wroth, T., & Dobson, L. A. (2008). Community care of North Carolina: Improving care through community health networks. *The Annals of Family Medicine, 6*(4), 361–367. https://doi.org/10.1370/afm.866

Thomas, P., Meads, G., Moustafa, A., Nazareth, I., Stange, K. C., & Donnelly Hess, G. (2008). Combined horizontal and vertical integration of care: A goal of practice-based commissioning. *Quality in Primary Care, 16*(6), 425–432.

U.S. Department of Health & Human Services, Center for Medicare & Medicaid Innovation. (2019). *CPC+ payment and attribution methodologies for program year 2020* (Vol. 1). https://innovation.cms.gov/files/x/cpcplus-methodology-py20.pdf

Veterans Administration (2009, June 10). *About VHA.* https://www.va.gov/health/aboutvha.asp

Whittington, J. W., Nolan, K., Lewis, N., & Torres, T. (2015). Pursuing the triple aim: The first 7 years. *The Milbank Quarterly, 93*(2), 263–300. https://doi.org/10.1111/1468-0009.12122

Wise, C. G., Alexander, J. A., Green, L. A., & Cohen, G. R. (2012). Physician organization-practice team integration for the advancement of patient-centered care. *The Journal of Ambulatory Care Management, 35*(4), 311–322. https://doi.org/10.1097/JAC.0b013e3182606e7c

PART III

Population Health Management Applications

CHAPTER 8

Alternative Payment Systems: Volume- to Value-Based Care

Anastasia Miller and Thomas B. Woodard

KEY TERMS

Alternative Payment System
Bundled Payments
Fee-for-Service (FFS)
MACRA
MIPPS

Pay for Performance
Shared Savings
Value-Based Care
Volume-Based Care

LEARNING OBJECTIVES

1. Articulate volume- and value-based care concepts.
2. Discuss legislative impact as a catalyst for alternative payment mechanisms.
3. Describe the types of value-based care arrangements.
4. Explain alternative finance payment models for accountable care organizations (ACOs) and patient-centered medical homes (PCMHs).
5. Examine population health managers' role in risk decision-making.

> Podcasts that exemplify the content of this chapter are available at Springer Publishing Connect™
>
> Podcast 8.1. What Do You Know About Risk and Financial Incentives?
> Podcast 8.2. Have ACOs Changed Over Time?

Access the podcast online at http://connect.springerpub.com/content/book/978-0-8261-4427-0/part/part03/chapter/ch08

INTRODUCTION

One of the key distinctions between the population health approach and population health management (PHM) is the latter's perspective demanding positive health outcomes. Various dashboards designed to measure the success of PHM have been developed over the years, and we can safely assume that "cost" and "quality" are included. The Population Health Alliance Framework contains financial outcomes in addition to four other key outcome metrics (psychosocial outcomes, behavior change, clinical and health status, and productivity, satisfaction, and quality of life) as part of its dashboard (Population Health Management Framework (PHA), 2018).

The healthcare sector's previous payment model, universally accepted by heathcare providers and payers alike, was restricted to single service interactions with a specific health care provider. Interactions could be characterized as being focused on acute care focus, quality indifferent, and involving no or little financial risk (Wagner, 2018). One of the major criticisms of the previous models of healthcare payment, including the managed care revolution of the 1980s and 1990s, is the system resulted in incentivizing providers to increase the number of patients and/or procedures performed to make a profit (Kwon, 1996). Known as **fee-for-service (FFS),** the entire payment process centered on recurring payments generated for a single service by each provider. But, as healthcare costs increased significantly, the administrative payment costs also escalated, as reimbursement standards became more complex along with preapproval processes. Increasing volume to offset these costs no longer appeared sustainable.

With the emergence of population health and a new focus on tailored interventions for groups of individuals and subpopulations, the opportunity to control separate costs and align them to positive outcomes encouraged the development of new financial payment strategies focused on value-based payment models. Two ideas formed the conceptual thinking supporting the proposed alternative payment systems. First, payment became tied to successful health outcomes. Second, the risk associated with the positive health outcome could be shared between the health provider, health agency (hospital), and the payer (proprietary insurance companies or state and federal health agencies). Both upside and downside risk are of importance to the population health manager (American Academy of Pediatrics, n.d.) Examples of these alternative payment systems are also known as **pay-for-performance systems** (NEJM Catalyst, 2018). An important characteristic of these new models was that risk segmentation and stratification approaches formed a solid foundation for the alternative payment mechanisms.

Value-Based Versus Volume-Based Care Applications for Population Health

**The two driving forces behind the alternative payment method:
Aligning payment to health outcomes
Sharing the financial risk between the provider, agency, and payer**

Common sense would suggest that population health managers seek value-based care for all their patients and consumers. But the entrenched

TABLE 8.1 Comparison Between Volume- and Value-Based Characteristics

Paradigm Shift: Volume (fee-for-service) to value (fee-for-value)	
Volume Based	**Value Based**
Incentives based on volume (fee-for-service only)	Payments used to incentivize health providers to deliver quality care and reduce cost
Reimbursement tied directly to cost of care	Manage higher patient volume and less out-of-network costs
Little or no emphasis on quality of care provided	Tailored to populations at risk, such as individuals with chronic conditions
Success is defined as achieving high-profit margins	Opportunity to increase market share based on outcome data

Shift from Volume-Based Care to Value-Based Care. (n.d.). University of Illinois Chicago. Https://healthinformatics.uic.edu/blog/shift-from-volume-based-care-to-value-based-care/

transactional, FFS model required a paradigm change to address the diverse and complex issues that underlie healthcare economics and payment systems in the United States. The transformation between the two approaches continues, as hospitals and payers gravitate toward the value-based alternative delivery model and learn to accept population outcome incentives (Shift from Volume-Based Care to Value-Based Care, n.d.). See Table 8.1.

Volume-based care, commonly described as FFS, refers to the payment a healthcare provider receives for services a patient might need. In the volume-based care model, the quality of service does not affect the payment received or impact the amount received. The only incentive available for healthcare providers is to increase the number of patients so that profits also increase as compared with cost. However, the primary goals of value-based care focus on quality services, positive health outcomes, and cost reduction. An additional emphasis is on providing preventive care, to further ensure quality of life, and managing social determinants of health risk factors.

The Benefits of Value-Based Care for Population Health Management

The challenges to implementing value-based care are significant and complex, as the goal is to transform a payment system that affects millions of American consumers and almost every element of the healthcare sector. However, insurance companies are obtaining significant reductions in cost that they are sharing with providers and consumers. A recent article, "*Humana Touts $4B in 2019 Savings due to Value-Based Care Agreements,*" shows a vivid example of the cost savings available and feasible (Leventhal, 2020). Individual health organizations may not accumulate these extraordinary savings, but the opportunity to adopt a new population health model offers a new financial sustainability strategy.

Once the healthcare sector recognizes the benefits of value-based care, the adoption and complexity of alternative payment mechanisms increases significantly. The Health Care Payment Learning & Action Network (HCP-LAN) developed The Alternative Payment Model (APM) Framework to help simplify the various alternatives for health organizations (HCP-LAN, 2017). Other reports refer to this model as the CMS HCPLAN Framework (AHA, 2019).

> **? DID YOU KNOW?**
>
> **Continuum of Risk: Alternative Payment Model**
>
> The APM (HCP-LAN, 2017) outlines and describes in detail a four-level continuum, with eight subcategories that captures clinical and financial risk for provider organizations. 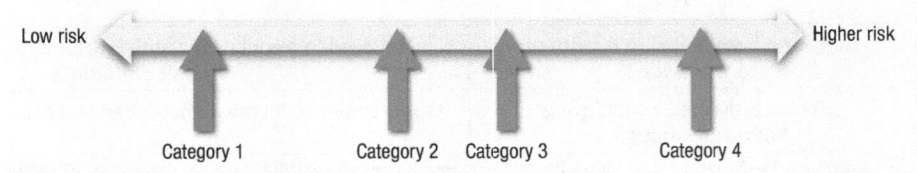
>
> Low risk ←———— Category 1 — Category 2 — Category 3 — Category 4 ————→ Higher risk
>
> **Source:** Adapted from APM Framework (2017)
>
> | Category 1 | Category 2 | Category 3 | Category 4 |
> |---|---|---|---|
> | Fee-for-Service | Fee-for-Service | Alternative Payment Systems | Population-Based Payment |
> | No Link to Quality & Value | Link to Quality & Value | Using Fee-for-Service Architecture | |
>
> The benefit of the APM is that it identifies core principles for APM design and provides a common standard for both payers and purchases (APM Framework: Overview [2017]).

Adopting and Aligning Alternative Payment Models for Population Health

The American Hospital Association's sponsored a recent Center for Health Innovation report: *Evolving Care Models: Aligning Care Delivery to Emerging Payment Models* (AHA Center for Innovation, 2019). This valuable document covered the following topics:

- Development of APMs
- The APMs Framework
- Common Alternative Care Delivery Models
- Transition to APM Challenges
- Maturity (Risk-Sharing Arrangements) Framework

Value-based care offers health organizations multiple adoption options, and over time, four common care approaches have emerged. Note which management arrangements offer internal versus external options for an organization (see Table 8.2).

For population health managers, the choice of value-based risk assessment will be influenced by the type of alternative care delivery model selected. The four most common alternative care delivery models, as outlined by the report are ACOs, PCMHs, integrated service lines, and provider-sponsored health plans (AHA, 2019). See Table 8.3.

TABLE 8.2 Descriptions of Value-Based Care Arrangements

Type of Value-Based Care Arrangement	Description
All departments share the risk	Involving all departments suggests a unified strategy and a total "risk" for all healthcare employees/providers involved.
Offer contracts to patients	Not quite as simple as capitated patients, but costs per person per month offer an option for a substantial and expected revenue source with a high accountability factor.
Bundle service offerings	Combining services by allowing to choose what is important to them and what services they do not need. This allows the patient to personalize their care, and it allows the healthcare provider to save money. With bundled payments, the total allowable acute and/or postacute expenditures (target price) for an *episode of care (EOC)* are predetermined. Participant providers share in any losses or savings that result from the difference between this target price and actual costs. Common examples include myocardial infarction, UTI, pacemaker, congestive heart failure, stroke, and sepsis.
Shared savings	Savings resulting from PHM payment mechanisms are shared across the organization and not just to health provider.

PHM, population health management; UTI, urinary tract infection.
Source: Adapted from The Shift from Volume-Based Care to Value-Based Care. (n.d.). University of Illinois Chicago. Https://healthinformatics.uic.edu/blog/shift-from-volume-based-care-to-value-based-care/

TABLE 8.3 Common Alternative Care Delivery Models for Value-Based Payment Options

Accountable care organizations	Networks of health providers jointly responsible for improving patient outcomes by reducing spending. May involve physician groups, behavioral health organizations, hospitals, and health systems.
Patientcentered medical homes	Integrated care team for primary care delivery, can seek accreditation, patient-centered.
Integrated service lines	Integrated services lines (disease states) across medical specialties and continuum of care. Uses bundled payments.
Provider-sponsored health plans	Health plans either sponsored or acquired by hospital—assume total risk for enrollees and involve capitation.

Accountable Care Organizations: Alternative Payment Mechanisms

> **Quality Payment Program (QPP)** includes both the **Merit-Based Incentive Payment System (MIPS)** and **Alternative Payment Model (APM)** value-based reimbursement models.

One of the major difficulties with managed care and previous integrated delivery networks (IDN) models was that they were lacking the technological and financial capabilities at the time for true clinical integration. Mechanisms such as reimbursement for coordination activities, shared-risk contractual agreements, and other reimbursement incentives were needed to make progress on population health (Croft & Parish, 2013). The ACA helped align these financial incentives with the Triple Aim for the first time. Although goals between an ACO and older managed care models are similar, such as **health maintenance organizations**, a vital difference is that ACOs must meet quality benchmarks in addition to saving money.

The ACA was not the only legislation to influence the financing of population health alternative payment systems by creating a pathway to fund innovative models, including ACOs. The **Medicare Access and CHIP Reauthorization Act of 2015 (MACRA)** was signed into law April 16, 2015, and finalized major details on ways to reimburse these agencies (Findlay, 2017). MACRA represented a fundamental shift in reimbursement for Medicare because it changed the basic billing system from FFS to a value-based reimbursement system. MACRA introduced the **Merit-based Incentive Payment System (MIPS)** and the **Alternative Payment Model (APM)**, for Medicare Part B providers, both of which are now collectively referred to as the **Quality Payment Program (QPP;** Sayeed et al., 2017). Both MIPS and APMs are payment models that incentivize high-quality and low-cost care, albeit through different methods. As of 2017, providers had to pick one of these payment plans, and with the 2-year lag between reporting and reimbursement, agencies were first reimbursed with the payment adjustments on January 1, 2019 (Sayeed et al., 2017).

The Primary Care First Act was passed in 2018 with the goal of improving the quality of and access to healthcare for all Medicare beneficiaries, particularly those with complex chronic conditions and serious illnesses. The legislation changes the reimbursement model and increases funding to primary care physicians (PCPs) to help facilitate better care, decrease the number of hospital visits for these patients, and improve outcomes.

Under MIPS, the performance of the individual or agencies seeking reimbursement is assessed by weighted percentages on four dimensions of quality, clinical practice improvement activities, advancing care information, and resource use (McWilliams, 2017). See Figure 8.1.

Agencies that score 70 or higher can get an Exceptional Performance Bonus up to a 5% payment and those that do not score at least a 15 will receive a up to a −5% payment adjustment while those scoring exactly 15 points

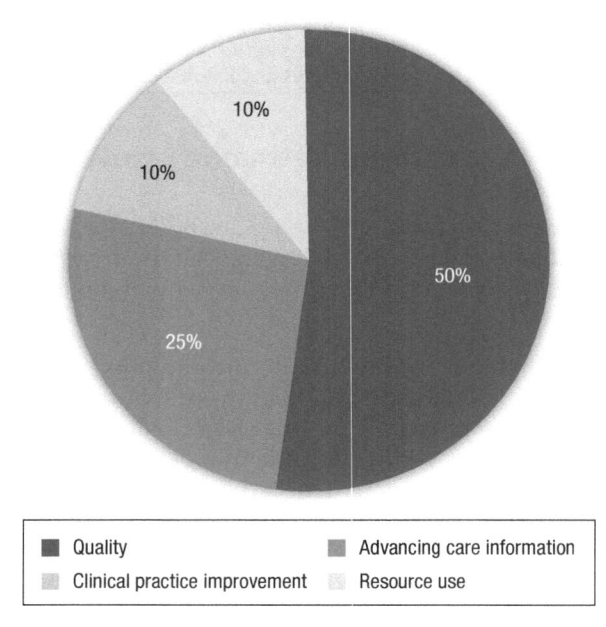

FIGURE 8.1 MIPS Scoring Criteria by Percentages

MIPS, Merit-Based Incentive Payment System.

receive no adjustment. The bonuses depend on the number of agencies scoring in the that range, as the CMS must be budget neutral. MIPS is the default program of Medicare Part B, and all providers not qualifying for APM will participate in MIPS. There are two exclusionary categories though of providers who do not need to participate in MIPS, in addition to those in APMs.

- The first are low-volume providers who bill less than $90,000 to Medicare each year or provider care to less than 200 Medicare beneficiaries per year.
- The second are new Medicare-enrolled providers, as they are exempt from MIPS requirements their first year.

As an added incentive for ACOs and their commitment to population health, Medicare ACOs in MIPS are considered MIPS APMs for reimbursement purposes and are given favorable benefits (NAACOS, n.d.).

> Merit-Based Incentive Payment System (MIPS) is the default reimbursement system of Medicare Part B.
>
> All providers not qualifying for Alternative Payment Mode (APM) will participate in MIPS.

MACRA requires that payments under an APM be based on quality measures that are comparable with those used in the MIPS program; however, there are notable differences. One of the requirements for APMs is that they must use certified EHR technology in addition to reporting on certain measures and bearing more of the financial risk. In exchange for these greater potential financial risks, there are greater potential financial rewards than with MIPS (Sampson, 2016). Under the APM reimbursement pathway, physicians, and/or agencies may be exempt from participation in the MIPS and be eligible to receive a 5% incentive payment. This pathway is also known as the **Medicare Shared Savings Program (MSSP)**, which was created in the final rule of the MACRA. The stated goal of this pathway is to "promote accountability for a patient population and coordinate items and services under Medicare Parts A and B and encourage investment in infrastructure and redesigned care processes for high quality and efficient service delivery (CMS, 2020)." See Table 8.4.

There are two tracks within the APMs: Basic and Enhanced. At a general level, the different tracks correspond to differing levels of potential risk and potential reward (the "shared savings" from improving the population health). One of the differences between MIPS and these MSSP tracks is that ACOs are required to maintain a certain level of financial responsibility, in the event costs increase past a predetermined benchmark (The Physicians Advocacy Institute, 2020).

On the Basic Track, the shared savings "bonus" is capped at 10%, whereas on the Enhanced Track, it is capped at 20%; however the shared loss is somewhere between 2% and 8% of the ACO revenue or 1% and 4% of the ACO

TABLE 8.4 Comparison of Basic and Enhanced APMs

APM Tracks	
Basic	Enhanced
Shared Savings Bonus ≤ 10% of savings	Shared Savings Bonus ≤ 20%
Shared Loss Penalty 2%–8% of ACO revenue	Shared Loss Penalty 15% of ACO revenue

TABLE 8.5 Comparison of MIPS and APMs Quality Program Tracks

QPP Tracks	
MIPS	**Advanced APMs**
Shared Savings Program Track 1	Shared Saving Program Track 2
BASIC Track Level A	Shared Saving Program Track 3
BASIC Track Level B	BASIC Track Level E
BASIC Track Level C	ENHANCED Track
BASIC Track Level D	Medicare ACO Track 1+ model

ACO, accountable care organization; APM, Alternative Payment Model; MIPS, Merit-Based Incentive Payment System; QPP, Quality Payment Program.

Source: Adapted from For Providers. (2020, September 11). https://www.cms.gov/Medicare/Medicare-Fee-for-Service-Payment/sharedsavingsprogram/for-providers

benchmark (depending on which of the three Basic levels the agency is participating in), but it is 15% on the Enhanced track. As of March 2020, 517 ACOs were participating in the MSSP pathway benchmark (Physicians Advocacy Institute, 2020). See Table 8.5.

Patient-Centered Medical Homes: Alternative Payment Mechanisms

Under the FFS payment structure, an incentive existed to increase patients and treatments, but Medicare and Medicaid did not provide financial incentives for patient-focused, long-term-oriented care. Care coordination efforts often failed, as these services were generally not reimbursable activities for most providers. To address this population health issue, the ACA included provisions to create Medicaid state plans and pilot programs. The biggest fundamental difference in the payment model between a PCMH and an ACO reflects the difference in the model for an individual agency versus a network.

PCMH providers are primarily accountable to themselves when investing in the development of patient-centered care while members of ACOs are rewarded or penalized based on their performance at regular intervals.

PCMH providers can participate in the value-based reimbursement models ACOs use, but there is not the same requirement of financial reform (Bresnick, 2017). They may or may not implement the same risk-based reimbursement arrangement as ACOs, depending on what makes the most sense for the PCMH.

The ACP suggests the most effective way to ensure the alignment of incentives with patient outcomes in PCMHs is to use a "three-part model": FFS for office visit, monthly risk-adjusted bundled care coordination fees, and a performance-based component (PCMH costs, benefits, and incentives, n.d.). Data do show that combining FFS and a care coordination fee can greatly improve the financial standing of a PCMH (Basu et al., 2016).

Medicare Access and CHIP Reauthorization Act of 2015

MACRA, legislation passed in 2015, also impacts PCMHs, specifically in the form of **Advanced APMs**. Advanced APM is another reimbursement category which includes both Advanced APMs and Other Payer Advanced APMs as defined by MACRA. These are like the APMs discussed in the ACO section, except there are additional requirements, because they must adhere to the **Medical Home Model**. The specific requirements for each model are as follows (Sampson, 2016):

Advanced APMs must

- require participants to use Certified EHR Technology;
- provide payments based on quality measures comparable to those used in MIPS; and
- require participants to adopt a Medical Home Model or accept more than a nominal amount of financial risk.

To qualify as an All-Payer Advanced APM, a commercial or Medicaid APM must

- require participants to use Certified EHR Technology;
- provide payments based on quality measures comparable to those used in MIPS; and
- require participants to adopt a *Medicaid* Medical Home Model or bear financial risk for more than a nominal amount.

The potential benefits of participating in these payment pathways are that they are excluded from MIPS requirements and can receive a 5% bonus as well as APM-specific rewards. There are multiple models of Advanced APMs, but one of the most talked about is the Comprehensive Primary Care Plus model.

Care Coordination Financing: Medicaid Health Homes

There are multiple financing structures related to chronic care management. In addition to PCMHs, both formal and informal financial approaches are possible. Often confused with PCMHs, **Medicaid Health Homes (MHHs)** were created as an optional Medicaid benefit for states to coordinate care for people with Medicaid who have chronic conditions (Shane et al., 2016). They are organizations for people with Medicaid, and who have two or more chronic conditions or a chronic condition and risk of a second one.

The job of the Health Homes is to provide an integrated and coordinator whole person care, which includes all primary, acute, behavioral long-term health services needed to treat the person. Chronic conditions stipulated in the ACA section, which authorized funding of MHHs (Sec. 2703), include mental health, substance abuse, asthma, diabetes, heart disease, and being overweight. States have the option of targeting health home services geographically, and they also have flexibility in designing the specific home health plan; however, they do not have the option of excluding dual covered individuals (those who have both Medicare and Medicaid coverage; Health Homes, n.d.). Under this statute, CMS helps states develop models to coordinate chronic healthcare. States that want to participate receive a 90% enhanced Federal Medical Assistance Percentage (FMAP) for the specific health home services; for the first eight quarters, the program is effective. The enhanced match does not apply to the underlying Medicaid services also provided to people enrolled in a health home, but only the chronic care management portion of the coverage (Health Homes, n.d.).

SUMMARY

Transforming the business of healthcare from individual patient to population outcomes remains an important management challenge. A 2018 report identified the top four reimbursement models for PHM in order as (a) pay-for-performance, (b) FFS + PHM fee, (c) shared savings with upside risk only, and (d) bundled payments (Healthcare Benchmarks, 2018). This trend continues as more organizations seek risk-based and alternative financial arrangements. **Value-based** contracts will reward providers who use innovative delivery models that improve a population's health and manage cost through risk-bearing arrangements.

DISCUSSION QUESTIONS

1. Differences between volume- and value-based payment systems are significant. Why do you think new alternative payment systems were necessary?
2. Why would bundled payments work for well for these two health services—myocardial infraction and hip or knee replacements?
3. Population health mangers assume accountability for selecting appropriate value-based payment arrangements. In upside risk models, the provider shares from the savings without the risks of loss. For example, if the total costs of care are less than budgeted, the savings are shared between payer and provider. If the total costs are more than budgeted, the provider is not at risk to pay. In the downside risk model, the provider shares savings if costs do not exceed the budgeted amount; however, they are at risk to pay if costs exceed the budget. However, under bundled payment models, both provider and payer share risks. The provider carries the utilization risk that the patient will utilize additional services than the bundled amount, whereas the payer carries the insurance risk. Can you provide examples of where each type of value-based payment would be appropriate?
4. Describe the impact of MACRA on payment systems.
5. Why do you think the Medical Home Models are required to use certified EHR technology?
6. Compare and contrast the differences between the Basic and Enhanced APM payment tracks. What are some of the reasons an ACO would pick the Basic track? The Enhanced?
7. Why might it make more sense for a PCMH to use the "three-part model" instead of the ACO payment models?

Toolkit Competency Application

Accountable Care Organization

Improving Quality and Reducing Expenditures: An ACO in Action

"What healthcare providers really want is to do is the right thing for their patients. They just need sustainable financial support for doing that," health economist Mark McClellan, MD, PhD, said at the start of an interview with RevCycleIntelligence.

"'Accountable care organizations' is jargon for the radical concept that when doctors and nurses actually talk to each other about shared patients, there will be fewer mix-ups, less duplication and patients will receive better, more convenient care at a lower cost," said Michael F. Cannon, director of health policy studies at the Cato Institute, in the opinion column "ACO Debacle Exposes Obamacare's Fatal Conceit" for Kaiser Health News (June 2011).

INTRODUCTION

With the launch of MSSP, established by the Patient Protection and Affordable Care Act under President Obama, population health leaders recognized the need to adopt new models of healthcare delivery. The development of this new healthcare delivery model is designed to reduce the national healthcare spending in ways to improve quality and outcomes across populations as noted in this illustration. See Figures 8.2 and 8.3.

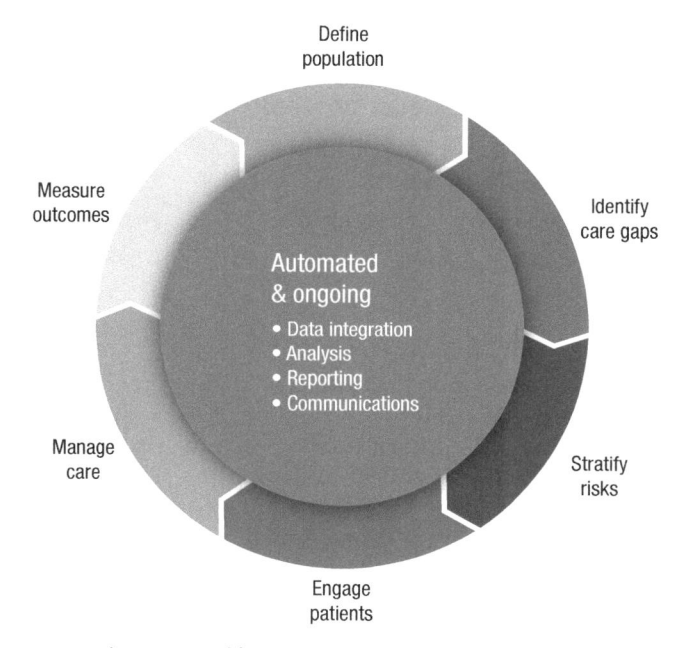

FIGURE 8.2 Population Health Process SPAC International—Population Health Management

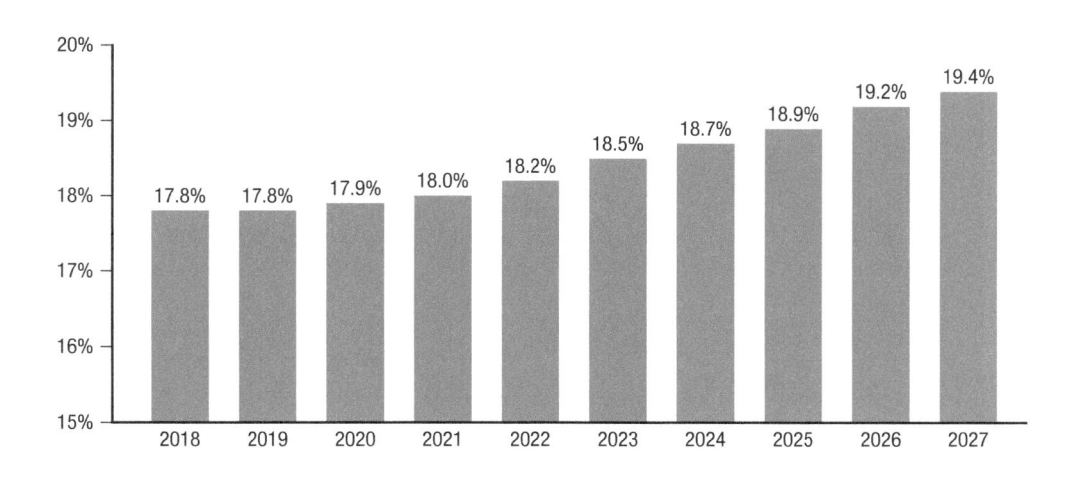

FIGURE 8.3 Projected U.S. Healthcare Expenditures as a Percentage of GDP, 2018–2027. From Center for Medicare & Medicaid Services

Results Speak Volumes

Today, we know how successful ACOs have been in reducing overall healthcare spend. Over 60% of healthcare payments are now linked to quality or value systems (Center for Medicare & Medicaid Services). ACOs in MSSP saved $739.4 million in 2018 after accounting for shared savings and losses that year—the savings were spread across 548 ACOs, which served about 10.1 million Medicare beneficiaries (Center for Medicare & Medicaid Services). Of those ACOs, 66% saved Medicare money by decreasing their costs compared with CMS set spending benchmarks and 37% saved enough to earn shared savings payments for its providers.

An Accountable Care Organization Example: Successful Preventive Care Reduces Healthcare Spend

The Atlantic ACO (AACO) was founded in 2012 as one of the first in MSSP. Such vision attributes that drive the AACO are

- improve individual and population health,
- improve the coordination and delivery of healthcare services,
- reduce the growth of health care expenditures, and
- participate in the transformation of care delivery.

For any ACO to be successful, all healthcare providers must work together to improve overall quality while at the same time at the reduced cost. The advancement of technology has lent itself to improve such quality through EMR coordination across providers to fully develop the "one medical record" for each patient. The AACO has coordinated such effort through the implementation of Epic (an enterprise wide EMR platform)—it has proven that the ability to coordinate patient care more effectively through one-medical record. All providers working together to achieve the best patient outcome while maintaining costs.

Coordination of care is critical for ACOs and population health success. The ability to manage our high-risk patients (diabetes, hypertension, vascular disease, heart failure, and coronary artery disease) is the primary focus to maintain expenditures and increase quality among these populations. Within the AACO patient population, the management of these high-risk populations reduced emergency room visits by 2.8% and inpatient admissions by 4.6%.

Another successful strategy for the AACO involved actively engaging physicians in meeting national benchmarks and monitoring their patient's outcomes. It focused primarily on the 33 quality indicators noted in Exhibit 8.1.

The purpose of any ACO Performance Improvement Incentive Program (Exhibit 8.2) is to engage providers to change behaviors in the overall care of patients that will enhance their population's outcomes.

	Preventive Health-Adult
1	Flu Shot
2	Pneumococcal Vaccine
3	Weight Screening and Follow Up

EXHIBIT 8.1 MSSP—33 Quality Indicators Developed by Medicare

MSSP, Medicare Shared Savings Program.

4	Tobacco Use Assessment and Intervention
5	Depression Screening
6	Colorectal Cancer Screening
7	Mammography Screening
8	Blood Pressure within 2 years
	At Risk Populations
	Diabetes
9	HGA1C < 8
10	LDL < 100
11	Blood Pressure < 140/90
12	Tobacco Non-Use
13	Aspirin Use
14	HGA1C < 9
	HTN
15	Blood Pressure Control
	Ischemic Vascular Disease
16	LDL < 100
17	ASA or Another Antithrombotic
	Heart Failure
18	B-Blocker for Systolic Dysfunction
	Coronary Artery Disease
19	Drug Therapy for LDL Lowering
20	ACE/ARB

	Care Coordination/Patient Safety
21	All Condition Readmissions
22	COPD Admissions
23	CHF Admissions
24	PCPs who Qualify for EMR Incentive
25	Med Reconcile after Inpatient Discharge
26	Fall Screening Done

	CAHPS: Patient/Caregiver Experience
27	Timely Care: Appointments and Information
28	Doctor Communication
29	Patient's Rating of Doctor
30	Access to Specialists
31	Health Promotion and Education
32	Shared Decision Making
33	Health Status/Functional Status

EXHIBIT 8.1 *(Continued)*
This sample spreadsheet example includes specific metrics used in the AACO to measure success.

Key Performance Indicators - Quarterly Report

PY2 Medicare Shared Savings Program (Attributed Data Sharing Members)
Claims: 12 months ending March 31, 2014, paid through May 2014
PMPY Cost - Risk Adjusted
Sort: By Region - By Practice
New 1st quarter 2014 practices have been excluded from the report due to immature claims data.

Region	Group Name	Beneficiary Data Sharing Count	Average Current Risk	Total Current Cost PMPY	Inpatient PMPY	Total IP Count Per 1,000	TIN ALOS	Total ER Count Per 1,000	Hospital Outpatient PMPY	SNF PMPY	Home Health PMPY	Hospice PMPY	Physician (Specialists & PCP) PMPY	DME PMPY
	Milliman Benchmark - Moderately Managed Market			$11,100	$2,780	277		335	$1,236	$1,200			$3,660	
	Milliman Benchmark - Highly Managed Market			$8,168	$2,568	224		212	$1,128	$840			$2,640	
		1	1.71	$87,443	$64,410	13,000	104.0	4,000	$9,580	$-	$1,617	$-	$16,834	$-
		59	0.94	$6,294	$1,251	85	0.7	186	$668	$72	$86	$-	$3,209	$124
		130	1.16	$19,900	$7,457	485	6.8	954	$2,376	$3,144	$718	$491	$5,165	$278
		34	1.65	$15,928	$3,525	529	6.6	1,118	$1,229	$1,785	$1,873	$1050	$5,307	$383
		1	0.17	$16,473	$-	-	0.0	-	$1,640	$-	$-	$-	$11,255	$-
		2	0.70	$18,086	$-	-	0.0	1,500	$8,813	$-	$-	$-	$6,572	$405
		39	1.14	$16,789	$4,262	385	3.7	359	$1,457	$4,849	$1,259	$1,257	$4,113	$130
		414	1.01	$3,574	$1,208	58	0.9	87	$539	$257	$110	$177	$1,286	$34
		168	0.81	$15,036	$4,864	220	1.9	387	$3,521	$256	$384	$55	$4,768	$186
		1	0.67	$16,954	$-	-	0.0	2,000	$2,487	$-	$-	$-	$11,191	$-
		297	0.82	$12,415	$3,058	209	1.9	492	$2,254	$1,504	$447	$488	$3,923	$203
		29	0.90	$9,165	$2,259	138	1.0	621	$1,598	$-	$369	$-	$4,228	$166
		81	1.17	$15,645	$4,886	568	4.6	1,407	$2,645	$1,416	$1,588	$78	$4,980	$302
		86	1.14	$10,859	$3,378	342	3.5	1,646	$2,056	$1,281	$553	$23	$3,455	$75
		20	1.02	$12,211	$2,634	50	2.8	400	$3,699	$-	$280	$-	$5,917	$205
		35	0.90	$12,454	$3,696	143	2.5	457	$2,600	$-	$127	$-	$4,830	$429
		101	0.95	$9,105	$3,411	69	2.0	257	$1,295	$69	$200	$-	$3,469	$122
		49	0.98	$18,062	$5,477	265	2.9	327	$1,832	$3,099	$702	$-	$6,037	$143
		78	0.58	$16,911	$9,338	256	3.4	333	$3,606	$-	$243	$1,045	$5,404	$271

EXHIBIT 8.2 AACO Key Performance Indicators
AACO, Atlantic ACO.
Source: ACO, used with permission

SUMMARY

These types of initiatives under the AACO tenure have saved the healthcare industry and Medicare more than $45 million. Quality management and aggressive preventive care initiatives will help maintain/reduce inpatient and SNF admissions, emergency department visits, while increasing primary care visits. To conclude, ACOs are "transformational" vehicles focused to move providers from a historical FFS payment methodology to a value-based/outcome payment model. Ultimately, ACOs will transform into "risk" initiatives and structures between healthcare providers and payers. See Figure 8.4.

CASE STUDY DISCUSSION QUESTIONS

1. Why do you think it took at least 3 years to achieve significant savings?
2. Given the five categories identified on the Performance Improvement Plan slide, why did AACO target patient engagement?
3. Where did AACO make its biggest gains in MSSP?
4. Where do we go from here? Is the ACO vision achievable in the long-term?
5. Can our healthcare system continue to achieve quality measures while reducing costs?
6. Why must we partner with our third-party insurance carriers to achieve success?

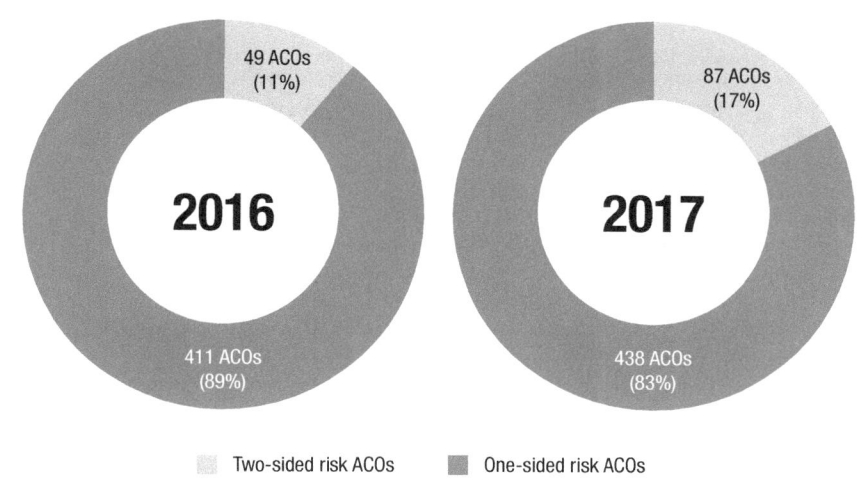

FIGURE 8.4 More Medicare ACOs Assuming Two-Sided Risk

ACO, accountable care organization.

REFERENCES

American Academy of Pediatrics. (n.d.) *Getting paid: Alternative payment models*. Retrieved May 18, 2021, from https://www.aap.org/en-us/professional-resources/practice-transformation/getting-paid/Pages/Payment-Models.aspx

American Hospital Association. (2019). *Evolving care models—Aligning care delivery with emerging payment models*. AHA Center for Health Innovation. https://www.aha.org/center/emerging-issues/market-insights/evolving-care-models/aligning-care-delivery-emerging-payment-models

APM Framework: Overview. (2017). *CMS health care payment-learning action network*. https://hcp-lan.org/apm-refresh-white-paper/

Basu, S., Phillips, R. S., Song, Z., Landon, B. E., & Bitton, A. (2016). Effects of new funding models for patient-centered medical homes on primary care practice finances and services: Results of a microsimulation model. *The Annals of Family Medicine*, 14(5), 404–414. https://doi.org/10.1370/afm.1960

Bresnick, J. (2017, July 17). *How does an ACO differ from the patient-centered medical home?* Health IT Analytics. https://healthitanalytics.com/news/how-does-an-aco-differ-from-the-patient-centered-medical-home

Centers Medicare and Medicaid Services. (2020). *For providers*. https://www.cms.gov/Medicare/Medicare-Fee-for-Service-Payment/sharedsavingsprogram/for-providers

Croft, B., & Parish, S. L. (2013). Care integration in the Patient Protection and Affordable Care Act: Implications for behavioral health. *Administration and Policy in Mental Health*, 40(4), 258–263. https://doi.org/10.1007/s10488-012-0405-0

Findlay, S. (2017). *Implementing MACRA*. Health Affairs. https://www.healthaffairs.org/do/10.1377/hpb20170327.272560/full/

Healthcare Benchmarks. (2018). *What are the leading reimbursement models for population health management programs? 2018 Healthcare Benchmarks: Population Health Management*. Health Information Network. www.hin.com/chartoftheweek/leading_reimbursement_models_for_population_health_management_programs_printable.html#.X-y_a-dOk2w

Health Care Payment Learning and Action Network (HCP_LAN). (2017). *Alternative payment framework*. The Mitre Corporation. https://hcp-lan.org/workproducts/apm-refresh-whitepaper-final.pdf

Health Homes. (n.d.). *Medicaid*. Retrieved August 12, 2020, from https://www.medicaid.gov/medicaid/long-term-services-supports/health-homes/index.html

Kwon, S. (1996). Structure of financial incentive systems for providers in managed care plans. *Medical Care Research and Review, 53*(2), 149–161. https://doi.org/10.1177/107755879605300202

Leventhal, R. (2020, October 8). *Humana touts $4B in 2019 savings due to value-based care agreement*. Healthcare Innovation. https://www.hcinnovationgroup.com/policy-value-based-care/medicare-medicaid/news/21157584/humana-touts-4b-in-2019-savings-due-to-valuebased-careagreements?utm_source=HI+Daily+NL&utm_medium=email&utm_campaign=CPS201008019&o_eid=6978A6266356F5Z&rdx.ident%5Bpull%5D=omeda%7C6978A6266356F5Z&oly_enc_id=6978A6266356F5Z

McWilliams, J. M. (2017). MACRA—big fix or big problem? *Annals of Internal Medicine, 167*(2), 122–124. https://doi.org/10.7326/M17-0230

NAACOS. (n.d.). Home. *National Association of ACOs*. Retrieved August 22, 2020, from https://www.naacos.com/

NEJM Catalyst. (2018, March 1). *What is pay for performance in healthcare?* https://catalyst.nejm.org/doi/full/10.1056/CAT.18.0245

PCMH Costs, Benefits and Incentives. (n.d.). *American College of Physicians*. Retrieved August 13, 2020, from https://www.acponline.org/practice-resources/business-resources/payment/delivery-and-payment-models/patient-centered-medical-home/pcmh-costs-benefits-and-incentives

The Physicians Advocacy Institute. (2020, July 13). *Shift from volume-based care to value-based care*. University of Illinois Chicago. Retrieved May 18, 2021, from https://healthinformatics.uic.edu/blog/shift-from-volume-based-care-to-value-based-care/

Population Health Management Framework (PHA). (2018). *Population Health Alliance*. https://populationhealthalliance.org/research/understanding-population-health/

Sampson, C. (2016, May 06). *Top 5 facts to know about MACRA alternative payment models*. Revcycle Intelligence. https://revcycleintelligence.com/news/top-5-facts-to-know-about-macra-alternative-payment-models

Sayeed, Z., El-Othmani, M., Shaffer, W. O., & Saleh, K. J. (2017). The Medicare Access and CHIP Reauthorization Act (MACRA) of 2015: What's new? *JAAOS, 25*(6), e121–e130. https://doi.org/10.5435/JAAOS-D-17-00151

Shane, D. M., Nguyen-Hoang, P., Bentler, S. E., Damiano, P. C., & Momany, E. T. (2016). Medicaid health home reducing costs and reliance on emergency department. *Medical Care, 54*(8), 752–757. https://doi.org/10.1097/MLR.0000000000000555

Wagner, S. L. (2018). *Fundamentals of medical practice management*. Health Administration Press/Association of University Programs in Health Administration.

CHAPTER 9

Population Health Models—Part II: Care Coordination Continuum, Behavior Change, Patient Engagement, and Telehealth

Anne M. Hewitt

KEY TERMS

Care and Case Management
Chronic Disease
Coordinated Care
Health Belief Model
Patient Engagement

Postacute Care
Self-Management Education (SME)
Transitions of Care
Transtheoretical (Stages of Change) Model
Virtual Care (Telehealth)

LEARNING OBJECTIVES

1. Discuss ways new population health models meet challenges for aligning medical and community resources.
2. Describe the strategies for implementing coordinated care for patients with chronic disease conditions.
3. Apply an evidence-based health behavior change model to a population at risk.
4. Assess virtual and face-to-face patient engagement techniques and models.

> Podcasts that exemplify the content of this chapter are available at Springer Publishing Connect™
>
> Podcast 9.1. Could You Identify Four New Patient-Centered Care Strategies?
> Podcast 9.2. Virtual Care or Telehealth?

Access the podcast online at http://connect.springerpub.com/content/book/978-0-8261-4427-0/part/part03/chapter/ch09

5. Compare care versus case management alternatives for postacute situations.
6. Analyze technological advances and options for providing telehealth/virtual health.

INTRODUCTION

Population health providers and professionals are generally familiar with health delivery models such as accountable care organizations (ACOs), patient-centered medical homes (PCMHs), and integrated delivery systems. This chapter presents the emerging models that address the challenges of today's health sector in preparation for the future. These innovative patient-centric, coordinated-care models, and strategies focus on the following:

- Chronic care in vulnerable and at-risk (Medicaid, Medicare) populations
- Telehealth, remote care monitoring, and wearables
- Expansion and enhancement of postacute care options to improve gaps and transitions of care
- Improving overall health outcomes via health behavior change and patient engagement models

Although there is tremendous diversity in these population heath management (PHM) approaches, they all address the challenge of improving access, quality, and cost for the most vulnerable and high-priority populations. The commonality is their innovative approaches that align patient centeredness, tailored interventions, community resources, and organizational cultural and environmental interventions. These exact concepts are depicted in the *Population Health Alliance Framework* (Figure 9.1).

In this model, note the highlighted intervention actions occur after completion of risk segmentation and stratification analyses showing the necessity of clearly identifying populations at risk for chronic care coordination.

Addressing the Coordinated Care Challenge

Despite the many important advances in how we provide care, there are still major gaps in our healthcare delivery system, which leads to unacceptable health outcomes. The stubborn issue of health disparities among the underserved and minorities remains prominent and a priority concern, along with another important driver of cost and poor outcomes—gaps in the transition of care system for those who need chronic care. As America continues to age, these individuals constitute a significant portion of the vulnerable health population. At least one in two Americans will suffer from chronic disease conditions in their lifetime (CDC, 2018). Medicare-eligible patients represent a population appropriate for developing value-based payment options.

The national health policy sector has responded to these challenges via implementation of the ACO and the PCMH models. To a certain extent, these strategies helped address chronic care transitions and coordination of care that involve multiple care settings for acute, specialty, primary, and **postacute care,** which includes all healthcare activities following acute (treatment) care. However, the revolving door of hospital readmissions within 30 days of discharge continues to cost the health system an inordinate amount of Medicare dollars (Healthstream, 2020). In 2015, the cost was 15 billion for Medicare readmissions (Healthstream, 2019). Given the tremendous impact of the COVID-19

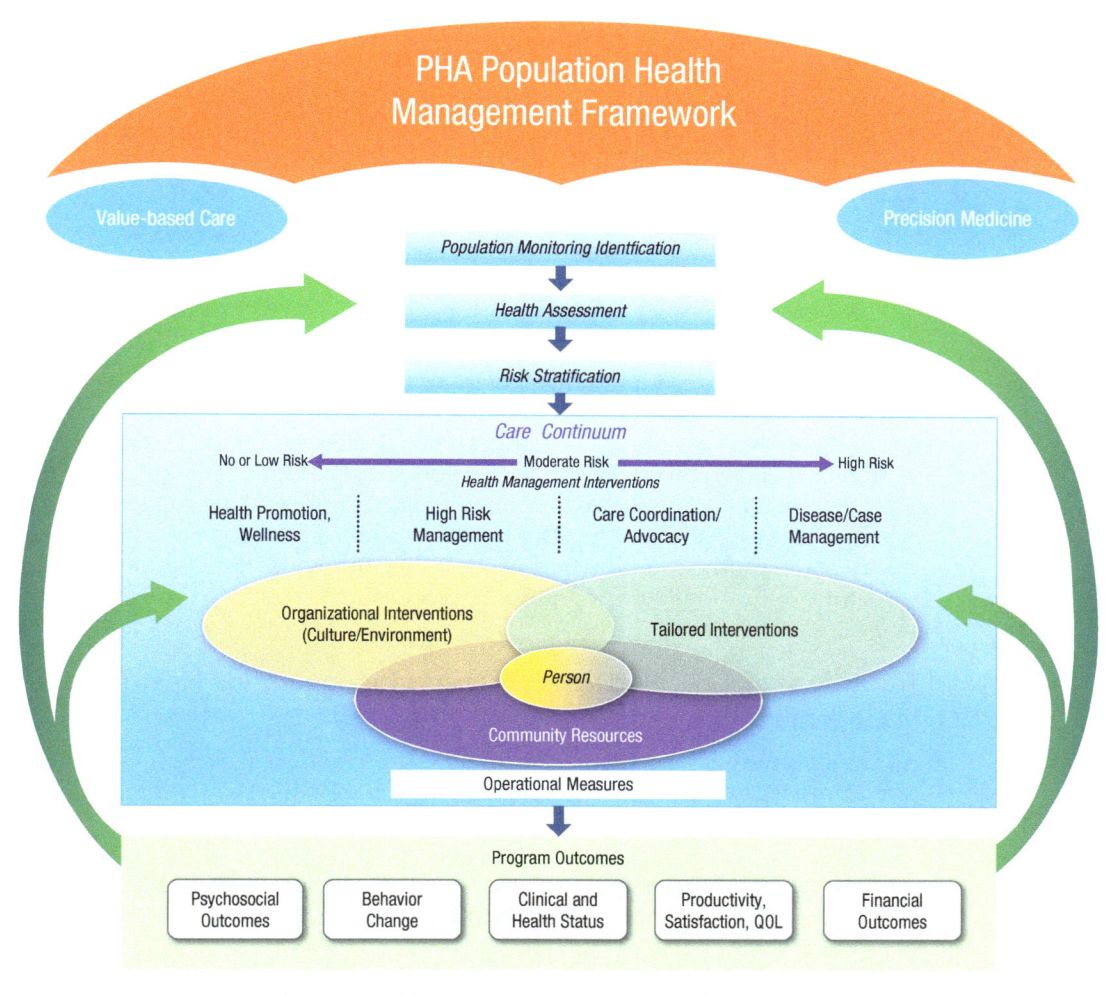

FIGURE 9.1 PHA Population Health Management Framework

PHA, Population Health Alliance.

Source: Population Health Alliance. (n.d.). *PHA—Population health management framework*. Population Health Alliance. Reprinted with permission © PHA PHM Framework 2010 PHA–PMH Umbrella for VBC 2018 RMaljanian. https://population healthalliance.org/research/understanding-population-health/

pandemic on the health sector, the gaps in care transitions become more prominent, as the public appears reluctant to take advantage of traditional health services due to fear of contracting the disease (Johns Hopkins Medicine, 2020). This "individual hesitancy" factor may result in regular checkups and routine care, for the most vulnerable, being postponed or ignored (McGinley, 2020).

Unlike acute disease, which is a condition that lasts a short time, comes on rapidly, and is accompanied by distinct symptoms, multiple definitions for chronic disease exist. A commonly used statement, from U.S. National Center for Health Statistics, defines chronic disease as one lasting 3 months or more," which generally cannot be prevented by vaccines or cured by medication, and does not disappear (MedicineNet, 2016).

Who are the most vulnerable chronic disease populations? Strong evidence suggests that individuals with any of these five major diseases/conditions constitute the chronic care subgroup that requires systematic and continuous healthcare and medical interactions (see Exhibit 9.1).

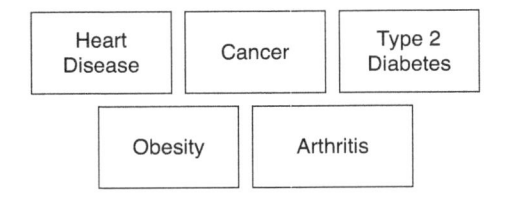

[Heart Disease] [Cancer] [Type 2 Diabetes]
[Obesity] [Arthritis]

EXHIBIT 9.1 Common Chronic Diseases/Conditions Associated With Mortality or Disability in the United States

Other chronic care conditions remain prevalent and are often mentioned: asthma, chronic obstructive pulmonary disease (COPD), and hypertension. Even AIDS can be considered a chronic disease, and one of the most forgotten categories is behavioral health conditions (Bernell & Howard, 2016). Currently, the CDC reports (CDC, 2020) 90% of the nation's 3.5 trillion in annual healthcare expenses are for people with chronic or mental health conditions. **Coordinated** care implies an established health plan that ensures access to appropriate providers and health services when needed. Regardless of the chronic disease type, the implications for continuous and coordinated care will be present.

Transitions of Care Model: Implications for Population Health Management

As the continuum of heathcare expands, the need for better transition of care approaches becomes evident. **Transitions of care** refer to the linkages between primary care, acute care, and multiple options for postacute care. Coleman's Four Pillars of Transition of Care provides an essential model for developing PHM workflows to assist chronic care populations (Coleman, 2007). The criteria include the following:

√ Medication self-management
√ Use of a dynamic patient-centered, personal health record that is patient-friendly
√ Timely primary care/specialty care follow-up based on evidenced-based research
√ Identification of signs or "red flags" that indicate a change in condition

While these goals were originally designed as inclusive criteria for ensuring appropriate transitions of care from acute to postacute, additional options are now available. PHM providers and managers may choose to adopt evidence-based **SME** programs as an additional transition strategy to address a patient's condition. SMEs are programs that educate patients in ways to help manage their chronic symptoms and diseases such as asthma, arthritis, diabetes, COPD, and chronic pain.

One of most popular SME is the Chronic Disease Self-Management Program, which features an interactive workshop for people with all types of chronic conditions (CDC, 2018). This evidence-based program helps people develop skills and gain confidence to manage their various chronic conditions. The beneficial impact is a reduction in demand for unnecessary primary care visits and more importantly fewer ED visits. State health departments began implementing chronic disease self-management programs (SMPs) as an effective PHM strategy for at-risk populations.

> **? DID YOU KNOW?**
>
> **State Health Self-Management Education Example**
>
> One public example of a population health approach is the adoption of general health promotion initiatives tailored to seniors who suffer proportionately from chronic diseases. New Jersey's Department of Human Services, Division of Aging Services publishes a monthly e-newsletter available to the public—"HealthEASE" (Office of Community Resources, Education and Wellness 2020). Provided here is a sample list of health promotion–inspired SMPs that were transferred to virtual formats due to the COVID-19 pandemic.
>
> **HealthEASE**
>
> A Matter of Balance: https://www.state.nj.us/humanservices/doas/documents/MOB%20Contact%20List.pdf
> Move Today: https://www.state.nj.us/humanservices/doas/documents/movetodaysites.pdf
> Project Healthy Bones: https://www.state.nj.us/humanservices/doas/documents/PHB%20sites%20and%20description%202014.doc
> Stress Busters for Family Caregivers: https://www.state.nj.us/humanservices/doas/documents/SB%20Contact%20List.pdf
> Tai Ji Quan: Moving for Better Balance: https://www.state.nj.us/humanservices/doas/documents/NJ%20TJQMBB%20Contact%20List%202.5.20.pdf
> Take Control of Your Health: https://www.state.nj.us/humanservices/doas/home/tchagencies.html
>
> This initiative is an excellent example of an evidence-based program that became a successful chronic disease model as the HealthEASE program facilitates the adoption of SMPs. HealthEASE aligns with PHM goals that emphasize access, quality of care, and value-based initiatives. (Shepard et al., 2021).

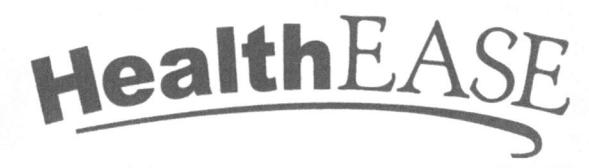

Postacute Care Strategies of Care

One of the most difficult hand-offs facing transition of care coordinators is the patient's journey from acute to postacute care, as options for these types of care require complex coordination.

Whether the care coordinator is based in the acute care setting (on-site) for face-to-face consultation, as part of a PCMH services, or accountable for hospital outpatient arrangements with patient and family, the health outcomes are dependent on well-executed delivery pathways. Embedded care managers are generally nurses (Hines & Mercury, 2013) and are being included in primary care practices as part of the transition from volume-based to value reimbursements systems.

Alternative sites for postacute care have expanded beyond traditional nursing homes to include skilled nursing facilities, rehabilitation options, and enhanced home-health programs. Palliative care and hospice care have also experienced greater interest by patients interested concerned with end-of-life care options. Improved electronic medical records with additional access for primary and acute care health providers and patient portal availability enhance the timely and useful flow of real-time data for both patients' transitions of care.

Hospital Without Walls: Population Health Innovation

In 2019, CMS expanded its acute hospital at home program (Raths, 2020a), and in March 2020, CMS announced a Hospital Without Walls program (Raths, 2020b), which includes regulatory flexibility for hospitals to provide services in locations beyond their existing walls. Hospitals receiving waivers to integrate this population health delivery care option can now provide acute healthcare services in the home setting and expand home health services into a full-service line. Treatment for over 60 acute conditions such as asthma, congestive heart failure, pneumonia, and COPD care is covered, which corresponds to those chronic conditions that impact population health's financial outcomes. Eligible patients must require acute inpatient admission to a hospital with at least daily rounding by a physician and monitoring conducted by a medical team. Recent research suggests that home hospital care can decrease healthcare costs significantly (<30%) compared with usual hospital care and decrease the number of readmissions by more than half (Levine et al., 2020). The enhanced monitoring of patients at home via virtual or in-person now lessens the chance of missing warning signs and dramatic changes in patient health status and reduces the number of hospital patients that could be successfully treated at home.

Population Health Management Comprehensive Care Models and Care Strategies

Behavior Change Models

The World Health Organization reports that 60% of factors related to individual health and quality of life are correlated to lifestyle (Farhud, 2015). Others report that lifestyle behavior accounts for 40%–50% of our health status (O'Neill-Hayes & Delk, 2018). Everyone's lifestyle reflects a collection of daily health behavior choices. Improving individuals' healthy behaviors is a primary component of any PHM intervention. We can all agree that health education alone often is not enough to change unhealthy behaviors although it is a required first step. *How do we encourage seniors to get vaccinations? How do we prevent obesity? How do we help smokers to quit?*

Tailored interventions, to assist positive behavior change, are often based on well-researched and evidence-based theories of change. Two commonly used health behavior theories targeting behavior change are the Health Belief Model (HBM) and the Transtheoretical/Stages of Change Model (TTM/SOC). The HBM, developed in the 1950s by a social psychologists from the U.S. Public Health Service, is a model that attempts to explain human health behavior (Champion & Skinner, 2008). This model suggests that individuals are motivated to change their health behavior by examining three major components: expectations, threats, and cues to action (Rosenstock et al., 1988). The model also integrates the concept of self-efficacy, which refers to an individual's perception of their capabilities for changing a behavior. Table 9.1 offers a quick example of how this theory would work for COVID-19.

Integrating messages and reminders into PHM programs that help people examines their own perceptions as outlined in the HBM will increase their likelihood of positive behavior change. But what if the chronic disease behavior that needs to be altered is more of a habit or an addiction?

Another useful behavioral change framework, the **Transtheoretical Model (TTM)** of behavior change, addresses the cycle of addictive behaviors and targets the broader issue of lifestyle behavior needing long-term change (Prochaska et al., 2008). There are five main core phases SOC: precontemplation,

TABLE 9.1 Application of the Health Behavior Model Theory

Health Behavior Model Theory Components	COVID-19 Example
Expectations	
Perceived Benefits of Action	• If I wear a mask, I will not be as likely to get COVID-19
Perceived Barriers to Action	• I do not breathe as well when I wear a mask and it is inconvenient
Perceived Self-Efficacy	• I am sure that I would wear a mask if I had one in the car or my purse. I can do that.
Threats	
Perceived Susceptibility	• Not everybody who does not wear a mask gets the disease
Perceived Severity	• Well, even if I get it, I will not be that sick
Cues to Action	
Media	• A TV message mention Stop the Spread "wearing a mask is the easiest thing you can do to protect yourself"
Personal Influences	• All my friends have started wearing masks now
Reminders	• The stores where I shop all require a mask.

TABLE 9.2 Application of the Transtheoretical Model (TTM): Stages of Change

Precontemplation—Individual may be unaware of problem behavior or devalue the need to change	"I'm fine. I don't drink more than anybody else."
Contemplation—Awareness and thinking about the near future 6 months	"What if I cut down how much I drink? Should I?"
Preparation—Individuals may start to take small positive action steps in the next 30 days	"Okay, I am ready to quit. I will not go to the liquor store next weekend."
Action—Behavior change has begun with intention to continue	"It has been six months since I cut down and finally quit drinking. Joining the gym really helped."
Maintenance—Evidence of positive behavior change for at least six months, but chance of relapse	"It wasn't easy to say no to my friend, but I'm not going to start drinking again".
Termination—A possible stage of no relapse indications, but rarely achieved.	"I know that I may want to drink again, but I don't intend to go back to that again."

contemplation, preparation, action, maintenance, and termination. We know that often individuals pass through a series of stages, as they seek to change their habits. Each stage of change can be identified by a health counselor/coach and appropriate support provided. This attention to specific detail and the ability to provide tailored messaging and reminders are key to the successful outcomes of this model. TTM is a cycle model of change meaning that an individual can skip over processes or need to cycle through one of them again (LaMorte, 2019). We all know how difficult these steps can be! In Table 9.2, an example shows TTM applied to a substance misuse situation with a student who wants to give up vaping, as they now recognize their addiction behavior.

Regardless of the type of health behavior theory integrated into and supporting a PHM continuation of care program, these interventions assist individuals to change negative lifestyles and are critical for successful outcomes.

Patient Engagement

One of the most common problems in healthcare is managing a nonadherent patient. In fact, the cost of non-compliance costs the U.S. healthcare system over $300 billion a year (Iuga & McGuire, 2014). Population health professionals now recognize that the term patient "compliance" is not an appropriate term to be used in the care process (Culberton, 2020), and the focus should be on an interactive relationship that is symmetrical between patient and healthcare provider. The population health challenge is to engage the individual patient or consumer in their own healthcare decision-making.

The success of PHM programs for comprehensive and coordinated care interventions requires patient engagement. Actively engaged consumers have better outcomes and lower costs (Scott, 2019).

Patient engagement is often described as activities or efforts to involve an individual in their own care (Graffigna & Barello, 2018) and is a very broad term to include all efforts for encouraging patients to participate in their personal care plans and work in partnership with health providers and team members. Patient engagement activities can be as simple as scheduling an annual wellness visit or more complex such as monitoring and daily management of diabetes

Patient engagement programs and initiatives constitute an important part of PHM's goals to assist individuals attain optimum health status. Note that health psychology findings suggests that not all chronic care patients want responsibility or accountability of their own care process.

The Patient Engagement Capacity Model, developed in 2019, aligns two sets of overlapping factors that impact a patient's capacity to engage (Sieck et al., 2019). In Figure 9.2, the triangular represents the reciprocal determinism component of interaction where the environment, person, and behavior all unite to determine behavior impact. The converging circle figure shows the conditions essential for the patient to develop the capabilities to engage. Together, they form a patient engagement capacity framework.

All population program return-on-investment reviews and evaluations will benefit from recognizing that lower patient participation rates and

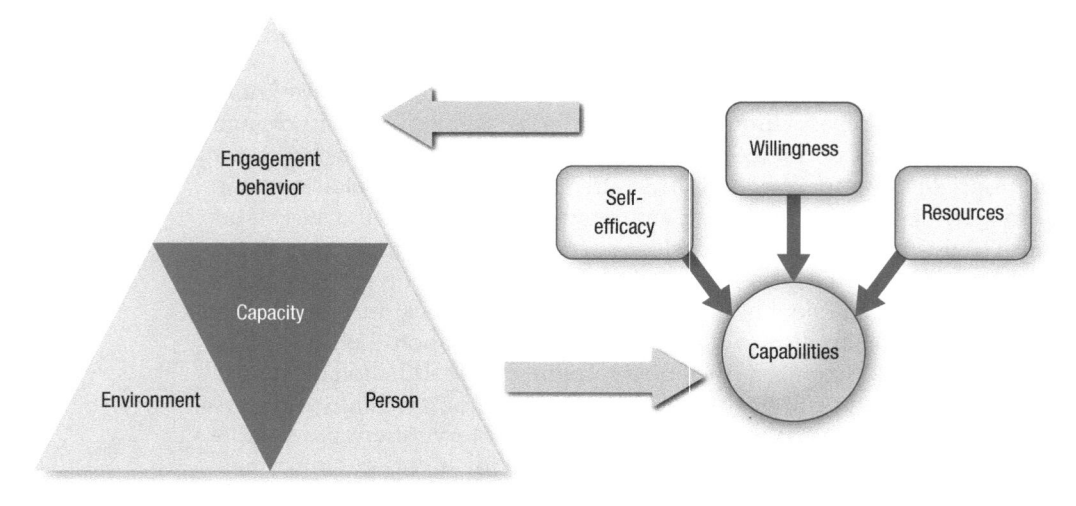

FIGURE 9.2 Framing Capacity for Patient Engagement
Adapted from Sieck et al., 2019

unfavorable outcomes may be linked to individual's level of engagement capacity. Hibbard and colleagues (2005) developed a Patient Activation Measure to assess an individual's level of engagement. An individual's score can help tailor interactions and communications that will encourage participation and strengthen their self-management capacities and ultimately lead to better health outcomes.

The Role and Components of Patient Engagement Programs

Patient engagement impacts not only the individual's health but also the success of population health interventions and programs, and the organization's ability to provide cost-appropriate care. If patients are not engaged, unhappy with their interaction experiences, or dissatisfied, the organization risks significant negative financial impact. Note that patient engagement differs from patient experience and satisfaction as shown in Figure 9.3.

Population heath managers are responsible for selecting and implementing various strategies and interventions that ensure patient engagement and this will directly contribute to improvements in quality healthcare and lower cost. Successful patient engagement is not an easy process and involves strategic decision-making based on population risk stratification and segmentation.

Patient engagement programs often include multiple components to achieve successful outcomes. A recent industry report (HIN, 2019) highlighted that successful health insurance companies include the following as part of their patient engagement strategy:

- Inclusion of patient/family/caregiver education on their chronic disease is one of the most common patient engagement strategies.
- In addition to the stakeholder education strategy, the use of embedded care coordinators is the second highest rated approach.
- Continued support for the use of care navigators is accountable for patient engagement, experience, and satisfaction.
- The use of patient-centered platforms and portals and mobile technologies is rated highly as effective PE initiatives.
- Recognition of the importance and usability of patient-generated data is becoming more evident.

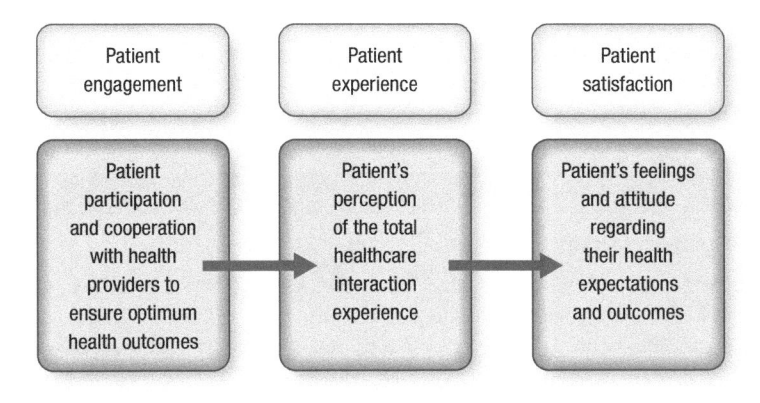

FIGURE 9.3 Definition Comparison of Patient Engagement, Experience, and Satisfaction

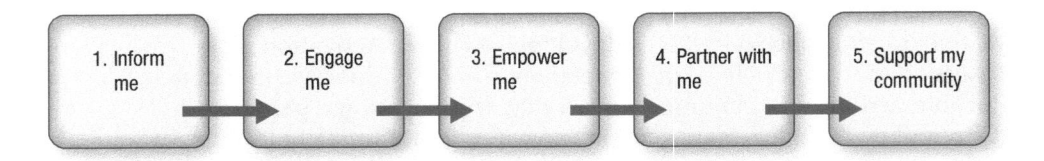

1. Inform me → 2. Engage me → 3. Empower me → 4. Partner with me → 5. Support my community

FIGURE 9.4 Five Phases of Patient Engagement

Social determinants of health remain the most common barrier to patient engagement. This finding highlights the role of including SDOH in electronic health medical records to ensure all health providers involved in a patient's transition of care recognize the potential negative impact of these conditions.

Aligning Technological Advances With Patient Engagement

Technological advances, especially the electronic medical record, have accelerated the adoption of patient engagement activities and strategies. An early patient engagement model, developed by the National Ehealth Collaborative (Perna, 2013). Figure 9.4 shows the patient engagement as a continuum framework with five phases.

Each phase focuses on engaging the patient through the healthcare delivery journey and suggests digital tools and strategies that are tailored for each stage. As the patient/consumer progresses along the continuum, the complexity of the interventions increases. While relatively easy to visualize, the actual execution of this PHM strategy is extremely difficult.

As technology supporting the health sector continues to expand and mature, more patient-health engagement service companies now offer mobile-based alternatives that meld health behavior theory with sophisticated health information technology infrastructures to provide real-time patient support and engagement. The m-health patient interactions may include the use of special apps or daily text reminders. The empowered patient is more likely to be fully engaged with their own healthcare when cues to action are present.

Why do patient engagement efforts fail? Often because individual patients are asked to assume too much individual accountability for changing behaviors and self-managing their own health issues (O'Keefe & Dunn, 2016). Adopting a dual and complementary strategy of both individual patient engagement interventions and addressing relevant socioeconomic factors will likely increase successful patient engagement outcomes for high-priority populations.

? DID YOU KNOW?

Case Management Versus Care Management

Case managers and care managers often have overlapping functions. Case managers have a broad role in tailoring care for individuals with complex needs, while care managers focus on ensuring coordinating less at-risk patient's routine care (Cuddeback & Fisher, 2016). Role differences may be directly associated with their accountability to either healthcare organization (hospital), health provider, or health insurer (Miller, 2013). Table 9.3 provides a basic comparison tool.

TABLE 9.3 Care and Case Manager Comparison Matrix

	Care Managers	Case Managers
Educational preparation	Social work, nursing, psychology, gerontology, and other health-related fields	Social workers and nurses primarily, with other health counselors when necessary
Typical employers	Primarily private for profit and (some nonprofits)	Insurance company, hospital, community mental health, and so forth Federal—vulnerable populations specific
Limits	Client defines the scope of work (based on a care plan that is developed with the client's input)	Agency defines the limits/scope of work, manages a specific disease, issue, condition or event, and adheres to regulations, policies, and funders
Focus	Holistic, client/family-centered approach with advocacy component for obtaining client needs to achieve maximum benefit	Client/patient-centered and considers medical/legal/financial issues that can involve stakeholders Focus on demand management of care and overutilization perhaps due to noncompliance
Primary stakeholder	Client	Can be a funding source (i.e., insurance company, entitlement, hospital, etc.)
Variable payment mechanisms	Client pays cost (occasionally some reimbursement from long-term care insurance but this is not typical)	Agency-specific funding (hospital system, insurance company, government program, for example)
Goal	Promote better quality of life, maintain independence to the extent possible	Improve health status, cost-effective outcomes, and efficiencies, and reduce overutilization of services

As you would imagine, **care and case management** roles differ in educational requirements, goals, and focus, as well as stakeholder involvement and payment methods. Care coordinators is a newer term for a hybrid role between case and care management. The Agency for Healthcare Research and Quality (AHRQ) defines the role of care coordination as involving deliberately organizing patient care activities and sharing information among all of the participants concerned with a patient's care to achieve safer and more effective care (AHRQ, n.d.) For PHM, coordinated care results in more successful health outcomes, the best use of resources for the patient both safely and efficiently.

Virtual Care or Telehealth? Technology Innovation across the Care Coordination Continuum

Population health managers readily recognize that technology has been the driving factor for health innovation in the past 20 years. The sophistication of IT platforms and data analytics supports the use of mobile technology for consumer healthcare and communication.

Technology integration throughout the healthcare continuum represents not only a daily operations challenge for population health managers but also a future opportunity for enhancing population health outcomes.

Whether you use the term **telehealth** or **virtual care**, you are probably referring to a digital interaction between a health provider and patient. Although confusion exists between the various terminology for telehealth, telemedicine, e-health, virtual, and mobile health, the common factor is the ability to interface with health consumers without them physically coming to a healthcare location where health providers are located. How important is virtual care? Experts suggest that digital health will reshape the healthcare sector, especially patient engagement, care delivery and payment models (Mohammed & Libby, 2020). Rather than create categories for types of virtual health, one management perspective is to develop ways to leverage digital applications, such as integrating virtual care into service lines, incorporating wearables and enhancing workflows.

Leveraging Digital Applications for Population Health Management

Evidence suggests that virtual visits increased significantly and, in some cases, doubled during the COVID-19 pandemic (O'Shea, 2020). Two service lines with the largest increases were behavioral health and chronic care (Landi, 2020). Health managers routinely face challenges in managing these two at-risk populations, and the rapid adoption of telehealth proved especially beneficial.

Behavioral health providers were among the first rapidly transitioned from bricks and mortar experiences to virtual care. A primary reason for the quick behavioral health delivery changeover was the need for of tele addiction visits due to rapid rise of substance misuse and abuse during the COVID-19 pandemic (Raths, 2020c). A recent study revealed that 80% of behavioral healthcare providers now deliver care virtually at least 60% of the time, and another 70% indicated at least 40% of their care will be virtual in the future (Qualifacts & NCBH, 2020). E-health and m-health initiatives appear to be very acceptable and accessible for behavioral health interactions that previously relied on continued relationships and the need for regular, face-to-face reinforcement visits with health providers. Virtual care visits should transition from an alternative care delivery option to an integrated component of coordinated care management for these populations.

Telemedicine has always served as a viable option for rural health where specialists were limited. During the pandemic, telehealth visits among rural residents peaked at 64% above baseline, which was 10% more than urban health consumers (Landi, 2020). Health planners can continue to enhance this virtual care strategy as opportunities for interstate care become available and access to specialty health providers expands.

Telehealth and telemedicine are part of an integrated **remote health monitoring (RHM) system.** RHMs can aid in reducing 90-day unplanned care, such as emergency department visits and admissions for chronic care populations (HIN, 2018). Health systems report relying on RHMs to follow up with COVID-19 patients (Minemyer, 2020). Remote patient monitoring (RPM) involves complex management decisions, as adoption requires patient selection and engagement, telehealth platform selection, in-house and external health provider training, and scheduling and workflow. Even more important for the population health managers is establishing enrollment, outcomes, and average cost of care planning (HIN, 2015).

Today, health systems report moving beyond the traditional patient conversations to virtual options at the convenience of the consumer. Patient portal reminders and medication adherence apps illustrate two additional virtual care options (Heath, 2019).

Now that Medicare billing is available for telehealth, both health providers and consumers should expect to see a continual increase, as these technologies lower cost delivery and can be just as efficient in their providing positive health outcomes and consumer satisfaction (CMS, 2020).

Integrating Wearables for Remote Care Monitoring and Wellness Populations

Consumers also have responded positively to "wearables" or devices that assist the individual in monitoring a health condition, symptom, or even a positive health lifestyle such as the number of steps taken in a day. Three common examples are as follows:

- Smartwatches and activity trackers can be used to improve lifestyle behaviors and monitor manageable chronic conditions.
- Continuous glucose monitors that transmit data via a digital device to help health providers connect relationships between eating, exercise, and blood sugar levels.
- Leveraging the use of basic wearables such as blood pressure cuffs, scales, and pulse oximeters can facilitate prevention of heart failure and avoid hospitalization (O'Shea, 2020).

The hospital-at-home concept incorporates both remote health monitoring and the wearables strategies. The home hospital concept attempts to reduce the costs of acute care episodes and reduce 30-day readmissions (Biofourmis, 2020). Early studies report significant progress in providing quality care at a lower cost, which also supports a value-based management strategy.

Impacting Population Health Management Workflows

Transforming any health delivery system requires technology expertise and resources and even more so when integrating digital applications to produce virtual health solutions. An obvious first step for population health managers is to leverage and align all efforts with current EMRs, which should provide access to real-time data for decision-making for both the healthcare provider and patients. As patients transition to a stronger consumer orientation, permitting access to appointment scheduling and selection of healthcare delivery sites and providers, virtual care options will be expected.

One of the primary steps in population health management remains the risk segmentation and stratification, and this process will require revision and criteria development to select those patients who would most benefit from a virtual care experience. Just as SDOH platforms have emerged to inform decision-making, preferred types of communication and interactions become an additional variable for increasing patient engagement, experience, and satisfaction.

Another important factor is the need for successfully implementing the various telehealth and app technologies which requires significant expertise, operations capability, and training for health professionals. All levels of health providers and staff benefit from basic instruction and coaching until virtual skills can become actual competencies. Simulations and virtual care checklists may help ensure a smoother patient and provider experience.

Finally, investing in virtual care capabilities may be organizational progression along the continuum of value-based care and facilitate success in risk-based contracts (O'Shea, 2020). Virtual health offers a complementary strategy for health promotion, disease prevention, better care coordination, and most importantly controlling population care costs. As health plans begin to support and encourage virtual care, adopting these strategies may have positive potential for financial outcomes and moving on the continuum of value-based care.

Virtual Care Caveats for Population Health

As with all innovations, questions inevitably arise as to the effectiveness of the new process, treatment, or intervention. Recent surveys suggest that specific applications provide improved access and patient/provider flexibility (HIN, 2018). The cliche "the doctor will see you now" has taken on new meaning! But, for populations with chronic health problems, this new accessibility to health providers should improve self-management and increase patient engagement. Health coaching continues to be offered by at least one-third of health delivery organizations adopting telehealth.

Virtual care will not be a panacea for lost revenue due to either COVID-19 or care provided at alternative ambulatory sites. During COVID-19, a survey found 64% of behavioral healthcare providers experienced revenue losses, accompanied by decreased no-show rates (Qualifacts & NCBH, 2020). Successful patient engagement will require a continuum focused strategy, which begins with adopting risk and finding appropriate quality metrics and value-based payment models. The role of technology integrates all processes and can also align outcomes.

The rapid rise of virtual care via telehealth and telemedicine will continue to be an additional care coordination model for health provider to patient contacts. Consumer surveys are reporting that 75% of patients who had never tried telehealth visits expressed an interest in participating, and recently industry experts suggest post-COVID-19 telehealth to be a quarter-trillion-dollar opportunity (Bestsennyy et al., 2020). The possibilities for virtual care are endless.

SUMMARY

As the health sector transitions to population health management applications, the focus remains on developing new models that prevent hospitalizations, reducing fragmented and uncoordinated care, and improving quality of life especially for chronic care patients. New models are emerging that improve transitions of care, through better care coordination such as expanding and enhancing postacute care option. Leveraging innovative health behavior change and patient engagement models can also improve health outcomes. And of primary importance is the rapid adoption of virtual care options and opportunities such as telehealth, remote care monitoring, and the use of wearables. Aligning technological advances with innovative new coordinated care models can result in improved value-based care.

DISCUSSION QUESTIONS

1. The original transitions of care model identified medical self-management as the first action step when assisting chronic care patients. What recent initiatives are currently available to address this issue?

2. Individuals are reluctant to change negative health behaviors and habits—especially those with chronic diseases. Which aspect of the Health Behavior Model do you believe would be most impactful for this population?
3. Discuss the relationship between patient engagement, experience, and satisfaction.
4. Why do chronic care patients pose such a major challenge for population healthcare coordination models and processes?
5. Why would the TTM be a favorite of insurance companies? What characteristics provide the most benefits?
6. The Patient Engagement Framework was originally developed for e-health—specifically mobile apps. Would this framework be appropriate for face-to-face interactions?
7. Virtual care includes a variety of options—telehealth, remote health monitoring, and the use of wearables. As a population health manager, which percent of the budget would you allot to each option and why?
8. Describe the benefits and challenges involved in developing a hospital without walls model.

Toolkit Competency Application
Strategic Decision-Making and Emerging Population Health Model Approaches

This chapter covers emerging models for improving population health management program and processes. One of the fastest growing models is virtual care, also referred to as telehealth. Review each of the following two articles and summarize the organization's digital health strategy. Next, compare the strategies based on the virtual care options available and the needs of chronic care patients.

Raths, D. (2020, December 21). *Scaling up the home hospital program at brigham and women's healthcare innovation.* https://www.hcinnovationgroup.com/population-health-management/remote-patient-monitoring-rpm/article/21203470/scaling-up-the-home-hospital-program-at-brigham-and-womens?utm_source=HI+Daily+NL&utm_medium=email&utm_campaign=CPS201221061&o_eid=6978A6266356F5Z&rdx.ident%5Bpull%5D=omeda%7C6978A6266356F5Z&oly_enc_id=6978A6266356F5Z

Wicklund, E. (2017, January 26). *Northwell health takes telehealth to the next level.* https://mhealthintelligence.com/news/northwell-health-takes-telehealth-to-the-next-level

REFERENCES

Agency for Healthcare Research and Quality. (n.d.). *Care coordination.* Retrieved May 19, 2021, from https://www.ahrq.gov/ncepcr/care/coordination.html

Bernell, S., & Howard, S. (2016). Use your words carefully: What is chronic disease? *Front Public Health, 4,* 159. https://www.ncbi.nlm.nih.gov/pmc/articles/PMC4969287/

Bestsennyy, O. G., Harris, A., & Rost, J. (2020, May 29). *Telehealth: A quarter-trillion-dollar post-COVID-19 reality?* McKinsey & Company. https://www.mckinsey.com/~/media/McKinsey/Industries/Healthcare%20Systems%20and%20Services/Our%20Insights/Telehealth%20A%20quarter%20trillion%20dollar%20post%20COVID%2019%20reality/Telehealth-A-quarter-trilliondollar-post-COVID-19-reality.pdf

Biofourmis. (2020). *Introducing BioVitals® hospital at home.* https://www.biofourmis.com/home-hospital/

CDC. (2018). *Managing chronic conditions: Self-management education programs for chronic conditions*. https://www.cdc.gov/learnmorefeelbetter/programs/general.htm

CDC. (2020). *Health and economic costs of chronic diseases*. National Center for Chronic Disease Prevention and Health Promotion (NCCDPHP). https://www.cdc.gov/chronicdisease/about/costs/

Centers for Medicare and Medicaid Services (CMS). (2020, March 17). *Medicare telemedicine health care provider fact sheet*. https://www.cms.gov/newsroom/fact-sheets/medicare-telemedicine-health-care-provider-fact-sheet

Champion, V. L., & Skinner, C. S. (2008). The health belief model. In K. Glanz, B. K. Rimer, & K. Viswanath (Eds.), *Health behavior and health education: Theory, research, and practice* (4th ed., pp. 45–66). Jossey Bass.

CMS. (2020, March 17). *Medicare telemedicine health care provider fact sheet*. https://www.cms.gov/newsroom/fact-sheets/medicare-telemedicine-health-care-provider-fact-sheet

Coleman, E. (2007). *Care transitions model*. John A. Hartford Foundation. https://www.johnahartford.org/ar2007/pdf/Hart07_CARE_TRANSITIONS_MODEL.pdf. https://www.mckinsey.com/industries/healthcare-systems-and-services/our-insights/telehealth-a-quarter-trillion-dollar-post-covid-19-reality

Cuddeback, J., & Fisher, D. (2016). Information technology. In D. Nash, R. J. Fabius, A. Skoufalos, J. Clarke, & M. Horowitz (Eds.), *Population health: Creating a culture of wellness* (2nd ed., pp. 231–256) Jones and Bartlett Learning.

Culberton, G. (2020, January/February). *Ethical community engagement: Lessons learned* (pp. 40–44). Healthcare Executive.

Farhud, D. D. (2015). Impact of Lifestyle on Health. *Iranian Journal of Public Health*, 44(11), 1442–1444. https://www.ncbi.nlm.nih.gov/pmc/articles/PMC4703222/

Graffigna, G., & Barello, S. (2018). Spotlight on the Patient Health Engagement model (PHE model): a psychosocial theory to understand people's meaningful engagement. *Patient Prefer Adherence*, 12, 1261–1271. https://www.ncbi.nlm.nih.gov/pmc/articles/PMC6056150

Health Information Network (HIN). (2015). *Remote patient monitoring for chronic condition management*. Health Information Network. https://hin.3dcartstores.com/Remote-Patient-Monitoring-for-Chronic-Condition-Management-a-45-minute-webinar-on-February-24-2015-now-available-for-replay_p_5012.html

Health Information Network (HIN). (2018). *Telehealth and remote patient monitoring in 2018*. Health Information Network. http://www.hin.com/library/registerTelehealthRemoteMonitoring2018.html

Health Information Network (HIN). (2019). *Patient engagement in 2019: Positive payoffs from patients activated in their healthcare*. Health Information Network. www.hin.com/library/registerPatientEngagement2019.html

Healthstream. (2019, July 8). *Reducing readmission rates in healthcare*. Healthstream. https://www.healthstream.com/resources/blog/blog/2019/07/08/reducing-readmission-rates-in-healthcare

Healthstream. (2020). *The economic and emotional cost of hospital readmissions*. Healthstream. https://www.healthstream.com/resources/blog/blog/2020/06/02/the-economic-emotional-cost-of-hospital-readmissions

Heath, S. (2019, March 1). *Patient engagement strategies for improving patient activation*. Patient Engagement HIT. https://patientengagementhit.com/features/patient-engagement-strategies-for-improving-patient-activation

Hibbard, J., Mahoney, E., Stockard, J., & Tusler, M. (2005). Development and testing of a short form of the patient activation measure. *Health Services Research*, 40, 1918–1930. https://doi.org/10.1111/j.1475-6773.2005.00438.x

Hines, P., & Mercury, M. (2013). Designing the role of the embedded care manager. *Professional Case Management*, 18(4), 182–187. https://alliedhealth.ceconnection.com/files/DesigningtheRoleoftheEmbeddedCareManager-1372337047139.pdf

Iuga, A. O., & McGuire, M. J. (2014). Adherence and health care costs. *Risk Management and Healthcare Policy*, 7, 35–44. https://doi.org/10.2147/RMHP.S19801

Johns Hopkins Medicine. (2020, April 30). *Don't avoid your doctor during the coronavirus pandemic*. Johns Hopkins Health. https://www.hopkinsmedicine.org/health/conditions-and-diseases/coronavirus/dont-avoid-your-doctor-during-the-coronavirus-pandemic

LaMorte, W. (2019). *Transtheoretical model of change/stages of change*. Boston University School of Public Health. https://sphweb.bumc.bu.edu/otlt/mph-modules/sb/behavioralchangetheories/BehavioralChangeTheories6.html

Landi, H. (2020, December 23). *Doctor on Demand, Harvard study finds telehealth surge driven by behavioral health, chronic care illness visits*. https://www.fiercehealthcare.com/tech/doctor-demand-study-finds-covid-19-telehealth-surge-driven-by-behavioral-health-chronic?mkt_tok=eyJpIjoiTWpneE1qVTJNV0prT1RWaSIsInQiOiJTbkpnOGltZXZOVjU1ZXBBTGV4TE5JNU1tVEhPOHpFSWNQODkyZFRJVEs0WVgxbUF4d3VvK1gwXC9JMFllM2N4ZlVjS0tocEdxTWNWWFN2Sko0MVBoS21DdzBMRlErOFZocVJqdHVEa3ZaTmxXRjUxcUg4NXpOXC9TMEhoMWxnRTZUIn0%3D&mrkid=931686

Levine, D., Ouchi, K., Blanchfield, B., Saenz, A., Burke, K., Paz, M., Diamon, K., Pu, C., & Schipper, J. (2020, January 21). Hospital-level care at home for acutely ill adults: A randomized controlled trial. *Annals of Internal Medicine, 172*, 77–85. https://doi.org/10.7326/M19-0600

MedicineNet. (2016). *Definition of chronic disease*. http://www.medicinenet.com/script/main/art.asp?articlekey=33490

McGinley, L. (2020, July 13). Patients are still denying essential care out of fear of coronavirus. *The Washington Post*. https://www.washingtonpost.com/health/wooing-patients-back-is-tricky-business-as-coronavirus-spikes-in-many-states/2020/07/13/b86d676e-bbb1-11ea-8cf5-9c1b8d7f84c6_story.html

Miller, C. (2013). *Care vs. care management: Seven structural differences*. Health Information Network. http://hin.com/blog/2013/12/12/care-vs-case-management-7-structural-differences/

Minemyer, P. (2020, June 11). *A look inside Geisinger's new remote monitoring program for COVID-19 patients*. Fierce Healthcare. https://www.fiercehealthcare.com/hospitals/a-look-inside-geisinger-s-new-remote-monitoring-program-for-covid-19-patients?utm_medium=nl&utm_source=internal&mrkid=931686&mkt_tok=eyJpIjoiT0dZM01UY3labVkwWVdGaSIsInQiOiJkQXJFZGs0N0lYUWhHUlN0c1NuOWFcL1FXZ2tHOFJxYkg1Zk4xbnkxOElqVGF3Rzd5YXpLMTU1TlNNbHNcL0FlUnFGT25pTXAxWElBbUpVZWJzMjJqZUVUR0ttN2JONmhkejZJTXUwdlwvbXhsaFQ0Zk9VWjFQbWU5cTRcL2NHV1BGcmwifQ%3D%3D

Mohammed, A. S., & Libby, D. (2020, November 18). *Digital health with reshape patient engagement, care delivery and payment models*. ECG Management Consultants. https://www.ecgmc.com/thought-leadership/whitepapers/we-believe-series-digital-health-will-reshape-patient-engagement-care-delivery-and-payment-models

Office of Community Resources, Education and Wellness. (2020). *HealthEASE Newsletter. Department of Human Services, Division of Aging Services*. Issue 247. Division of Aging Services. https://www.state.nj.us/humanservices/doas/services/healthease/. https://www.state.nj.us/humanservices/doas/contact/

O'Keefe, O., & Dunn, M. (2016, October 18). *Improve patient engagement with five public health-inspired principles*. Health Catalyst. https://www.healthcatalyst.com/successful-patient-engagement-with-5-public-health-principles

O'Neill-Hayes, T., & Delk, R. (2018, September 4) *Understanding the social determinants of health*. American Action Forum. https://www.americanactionforum.org/research/understanding-the-social-determinants-of-health/#ixzz6inF2ELq2

O'Shea, D. (2020, December 18). *How health care providers can use technology to help improve patient care and their practices*. Modern Healthcare. https://www.modernhealthcare.com/technology/how-health-care-providers-can-use-technology-help-improve-patient-care-and-their

Perna, G. (2013, April 10). *5 steps to patient engagement, a NeHC framework is created*. https://www.hcinnovationgroup.com/clinical-it/clinical-documentation/article/13020460/5-steps-to-patient-engagement-a-nehc-framework-is-created

Population Health Alliance. (n.d.). *Population health alliance framework*. Retrieved May 19, 2021, from https://populationhealthalliance.org/research/understanding-population-health/

Prochaska, J. O., Redding, C. A., & Evers, K. E. (2008). The transtheoretical model and stages of change. In K. Glanz, B. K. Rimer, & K. Viswanath (Eds.), *Health behavior and health education: Theory, research, and practice* (4th ed., pp. 97–121). Jossey Bass.

Qualifacts and National Council of Behavioral Health (NCBH). (2020). *The new role of virtual care in behavioral healthcare.* Qualifacts and National Council of Behavioral Health. https://naccme.s3.amazonaws.com/Qualifacts+August+2020+WP/The_New_Role_Of_Virtual_Care_In_Behavioral_Healthcare__Qualifacts.pdf?__hstc=233546881.9eaa5e568f758a79e21a1a75923e4184.1603991852815.1603991852815.1603991852815.1&__hssc=233546881.1.1603991852816&__hsfp=3055432663

Raths, D. (2020a, November 25). *CMS Expands Hospital-at-Home Program.* Healthcare Innovation. https://www.hcinnovationgroup.com/population-health-management/remote-patient-monitoring-rpm/news/21164286/cms-expands-hospitalathome-program

Raths, D. (2020b, December 21). *Scaling up the home hospital program at brigham and women's healthcare innovation.* https://www.hcinnovationgroup.com/population-health-management/remote-patient-monitoring-rpm/article/21203470/scaling-up-the-home-hospital-program-at-brigham-and-womens?utm_source=HI+Daily+NL&utm_medium=email&utm_campaign=CPS201221061&o_eid=6978A6266356F5Z&rdx.ident%5Bpull%5D=omeda%7C6978A6266356F5Z&oly_enc_id=6978A6266356F5Z

Raths, D. (2020c, December 28). *Highmark adds tele-addiction, peer support services to SUD recovery approach.* https://www.hcinnovationgroup.com/population-health-management/behavioral-health/article/21204045/highmark-adds-teleaddiction-peer-support-services-to-sud-recovery-approach?utm_source=HI+Daily+NL&utm_medium=email&utm_campaign=CPS201231003&o_eid=6978A6266356F5Z&rdx.ident%5Bpull%5D=omeda%7C6978A6266356F5Z&oly_enc_id=6978A6266356F5Z

Rosenstock, J. M., Strecher, V. J., & Becker, M. H. (1988). Social learning theory and the Health Belief Model. *Health Education Quarterly, 15,* 175–183. https://doi.org/10.1177/109019818801500203

Scott, D. (2019, July 11). *Patient engagement in 2019: Will it impact patient outcomes?* https://www.spok.com/blog/patient-engagement-in-2019-can-it-impact-patient-outcomes/

Shepard, V., Park, M., & Lee, B. (2021). Policy and advocacy. In D. Nash, A. Skoufalos, R. Fabius, & W. Oglesby (Eds.), *Population health: Creating a culture of wellness* (3rd ed., pp. 251–273). Jones & Bartlett Publishing.

Sieck, C., Walker, D., Sheldon, R., & McAlearney, A. (2019, March 13). *The patient engagement capacity model: What factors determine a patient's ability to engage?* NEJMCatalyst. https://nam05.safelinks.protection.outlook.com/?url=https%3A%2F%2Fcatalyst.nejm.org%2Fpatient-engagement-capacity model%2F&data=01%7C01%7Canne.hewitt%40shu.edu%7C9ae44a0dba4c46706a1208d6b513b4c5%7C51f07c2253b744dfb97ca13261d71075%7C1&sdata=OSbrk3NbO1dierYT%2BcONz6RZmTXpk6%2BsOzxEAtI%2BOZc%3D&reserved=0

Wicklund, E. (2017, January 26). *Northwell health takes telehealth to the next level.* https://mhealthintelligence.com/news/northwell-health-takes-telehealth-to-the-next-level

CHAPTER 10

Consumerism: Population Health Marketing Applications

Julie L. Mascari, Moses O. Salami, and Anne M. Hewitt

KEY TERMS

Behavioral Economics
Consumerism
Digital Marketing
Heuristics
Influencers
Loss Aversion
Marketing
Marketing Mix

Marketing SWOT
Meaningful Consumerism
Mental Accounting
Nudges
Relationship Marketing
Social Marketing
Social Media
Social Networks

LEARNING OBJECTIVES

1. Explain the role of consumerism and its impact on population health management (PHM).
2. Identify the differences between consumer and patient experience.
3. Align basic consumer behavior concepts with population health (PH) applications.
4. Discuss the role of marketing in PHM.

> 🔊 Podcasts that exemplify the content of this chapter are available at Springer Publishing Connect™
>
> Podcast 10.1. How Did You Find Your Doctor?
> Podcast 10.2. Think of the Last Item You Purchased—Why Did You Buy It?

Access the podcast online at http://connect.springerpub.com/content/book/978-0-8261-4427-0/part/part03/chapter/ch10

5. Distinguish between basic health marketing and social marketing fundamentals.
6. Demonstrate an application of PH marketing for a population of interest.

INTRODUCTION

We are all consumers. When you make a decision, do you follow a process? Healthcare **consumerism** is people proactively using trustworthy, relevant information and appropriate technology to make better informed decisions about their healthcare options (Carman et al., 2019).

Today's health sector offers many diverse services to multiple populations and follows the standard exchange system between a health organization/agency or provider (supply) and the patient or consumer (demand). Although patients may now be referred to as consumers, this basic economic principle continues. The difference between the previous unbalanced relationship of a healthcare provider dictating to their patients and today's 21st-century consumer autonomy in which the individual chooses services and locations is transformational. Consumer-informed decision-making with clear expectations is rapidly changing health marketing. The current healthscape is now cluttered and saturated with marketing campaigns and advertisements.

Increased interaction and thoughtful exchanges between healthcare providers and patients/consumers offer multiple opportunities for enhanced and expanded communication with the goal of creating shared engagement. Based on research by the Patient-Centered Outcomes Research Institute (PCORI), the phrase **meaningful consumerism** encompasses five important requirements for PH managers as shown in Figure 10.1 (PCORI, 2019).

Healthcare consumerism involves satisfying individual consumer preferences including offering multiple options for communication. E-commerce technology has clearly served as a catalyst for the increased rise in healthcare consumerism, as individuals, now familiar with banking and retail interactions using online and mobile devices, have come to expect the same type of seamless service from healthcare providers (Accenture, 2019). Health management experts also suggest that the COVID-19 pandemic has also accelerated the transition to much more consumer-oriented care (Hegwer, 2020). Healthcare consumerism can be a valuable strategy for PH managers, as they continually strive to engage all consumers and facilitate better health outcomes at lower costs.

Consumer and Patient Experience

Increased consumer participation in healthcare decision-making requires PH managers to assess their abilities to meet consumer demands and expectations. A recent study found that consumers' top three health concerns were cost, transparency, and a satisfactory consumer and patient experience (HEGT, 2019). **Consumer experience** refers to a buying/retail or similar expectation where overall convenience is key. **Patient experience** differs

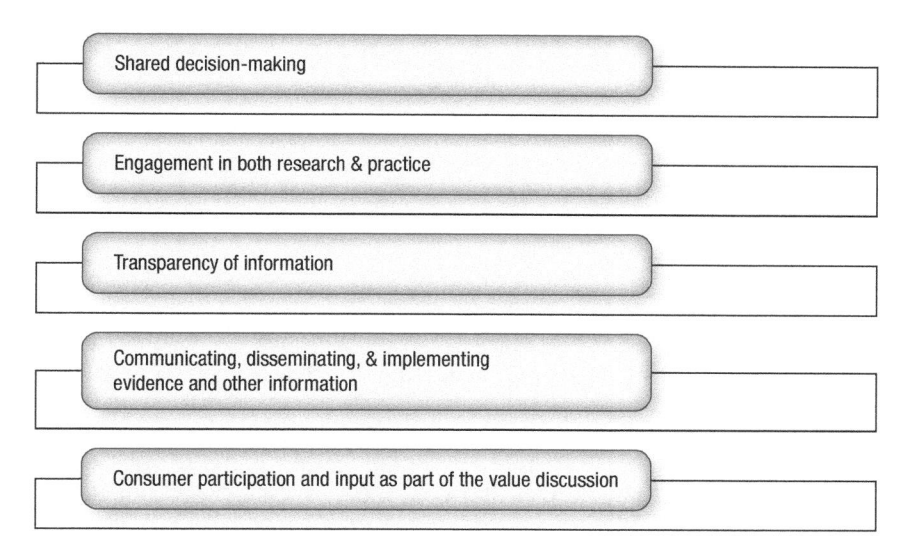

- Shared decision-making
- Engagement in both research & practice
- Transparency of information
- Communicating, disseminating, & implementing evidence and other information
- Consumer participation and input as part of the value discussion

FIGURE 10.1 Elements of Meaningful Consumerism

Adapted from PCORI, 2019

significantly, as the emphasis is less on a two-way transaction of services and more on the emotions generated from an entire set of health experiences. See Figure 10.2.

Note that both sets of expectations require PH managers to provide quality experiences. Consumer experience challenges may be more technological and process oriented, while patient experience activities include many subjective elements related to personal interactions and perceptions. This dichotomy of focus simply means that PH delivery processes should be concerned with the ease of use as well as patient-centered care.

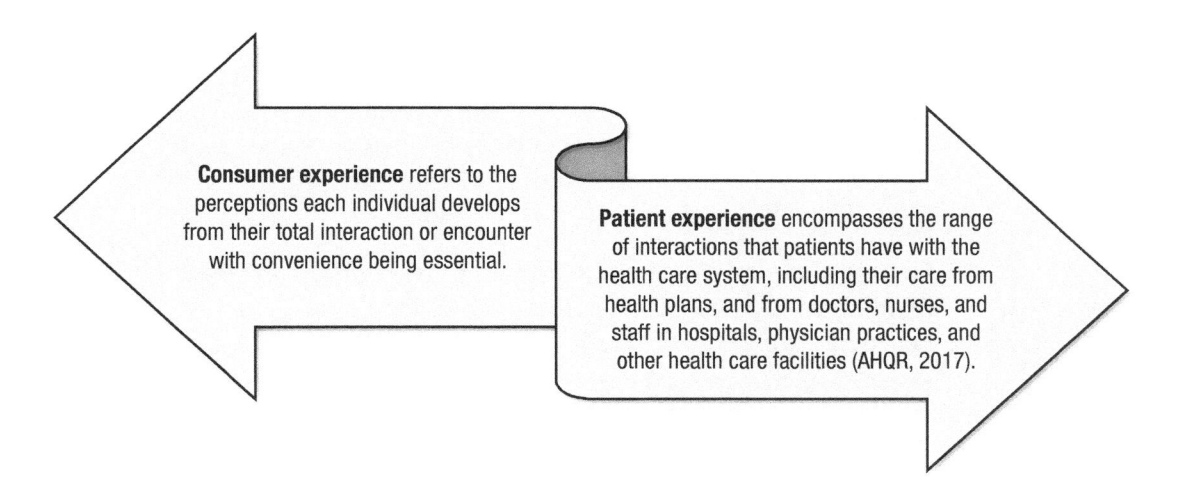

Consumer experience refers to the perceptions each individual develops from their total interaction or encounter with convenience being essential.

Patient experience encompasses the range of interactions that patients have with the health care system, including their care from health plans, and from doctors, nurses, and staff in hospitals, physician practices, and other health care facilities (AHQR, 2017).

FIGURE 10.2 Consumer and Patient Experience Definition Comparison

> **DID YOU KNOW?**
>
> **Consumer Behavior and Patient Experience**
>
> Here are two fictitious examples of consumers in their late 20s who work for the same computer software company as web designers:
>
> Narrative #1: Stephanie is expecting her first baby and has completed an extensive online review of obstetricians. She has even outlined criteria including physician credentials, hospital ratings, and ancillary services (midwife and doula). She virtually arranges a previsit with the practice obstetrics group's nurse practitioner, where they discuss her wishes for the experience and review the preprofile Stephanie completed via a mobile survey. She adds the "I'm Expecting" app to her phone for any potential follow-up questions she may have. Together they arrange a prenatal class for she and her husband.
>
> Narrative #2: Melissa has confided in her family the baby's due date. Together, they discuss steps she should take. Melissa is quiet and unsure as this is her first pregnancy, and her Mom seems to have all the answers including recommending her former obstetrician. They are both so excited, and her Mom starts talking about a baby shower. A week later, Melissa still has not reached out to any health provider or talked over any details with her significant other. She knows she should be taking vitamins but does not know what to take, and her morning nausea seems to be becoming more persistent. On her lunch hour, she schedules and completes a telehealth visit on her computer through her company's insurance plan. The health adviser, after listening to her situation, immediately schedules an appointment with a local obstetrician, provides her with e-resources, and sends her a podcast on morning sickness. Melissa is relieved.

These brief narratives highlight consumer's expectations for transparency, high standards for convenience, and the need for online and digital engagement (Hegwer, 2020). As both examples illustrate, digital engagement appears to be both a nonthreatening and convenient pathway to reach consumers who may be reluctant to take the first step toward a needed health interaction. The challenge for PH managers will be to quickly move beyond patient portals and the use of patient engagement apps to new innovations, such as consumer self-service, which can also support value-based healthcare.

Consumer healthcare decisions differ from regular shopping experiences, as the issue of physician influence needs to be considered. This shift from the primary care provider as gatekeeper to the individual patient with a consumer mentality significantly alters the previous service transaction between health provider and patient, as this population represents the health sector's future patients.

Linking Consumer Behavior Concepts to Population Health Applications

Health organizations market their services to meet the needs of the consumer fulfilling an essential component of marketing. Consumers are inundated with various marketing tactics several times a day from advertisements on their mobile phone, roadside billboards, television commercials, radio, and all the various social media platforms. Understanding the way consumers absorb information and complete decision-making is clearly a PH management competency (see Figure 10.3).

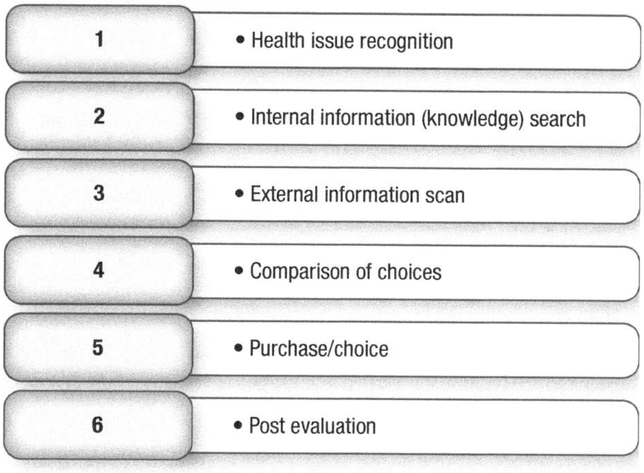

1	• Health issue recognition
2	• Internal information (knowledge) search
3	• External information scan
4	• Comparison of choices
5	• Purchase/choice
6	• Post evaluation

FIGURE 10.3 Consumer Health Decision-Making Process

The consumer decision-making model is comprised of the five steps: problem recognition, internal search, external search, purchase, and postpurchase evaluation (Berkowitz, 2011; Engel et al., 1993). The first step of the decision-making model is problem recognition. This is where a consumer recognizes that there is a health issue that needs to be solved. This could be a consumer who is having a hard time finding a primary care physician who accepts their insurance near where they live, or a physician practice who seems to have a long wait time to see the doctor or finding a specialist. The consumer experiences a health problem with a level of personal discomfort or inconvenience and needs a solution. This initial step is followed by an interpersonal search for previous information and knowledge, and then an external scan for available information. At this point, the consumer weighs their options and makes a choice. The final step is evaluation of the healthcare decision by the consumer. At each step, the PH manager has opportunities to influence the consumer's decision making and behavior.

Consumer Marketing: Behavior Economics

Consumers may follow a decision-making pathway as presented above, but their behavior still may not be economical, rationale, or even predictable. **Behavioral economics** is a field of study that describes the "how" and "why" health consumers and patients make important health decisions. The focus is on integrating individual's decisions that are influenced by both economic and social psychology ideas and concepts (Lin, 2016).

Everyone is aware of the dangers of smoking, substance misuse and abuse, and not wearing seat belts for injury protection, and yet individuals often make decisions that put themselves at a health risk. PH management is concerned with behavior economics, as these choices impact health outcomes. The goal is to influence health choices in a positive way that includes and engages the consumer. Understanding these behavioral economic strategies is especially important for the PH managers, various health payers (insurance companies and employers), and other stakeholders. Commonalities do exist among various consumers and are directly related to how choices are made regardless of the type of choice.

- Health decisions are often made following a "rule of thumb" known as a **heuristic** (Lin, 2016). Patients and consumers may make choices based on short-cut thinking from past experiences.

Consumer example: "This medication helped take my knee pain away, I'll try it for my sore shoulder."

- Other decision-making factors include how and when the decision is made, and the way the decision is presented and described. Patients often use a **mental accounting** system of weighing pros and cons of a health action and might ask the health provider for a "probability" of an event so they can place the choice in their own personal situation.

Consumer example: "Maybe I'll be one of the lucky COVID-19 patients and not get too sick. I don't get the flu very often so the probability is probably not that high.

- Workplace wellness programs may rely on a behavioral economic strategy known as loss aversion. **Loss aversion** means that an employee's personal preference is for loss avoidance as compared with acquiring gains.

Consumer example: "If my company wants me to select either attending smoking cessation meetings or participating in a wellness program that covers nicotine gum and/or patches, I'll go to the meetings and keep my health insurance deductible low."

PH managers consistently struggle with issues related to medication adherence or compliance especially for chronic care populations. Although these terms unfortunately present an asymmetrical power relationship between the health provider and consumer/patient, the goal remains to attain a positive health outcome. The importance of practicing health promotion lifestyle activities and maintaining a positive health status by following through with medication consistently cannot be overstated. Population health managers are accountable not only for health implications, but also for financial outcomes of these populations at risk. For example, using behavioral economics principles and strengthening the convenience factor for medication refills can result in significant adherence and overall improvement (Costa et al., 2015).

A patient engagement strategy that can impact a patient's decision-making process is based on behavioral economics. The concept of **nudges** relies on targeted and tailored information that can be used to engage consumers/patients to participate in healthy actions and activities. For example, in addition to an individual receiving a yearly referral from a primary care practitioner at a wellness visit, they might receive a follow-up email or text reminder 2 weeks later asking if they have made an appointment or would like assistance.

Health Marketing Strategies for Population Health Managers

Despite the existence of consumer decision-making pathways, behavioral economic models, and consumer and patient experience initiatives, PH management will not be successful without a marketing strategy appropriate for the specific population of interest.

Marketing is viewed as multiphase essential process for creating health sector value. The American Marketing Association (AMA) definition includes many of the diverse elements of marketing as the activity, set of institutions, and processes for creating, communicating, delivering, and exchanging offerings that have *value* for customers, clients, partners, and society at large (AMA, 2017).

Another second marketing definition focuses on the operational process including the steps such as planning and executing the conception, pricing, promotion, and distribution of ideas, goods, and services (Bennett, 1995). PH managers will need to oversee these processes and assess their impact on various population of interest's health outcomes.

One of the most essential marketing strategies is the development of the four Ps (product, place, price, and promotion), also referred to as the marketing mix (Berkowitz, 2011). Without this operational approach, health promotion and disease prevention interventions may fail to reach the desired population.

Marketing mix is a commonly used term that refers to four key management decisions when planning a marketing plan or project. They include what are known as the four Ps and cover these categories: product, place (distribution), promotion, and price (positioning); (Wagner, 2018, p. 142). Without successful marketing campaigns based on the marketing mix, any PHM program or initiative will not reach its full potential or create the desired health outcomes.

These four marketing variables form the basis for health marketing initiatives (see Table 10.1).

Of the four marketing mix components, the choice of place may represent the most significant challenge for current PH planners. Exhibit 10.1 shows the five traditional marketing placement outlets that have been used successfully over the years.

Today's opportunities now include the complex array of marketing options that fall under the category of digital marketing. Most individuals are familiar with Facebook, Instagram, Twitter, Pinterest, Google, and many more commonly used sharing platforms. See Exhibit 10.2.

Digital marketing refers to any marketing strategy that uses an electronic device that may or may not be connected to the internet, and these strategies represent complex decisions as to the purpose and type of consumer and the best digital approach to reach the consumer (Simplilearn, 2021).

PH managers may want to familiarize themselves with the various applications of each one of these strategies. The American Marketing Association offers a complete overview on their website at https://www.ama.org/pages/what-is-digital-marketing (AMA, 2021). Although the development, implementation, and eventual assessment of the marketing plan may be outside the PH manager's direct scope of work, they can expect to be held accountable on the overall impact on the population of interest's health status and specific to acquisition cost per consumer per program.

TABLE 10.1 Four-P Marketing Application: A Population Health Initiative

Four-P Elements of Marketing	Population Health Management Application
Product: What do you want to market? Is it a service, a good (type of product), or even an idea? Is it a special procedure (colorectal screening?) or a self-management program for seniors with diabetes?	Telemedicine program: providing care to patients via a smartphone, tablet, or laptop.
Price: What will your consumers expect to spend for your product? Does it include time, after-care, additional medications, and other expenses? Consumerism is increasing the necessity for transparency of overall cost.	Most copays will be accepted. Concern exists over what amount insurances will cover.
Place: Do you know the best strategy to distribute your good product or idea? Would your consumer prefer it to be available online or in-person? Mass distribution or tailored to specific individuals and/or populations?	Available virtually to all patients in the service area with insurance and have a working camera on a laptop, iPad, or smartphone.
Promotion: What are the elements of your marketing plan? Do your promotion activities include publicity, advertising, or even personal consultation?*	Advertising in magazines, on billboards, and digitally/social media continues to be emphasized to reach populations of interest. Public relations activities developed to aide public adoption of new form of providing clinical care. Use of patient testimonials to help show ease of use with the program.

*Adapted from Berkowitz, 2011

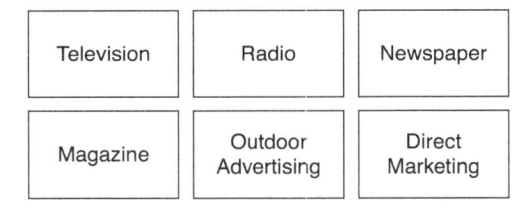

Television	Radio	Newspaper
Magazine	Outdoor Advertising	Direct Marketing

EXHIBIT 10.1 Traditional Health Marketing Advertising Options

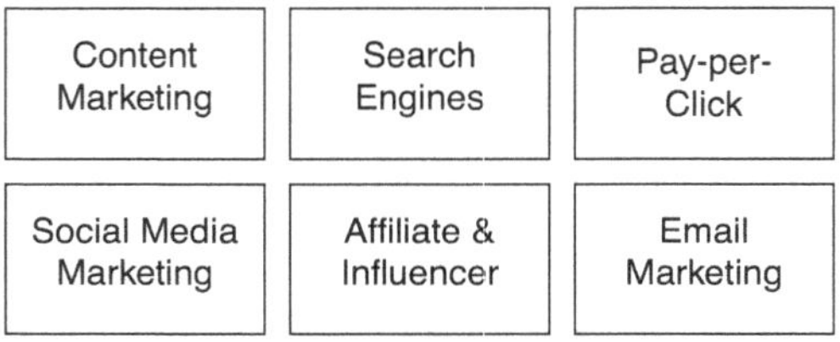

Content Marketing	Search Engines	Pay-per-Click
Social Media Marketing	Affiliate & Influencer	Email Marketing

EXHIBIT 10.2 Common Types of Digital Marketing

Social Marketing

PH managers provide a continuum of care for their patients/consumers. For example, chronic care populations benefit from virtual reminders and telehealth visits, and postacute populations may receive monitoring follow-up calls and/or specific at-home, short-term follow-up coordinated care. But healthy populations require general health promotion and disease prevention support, such as reminders for annual physicals and screenings for colorectal cancer. The marketing goal for this population is to promote an idea and approach such as "Take care of yourself and stay healthy." Social marketing can be thought of as the selling of an idea, such as wellness, as compared with a product. Social marketing messages can focus on prevention risky health behavior through education or the promotion of healthier lifestyle alternatives (Evans, 2006).

Social marketing can be described as the application of proven concepts and techniques drawn from the commercial sector to promote changes in diverse socially important behaviors such as drug use, smoking, and sexual behavior (Andreasen, 1995). One of the primary differences between traditional marketing and social marketing, besides the selling of an idea versus a product, is that social marketing is for the "greater good."

Social marketing is a concerted effort to influence groups, communities, and society as a whole (Cellucci et al., 2014, p. 102) and extremely appropriate for PHM initiatives. There may be no clear "payer" for these types of messages, as all populations benefit and as social marketing does not sell a particular brand. See the following two exemplary social marketing campaigns that also introduce another concept—the use of social media as a channel to carry the social marketing message.

DID YOU KNOW?

Social Marketing

One of the most famous examples of social marketing was created by the 80s Partnership for Drug Free America, titled "This is your brain. This is your brain on drugs" (https://www.youtube.com/watch?v=GOnENVylxPI; Huhn, 2019; Partnership to End Addiction, 2021). Countless other public health success stories using social marketing techniques to sell an idea and change behavior exist such as the adoption of children's car seats and those that focus on environmental issues such as clean air and water.

Recently, Proctor and Gamble partnered with a TikTok celebrity to create a video #DistanceDance to encourage people to social distance due to the COVID-19 pandemic. The video received worldwide 8 billion views and 1.7 million iterations, with endorsements by celebrities and sports teams (Cyca, 2020).

Social Media Marketing

The term **social media** describes many diverse e-platforms selected to convey tailored PH messages. Common digital communication channels include Facebook, Google, Instagram, Pinterest, Snapchat, Twitter, and YouTube.

Healthcare marketers are trending toward using more digital focused advertising, as results are easier to track and a less expensive outlet than traditional advertising activities. Social media differs from **social networks,** which are groups of individuals who want to connect and build relationships (Hausman, 2011). Social networks can be exceptionally persuasive and valuable to participants. The concept of **influencers** refers to the role of trusted individuals to promote an idea or a cause, such as wellness. Influencers encourage populations of followers to adopt suggested preferences with the purpose of shaping behaviors (Nash et al., 2021).

With the rise of social media, health marketers can reach more groups of individuals and populations at risk. Healthcare marketers should remember that the communication channel selected depends on the type of content you need to post. Twitter, for example, has a 280-character limit, and content placed on that channel should be direct to the point. Additionally, a marketer must keep in mind the age groups most likely to use the communication channel. For example, a healthcare marketer could try and target a population subgroup such as millennial mothers to advertise OB/GYN and pediatric services. You need to know which channels appeal to a majority of millennial mothers. According to the American Marketing Association, Snapchat, although a large platform with more younger viewers, than most, has only 8% of millennial mothers on that platform. But in 2016, Facebook reported about 26.3% of millennial mothers were using the platform and would appear to offer a better choice today. Facebook allows marketers to target locations, age, gender, education, interest, hobbies and much more. See Figure 10.4.

In today's world, the use of traditional marketing combined with social and digital marketing allows for integrated marketing plans where the organization's online strategy and presence mirrors communications placed through traditional channels. Healthcare organizations benefit from having more touch points for patients and populations of interest to interact with the organizations content.

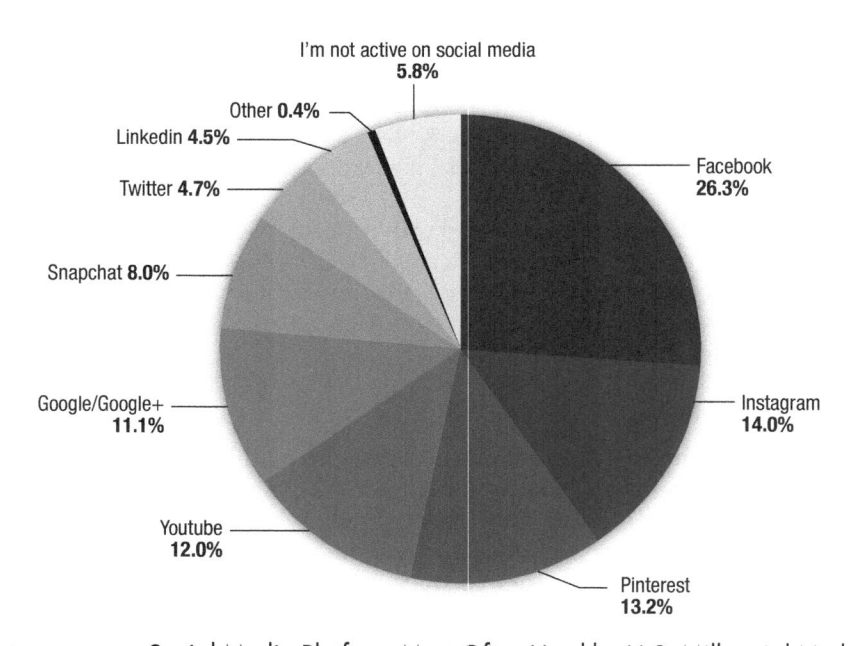

FIGURE 10.4 Social Media Platform Most Often Used by U.S. Millennial Mother Internet Users, September 2016

Data from Roth Capital Partners (ROTH), "2016–2017 Millennial Mom Survey" conducted by Research Now, Oct 13, 2016

❓ DID YOU KNOW?

Marketing Segmentation by Generational Differences

PH managers regularly segment populations by risk factors, behaviors, and acuity. Marketers segment populations by many different characteristics, some of them similar to shopper preferences and behavioral economic principles that are components of consumerism. But especially important to PH marketing is the need to specifically tailor messages not only to health condition but also to age, generational differences, and communication preferences.
- Traditionalists/Silent Generation: born 1928–1945
  - Baby Boomers: born 1946–1964
    - Generation X: born 1965–1980
    - Millennials: born 1981–1996
  - Generation Z: born 1997–onward (Dimock, 2019)

Key differences between social and commercial marketing revolve around a populations-of-interest unique characteristics. These consumers are often difficult to reach patients, have inconsistent and challenging consumer engagement patterns, and require tailored messages that nudge each member to seek care at right place and right time. An important social marketing task is to develop a sustained relationship between your organization and the population-of-interest. The concept of **relationship marketing** builds on seeking loyalty among consumers and can build a sense of trust and encourage patient engagement (Cellucci et al., 2014). As other industries have demonstrated consistently over the years, trust generated from continuing relations can benefit both consumer and provider.

Aligning Marketing Fundamentals to Population Health Management

SWOT Analysis

Healthcare marketers should be progressive in their marketing plans and strategies and, on a regular basis, evaluate the organizations product/service line offerings and their respective population target markets. The Strengths, Weaknesses, Opportunities and Threats (SWOT) analysis tool helps health organizations assess their current internal and external situations in relationship to the entire organization's products/service line provided to prospective patients/customers. Using a SWOT analysis for marketing decision-making involves identifying the organizations strengths, weaknesses, opportunities, and threats. To create a **marketing SWOT,** first determine your marketing objective and then identify the strengths, weaknesses, opportunities, and threats. The **strengths** are the positive attributes and qualities of the product or organization. Excellent patient experience, low ED wait times, strong brand identity, and great customer service are all examples of strengths. Using these strengths to the organization's advantage helps marketers make great progress in achieving marketing goals. The **weaknesses** are negative attributes related to the product or organization and can unfavorably impact the success of the product such as expensive out-of-pocket expenses, less appointment availability to see the physician, no online appointment booking capabilities, and low advertising budget. Steps to improve the weakness must be taken, as the weakness can affect the product usage, revenue, and

TABLE 10.2 Fundamental Marketing Concepts, Skills, and Competencies Useful for Population Health Management

✔	Fundamental Marketing Concepts, Skills, and Competencies Useful for Population Health Management
	Marketing research
	Population segmentation
	Message alignment
	Branding
	Advertising
	Public relations
	Milestones and budget
	Campaign effectiveness evaluation

customer satisfaction. **Opportunities** are the potential avenues to positively impact, and the marketer's role is to identify and take advantage of opportunities to improve financial success and viability. Examples of population health opportunities might include new technology to improve the delivery of product, introduction of a novel target market population, and revised federal regulation in favor of product services that include reimbursement such as the recently enacted mandates to support telemedicine initiatives. **Threats** have the potential to negatively impact your product. Threats might include new competitors entering your market or expanding because of innovative technology, federal and local legislation changes, or an increase in healthcare organizations entering market with innovative business models.

Although many traditional marketing tasks are completed by different health organizational units or outsourced to consultants, PH managers still need to develop marketing competencies to assess the success of any communication campaigns. This role includes oversight of the following areas related to any marketing plan as outlined in Table 10.2.

Marketing is an important tool to use in conjunction with population behavioral change strategies to positively impact the health of any population whether in a rural, suburban, or urban environment through marketing healthcare services that lead the community to utilize appropriate services.

SUMMARY

The rise of consumerism for the healthcare sector represents another 21st-century challenge impacting the relationship between current and future patients and the health system. Addressing consumer expectations requires PH managers to demonstrate competencies in both behavioral economics and the fundamental concepts of marketing as applied to specific populations of interest. Successful PH programs will depend on the organization's capabilities for applying consumer behavioral concepts such as meaningful consumerism and decision- pathways influencing both patient expectations and choices. The complexity of marketing fundamentals and options now includes not only the four Ps but also social marketing and digital marketing, including social media. The competency to oversee the development of innovative marketing plans capable of increasing patient engagement, improving outcomes, and aligning with strategic financial goals to achieve value over volume is paramount.

DISCUSSION QUESTIONS

1. Discuss the ways technology has enabled the concept of consumerism to impact the healthcare sector.
2. Explain the term "meaningful consumerism" and provide a relevant example.
3. Marketing managers often discuss that "placement" is the most difficult concept of the four Ps to implement. Provide a brief explanation of why this would be true in today's health environment?
4. Construct a SWOT analysis grid and describe the importance of completing the analysis before designing and implementing a PH marketing plan.
5. Select one of the five population age cohorts and discuss how the characteristics of this group might impact a marketing campaign.
6. Articulate the differences between marketing and social marketing? What is the relationship of social marketing to social media?

Toolkit Competency Application: Mini Case Study

Garden State Regional Medical Center

Garden State Regional Medical Center (GSRMC) is the fifth largest hospital in the State of New Jersey. The cases of COVID-19 in the United States were first reported in January 2020. GSRMC was one of the first and hardest hit hospitals in the state with COVID-19 patients. From March through May, the medical facility saw a major increase in COVID-19 patients. To accommodate this new population at risk, multiple hospital operating processes changed dramatically during this time. Visitor restrictions for inpatients were limited, staff was mandated to wear facemasks at all time, personal protective equipment was used following strict protocols, and elective procedures were postponed till June. In the medical centers, patient volume for outpatient services decreased drastically and with negative financial pressures. The medical center sought a rapid solution for continuing services to non-COVID-19 patients.

In April, the clinical leadership and information technology team began investing in a telemedicine program. A third-party vendor was selected, and the marketing department charged with developing a rollout plan quickly for this timely product. The marketing manager with the administrative director of the newly created program assessed the future telemedicine programs from the competitors' perspective by completing a SWOT analysis. See Table 10.3.

Once the SWOT analysis was complete, the marketing team and administrative director developed a campaign with an emphasis on digital and social media advertising. With a reduced number of the workforce commuting to work or handling normal routines, digital and social media advertising clearly became the ideal advertising avenue, as online engagement rapidly increased following quarantine orders. Specific marketing components included Facebook, Instagram, Streaming Radio Advertising, and Television.

TABLE 10.3 SWOT Analysis of Telemedicine Program

SWOT Analysis of Telemedicine Program	
Strengths – Timely product with demand at the onset of launch. – Only one other medical center in area offering telemedicine. – Patients can conveniently make telemedicine appointments on their own schedule.	Weaknesses – Third-party telemedicine will be integrated for the first time with GSRMC's clinical system. Likelihood for troubleshooting needed at launch time. – Multiple and diverse providers will need to be encouraged to use this method for patient interaction suggesting a time lag of adoption. Some long-standing outpatient physician practices may need laptops and iPads to offer this service.
Opportunities – Telehealth can reduce the number of patients coming to the hospital for medical care. Medical staff can continue to focus on COVID-19 patients. – Also supports COVID-19 treatments, and patient can self-quarantine at home.	Threats – When the peak of the pandemic is over, patients may choose to not use these services any longer. Uncertainties exist in regard to reimbursement for telehealth services. – A nearby competitor has been using telehealth previously with more features available than what GSRMC can offer at this moment.

GSRMC, Garden State Regional Medical Center.

TABLE 10.4 Components of the GSRMC's Telemarketing Campaign

Telemedicine Marketing Campaign Execution April–May	
Facebook Instagram Streaming Radio (Pandora and Spotify) Television	All marketing channels permit a wider reach in advertising to prospective patients on various platforms directly.

This permitted a wide variety of prospective patients to view Garden State Regional Medical Center's new product offering. After 2 months, following the telehealth program's April launch, GSRMC had completed more than 15,000 telehealth appointments. The telehealth program proved to be a significantly useful clinical offering and met the needs of two targeted populations—non-COVID-19 patients and COVID-19 patients appropriate for virtual care and follow-up. See Table 10.4.

GSRMC, Garden State Regional Medical Center.

With 2 months of data now available, the marketing team was able to segment the age groups that utilized the telehealth platform. 55% of the telehealth users were women, with a priority age range between 30 and 45 years old. After reviewing the patient experience survey statistics, three areas of improvement were identified.

1. Access: Additional telemedicine appointment times were required, as patients requested more options to accommodate their lifestyles.

2. Information: Patients expressed confusion as to which types of medical care were available and appropriate via telehealth. One example was concern over visiting an ED or via telehealth.

3. Privacy concerns: Patients expressed lack of confidence in the safety and security of care provided via telehealth.

From the month of June onward, GSRMC focused on addressing the three concerns expressed on the patient experience survey and also looked to further leverage engagement with the strong base of women patients. First, GSRMC expanded the number of hours available for telemedicine appointments by increasing additional providers such as Nurse Practitioners (NAs), Personal Assistants (PAs) and extra physicians across a few specialties. The new hours were highlighted on revised marketing collateral and other informational components. Secondly, GSRMC focused on developing content pieces such as blogs, social media posts, and articles for new sites explaining the benefits of telemedicine and clarifying what types of appointments were appropriate compared with conditions that should be seen in person by a physician. Further information regarding the types of telemedicine appointments accepted were added to the website. Lastly, all marketing collateral were revised to affirm that telemedicine visits are HIPPA compliant.

As society adjusted to the new normal with COVID-19, GSRMC reopened the medical center campus fully following a thorough disinfection of the facility, temperature checks at all entrances, and questionnaires completed by all patients and visitors regarding their interactions and/or potential exposures to COVID-19 at-risk individuals. Despite a strong public relations campaign, GSRMC experienced a low number of returning patients for routine medical care, postponed surgeries, and infusion services. The organization recognized the need for rebuilding consumer trust and reducing fears concerning coronavirus exposure. A content building campaign was developed in conjunction with the continuing marketing push for telemedicine. Marketing and service line leaders utilized educational pieces from clinical physicians to develop blogs on healthcare topics that people may have overlooked during the pandemic such as exercising from home, maintaining mental health and nutrition, and viewing consistent hospital updates. With consistent content now available on all platforms, GSRMC's brand identity continued to grow, consumers became stronger, and over time patient volume at the medical center started to increase. Administration affirmed that the full recovery process may take more than a year for patient volume to return to pre-COVID-19 levels, but the increases over several months are trending in a positive direction.

GSRMC CASE STUDY DISCUSSION QUESTIONS

1. Identify the reasons why the adoption of telehealth was the appropriate solution for GSRMC's dilemma.
2. What insights did the marketing director glean from the SWOT analysis?
3. Suggest an additional marketing strategy for the new base for women users participating in the telehealth initiative.
4. Propose one other marketing option for promoting the telehealth initiative.
5. Describe the responses to the three issues identified as concerns from the initial users.
6. Provide additional marketing solutions for more former and new patients to use telehealth and stop delaying regular or routine care.

REFERENCES

Accenture. (2019, February 12). *Today's consumers reveal the future of healthcare*. https://www.accenture.com/us-en/insights/health/todays-consumers-reveal-future-healthcare

Agency for Healthcare Research and Quality (AHRQ). (2017, March). *What is patient experience?* Agency for Healthcare Research and Quality. https://www.ahrq.gov/cahps/about-cahps/patient-experience/index.html

American Marketing Association (AMA). (2017). *Definition of marketing.* https://www.ama.org/the-definition-of-marketing-what-is-marketing/

American Marketing Association (AMA). (2018). *Marketing mix.* AMA Dictionary. https://marketing-dictionary.org/m/marketing-mix/

American Marketing Association (AMA). (2020). *Definition of social marketing.* Common Language in Marketing Project. https://marketing-dictionary.org/s/social-marketing/

American Marketing Association (AMA). (2021). *What is digital marketing?* https://www.ama.org/pages/what-is-digital-marketing/

Andreasen, A. (1995). *Marketing social change.* Jossey-Bass.

Bennett, P. D. (Ed.). (1995). *Dictionary of marketing terms* (2nd ed.). American Marketing Association.

Berkowitz, E. (2011). Buyer behavior (Chapter 4). In *Essentials of health care marketing* (3rd ed., pp. 125–160). Jones & Bartlett Learning.

Carman, K., Lawrence, W., & Siegel J. (2019, March 5). *The "New" health care consumerism.* Health Affairs Blog. https://www.healthaffairs.org/do/10.1377/hblog20190304.69786/full/10.1377/hblog20190304.69786

Cellucci, L., Wiggins, C., & Farnsworth, T. (2014). *Healthcare marketing: A case study approach.* Health Administration Press/AUPHA.

Costa, E., Giardini, A., Savin, M., Menditto, E., Lehane, E., Laosa, O., Pecorelli, S., Monaco, A., & Marengoni, A. (2015). Interventional tools to improve medication adherence: Review of literature. *Patient Preference and Adherence, 9,* 1303–1314. https://doi.org/10.2147/PPA.S87551. https://www.ncbi.nlm.nih.gov/pmc/articles/PMC4576894/

Cyca, M. (2020, August 19). *7 of the best social media campaigns (and what you can learn from them).* https://blog.hootsuite.com/social-media-campaign-strategy/

Dimock, M. (2019, January 17). *Defining generations: Where millennials end and generation Z begins.* https://www.pewresearch.org/fact-tank/2019/01/17/where-millennials-end-and-generation-z-begins/

Engel, J., Blackwell, R., & Miniard, P. (1993). *Consumer behavior* (7th ed.). They Dryden Press.

Evans, W. D. (2006). How social marketing works in health care. *BMJ, 332*(7551), 1207–1210. https://doi.org/10.1136/bmj.332.7551.1207. https://www.ncbi.nlm.nih.gov/pmc/articles/PMC1463924/

Hausman, A. (2011, March 14). *Social media is a communication channel: Social networks are NOT.* https://www.hausmanmarketingletter.com/social-media-is-a-communication-channel-social-networks-are-not/#.X-IPDOdOk2w

Healthcare Executive Group Team (HEGT). (2019, December 5). *Healthcare 'costs & transparency' and 'consumer experience' – Top of mind for 2020 & beyond.* https://hceg.org/healthcare-costs-transparency-consumer-experience-top-of-mind-2020-predictions/

Hegwer, L. (2020, September/October). *Narrowing the digital divide: Connecting Americans in a post COVID-19 era* (pp. 18–26). Healthcare Executive.

Huhn, J. (2019, September 5). *What is social marketing? (with 7 stellar examples).* https://www.business2community.com/digital-marketing/what-is-social-marketing-with-7-stellar-examples-02236451

Lin, J. (2016). Behavioral economics (Chapter 8). In *Population health management: Creating a culture of wellness* (2nd ed., pp. 153–165). Jones and Bartlett Learning.

Nash, D., Skoufalos, A., Fabius, R., & Oglesby, W. (Eds.) (2021). *Population health: Creating a culture of wellness* (3rd ed., pp. 188–190). Jones and Bartlett Learning.

Partnership to End Addiction. (2021). *Our history.* https://drugfree.org/article/our-history/

Patient Centered Outcomes Research Institute (PCORI). (2019, November 12). *By consumers, for consumers: Building capacity and partnerships to enhance patient-centeredness.* PCORI. https://www.pcori.org/research-results/2015/consumers-consumers-building-capacity-and-partnerships-enhance-patient

Simplilearn. (2021, January 6). *Types of digital marketing: When and how to use them?* https://www.simplilearn.com/types-of-digital-marketing-article

Wagner, S. L. (2018). *Fundamentals of medical practice management.* Health Administration Press.

PART IV

Population Health
Management: Outcomes
and Accountability

CHAPTER 11

Population Health Management: Quality Outcomes and Accountability

Stephen L. Wagner

KEY TERMS

Comparative Effectiveness Research (CER)
Cost–Benefit Analysis
High-Reliability Program
Lean
PDSA

Quality
Quality Improvement
Six Sigma
Value Stream Mapping

LEARNING OBJECTIVES

1. Describe the major quality tools (control charting, 5 Whys, Lean, and Six Sigma) that form the foundations of quality management Plan, Do, Check, Act (PDCA).
2. Select and apply appropriate quality tools to determine population health (PH) intervention effectiveness and validate decision-making processes.
3. Analyze and evaluate PH interventions using comparative effectiveness research (CER) strategies.
4. Identify the components of a high-reliability organization (HRO) and describe applications for population health management (PHM).
5. Align PHM to **quality improvement (QI)** and safety issues.

> 🔊 Podcasts that exemplify the content of this chapter are available at Springer Publishing Connect™
>
> Podcast 11.1. What Is the Real Purpose of Quality Improvement?
> Podcast 11.2. Moving to Become a High Reliability Organization

Access the podcast online at http://connect.springerpub.com/content/book/978-0-8261-4427-0/part/part04/chapter/ch11

INTRODUCTION

I want to talk to you about one of the biggest myths in medicine, and that is the idea that all we need are more medical breakthroughs and then all of our problems will be solved.

—Quyen Nguyen

Managing the benefits of PHM (and health promotion) strategies is often difficult because in some cases it may take years to show the positive effects of an intervention (Slabaugh et al., 2017b). Heart disease, for example, may take decades to reveal. People often "front-load" their lives by ignoring healthy behaviors when they are young, only to face more serious illness and disability as they age. Andrew Weil discusses the idea that humans are intended to live a long healthy life until they are in there later years, and then decline quickly into death (Weil, 2008). It is unnatural for us to face many years of slow decline, often due to lifestyle issues that can be mitigated by population health strategies (Ramos, 2016).

According to the Centers for Disease Control and Prevention (CDC), as much as 75% of our healthcare cost, not to mention the disability and suffering, comes from preventable conditions, such as obesity, diabetes, high blood pressure, unintended injury, that are large due to or exacerbated by our modern lifestyles, eating habits, lack of exercise, and stress (CDC, 2018). There has been provider resistance to measurement of outcomes and tying it to reimbursement, but that seems inevitable, and it is in the best interest of providers to be involved in the process of determining appropriate allocation of resources to prevent arbitrary or political processes from determining how resources are spent (Goitein, 2014; Mandal et al., 2017; Merkley & Bickmore, 2017; Wen et al., 2016).

PHM and health promotion are uniquely suited to address the issues related to chronic disease, such as heart disease, because it stratifies and targets populations with similar needs and introduces strategies that are applicable and proven to all members of the population group, without relying solely on individual interventions (Kent, 2018). PHM approaches also allow for systematic application of home-based communication interventions to improve compliance and patient literacy (Gaikwad & Warren, 2009).

Much of the reform to payment structures has emphasized accountability of providers to do more to manage health instead of just providing services once illness has occurred. Capitation and similar payment structure encourage the active management of a patient's health as a means of reducing cost and improving health outcomes. Because of this new realization on how reform will likely take shape, PH has become a management imperative for healthcare organizations, as they take on more risk and assume more accountability for patient care and outcomes (Quinn, 2015).

The Key Concerns: Quality Does Matter

Managing the quality of PH program is vitally important to maximize the benefits of these programs and to increase their recognition as important aspects of healthcare and community well-being and at the same time demonstrate the value they provide (Deloitte Development, 2017; Smith, 2006). This chapter focuses on providing the evidence to overcome the recognized barriers to investing in PH initiatives and support the need for greater cost-effectiveness evidence. Some of these barriers include the misguided belief that in the long run prevention may cost more than treatment, the "identifiable victim effect," the influence of special interest groups, and the reality that evidence alone does not drive health policy or funding (Richardson, 2012). The identifiable victim effect refers to the tendency of individuals to provide more aid when a specific, identified person is observed in an adverse situation, as compared with a large, vaguely defined group with the same condition or circumstances (Jenni & Loewenstein, 1997).

What Is Quality?

Quality has many definitions depending on one's perspective. Are we asking about quality of healthcare? Quality of Life? Well-being? Another view is value, what we get for the money we spend, or in the case of healthcare, the money society spends (NEJM Catalyst, 2017). A complex question indeed. In the landmark work by the Institute of Medicine (IOM) published in 2001, quality in healthcare has 10 components, many of which are relevant to PH.

DID YOU KNOW?

What Are the Components of Quality Care?

The IOM states that private and public purchasers, healthcare organizations, clinicians, and patients should work together to redesign healthcare processes in accordance with the following rules. The components of quality care are as follows:

1. **Care should be based on continuous healing relationships.** Patients should receive care whenever they need it and, in many forms, not just through face-to-face visits. The healthcare system should always be responsive (24 hours a day, every day), and access to care should be provided over the Internet, by telephone, and by other means in addition to face-to-face visits.
2. **Care should be customized based on the patient's needs and values.** The system of care should be designed to meet the most common needs but should have the flexibility to respond to an individual patient's choices and preferences.
3. **The patient should be in control.** Patients should be given necessary information and the opportunity to exercise as much control as they choose over healthcare decisions that affect them. The health system should be able to accommodate differences in patient preferences and should encourage shared decision-making.
4. **The system should encourage shared knowledge and the free flow of information.** Patients should have unfettered access to their own medical information and to clinical information. Clinicians and patients should communicate effectively and share information.
5. **Decision-making should be evidence based.** Patients should receive care based on the best available scientific knowledge. Care should not vary illogically from clinician to clinician or from place to place.
6. **Safety should be a property of the system.** Patients should be safe from injury caused by the care system. Reducing risk and ensuring safety will require systems that help prevent and mitigate errors.
7. **The system should be transparent.** The healthcare system should make information available to patients and their families, which allows them to make informed decisions when selecting a health plan, a hospital, or a clinical

practice or when choosing among alternative treatments. Patients should be informed of the system's performance on safety, evidence-based practice, and patient satisfaction.
8. **The system should anticipate patients' needs.** The health system should be proactive in anticipating a patient's needs, rather than simply reacting to events.
9. **The system should constantly strive to decrease waste.** The health system should not waste resources or patients' time.
10. **The system should encourage cooperation among clinicians.** Clinicians and institutions should actively collaborate and communicate with each other to ensure that patients receive appropriate care (Institute of Medicine, 2001).

Others define health more generally and take a more inclusive approach. According to Health Quality Ontario, "Health quality is best shaped by understanding the experiences and wisdom of patients, families, caregivers, and the public" (Health Quality Ontario, 2020). This is a much more of a coproduction model of health and healthcare.

Leadership, Governance, and Quality

As a starting point, there must be a strong leadership group and a governing structure for any PH initiative to reach its potential. These programs have many potential challenges given the number of people, groups, and organizations involved and the nature of the undertaking (Arnwine, 2002; Baicker & Levy, 2013; Blendon et al., 2006; IOM, 2001; Leape & Berwick, 2005; National Academies of Science, 1999; Porter, 2010; Thompson, 2011). Without effective leadership and management of PH programs, the results will be suboptimal at best, and failure to reach important goals is likely. Leadership sets the stage for innovation and establishes a culture of quality in addition to providing a completing vision of what the program will accomplish and why it is important (Bahensky et al., 2005; Bielaszka-DuVernay, 2011; Fillingham, 2007; Institute for Healthcare Improvement, 2005; Juran & De Feo, n.d.; Mazzocato et al., 2014; McConnell et al., 2014; Seidl & Newhouse, 2012; Toussaint, 2009; Vest & Gamm, 2009; Weick & Sutcliffe, 2015).

Important Tools for Quality Improvement

QI represents the ongoing efforts and activities to upgrade organizational operations. Although multiple QI tools are appropriate for diverse PHM applications, we can categorize them into two groups. Process models focus on a flow of tasks, while program models assess the overall impact of a PH program and the outcomes (see Figure 11.1).

Lean and Six Sigma and Other Quality Improvement Tools

There are literally hundreds of books and thousands of articles written about QI and the various tools and processes needed to achieve this end. Countless businesses have arisen in the past 30 to 40 years focused on QI. Some of the most used tools are Lean, Six Sigma (Coleman, 2012; Kang et al., 2005; Vest & Gamm, 2009; Viau & Southern, 2007), and a combination of the two known as Lean Six Sigma. Both Six Sigma and Lean have the same goal of improving quality with somewhat different approaches. Lean focuses on waste reduction, while **Six Sigma** emphasizes variation reduction. Lean uses fewer

Process models
- Lean
- Six Sigma
- 5 Whys
- PDSA

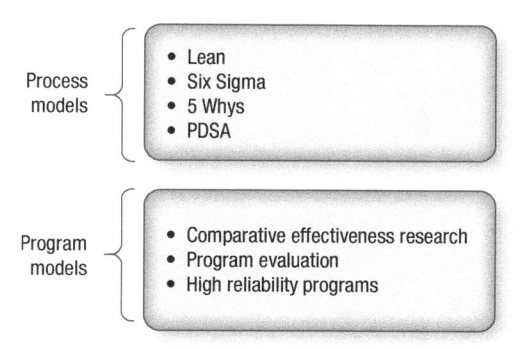

Program models
- Comparative effectiveness research
- Program evaluation
- High reliability programs

FIGURE 11.1 Process and Program Models of Quality Improvement

TABLE 11.1 Comparison of Quality Improvement Tools Lean and Six Sigma

Comparison of Lean and Six Sigma	
Lean = improvement focused on improving patient flow and eliminating the eight deadly wastes.	*Six Sigma* = process breakthroughs, design, or improvement. Teams focused on eliminating chronic problems and reducing variation in processes.
• Define value	• Define
• Measure	• Measure
• Analyze process	• Analyze
• Improve process	• Improve
• Create new standard work (for the improvement)	• Control
Which is better? It depends.	

technical tools and visual controls. Six Sigma uses much more statistical data analysis, experimental design, and hypothesis testing than Lean (ASQ, n.d.). It is important to note that anyone seeking to engage in the application of Lean, Six Sigma, or the combination of these QI strategies must gain sufficient training on using the many techniques and tools necessary to fully benefit from their use. Such training is beyond the scope of this chapter, which is intended to provide an overview. Other process tools that population health managers may consider are the 5 Whys.

As shown in Table 11.1, Lean and Six Sigma have similar goals. QI practitioners often begin by using a Lean approach to reduce waste and create value stream maps to improve understanding of the process. At that time, it may be appropriate to incorporate some of the statistical tools used in Six Sigma (Smith, 2006).

Which is a better choice would depend on the manager's perspective and the level of training they may have developed in statistical techniques. As noted in the Table 11.1, Six Sigma represents six standard deviations from the mean, presenting the number of errors that occur in a process. For such things, as PHM expecting defects or errors at 3.4 per million occurrences of the activity is rather daunting and can be very discouraging to those finding that their error rates fall more in much lower Sigma ranges. Lean on the other hand focuses on improving the process more so than a specific numerical level of performance; however, it does seek perfection. Seeing steady

What Does Six Sigma Means?

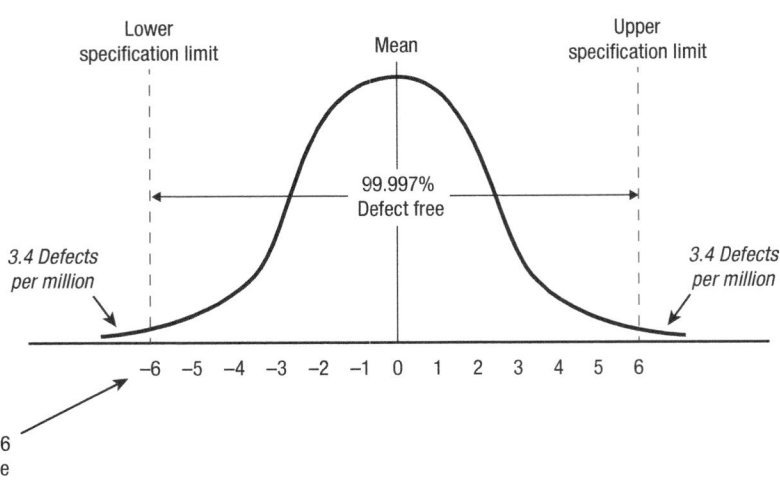

FIGURE 11.2 Six Sigma Curve of Variation

improvement without it being labeled as having achieved a statistical goal (Six Sigma) can be very motivating to those working to improve a process (see Figure 11.2).

Lean

Lean was created by the Toyota Motor Company and is heavily process-oriented. Dr. Deming often posited the notion that most of the outcome seen in an activity was the result of the process not simply the efforts of the people involved. A bad process will beat a good person every time (Deming, 1986). The eight common and ubiquitous wastes that Lean seeks to eliminate are as follows:

- *Overproduction,* which is doing more than is required earlier than needed.
- *Waiting,* which can be waiting for people, supplies, or other activities to occur, and this may happen at any stage of a process.
- *Transportation,* getting people and things to where they belong.
- *Inventory,* having more supplies or unfinished work that is needed to carry out the task.
- *Motion,* having a process that requires unnecessary physical or process steps due to inefficient layouts of the process or activity.
- *Defects,* having to redo things because of errors. Expensive and wasteful.
- *Underutilized people,* which is having people work beneath their skill levels and not listening to their ideas (Joosten et al., 2009; Juran & De Feo, n.d.).

TABLE 11.2 Common Factors Contributing to Lean Project Failures

Factor	Lessons Learned
Leadership	Loss of a process owner following can lead to poor follow-through in implementing and revising process changes. Lack of staff accountability by the process owner and leadership for changes made to activities on the action plan can derail success. Lack of outward support from all team leaders creates a climate where lack of adherence to process changes by all members is tolerated.
Scope	Failure to review the evidence base may lead to a focus on improving processes that are unrelated to targeted outcomes. Attempting to improve too many processes can overwhelm the team. Failure to complete all steps of the improvement process can derail the effort.
Resources	Without resources being allocated for data collection, it is difficult to determine the impact of Lean on efficiency of the targeted activities that are not working. Lean events are time consuming for team. Team turnover might make it difficult to make and sustain process changes and to develop a Lean culture.
Communication about Lean	There is not always effective communication about events and solutions to the team who do not participate in the event, especially large diverse teams.
Lean team composition and size	Using the same team members repeatedly on Lean events might lead to burnout.

Adapted from: Exhibit 4.19. Major Factors that Inhibit Lean Success. Agency for Healthcare Research and Quality, Rockville, MD. Http://www.ahrq.gov/professionals/systems/system/systemdesign/leancasestudies/lean-exhibit4-19.html

The aforementioned list represents potential gaps in care for various populations-of-interest. Addressing these types of quality issues can not only improve health outcomes but also result in significant cost savings.

QI models help provide frameworks and guide PH managers through the process of improving healthcare outcomes. Not all Lean projects are successful, and Table 11.2 describes the most common factors that contribute to potential failures.

Lean Tool Options: Value Stream Mapping, Kaizen, and 5 Whys

Value Stream Maps

Most Lean process improvement initiatives begin with a **value stream map (VSM)**. Lean is about creating patient or community value by eliminating waste (Toussaint & Berry, 2013). Mapping the process visually depicts the steps necessary to produce a service. As shown in Figure 11.3, mapping represents a good starting point for process improvement. The VSM defines each step as well as the time taken to complete the step. This is known as the Take time.

In our example of providing screenings for blood pressure, body mass index (BMI), a measure of obesity and blood glucose, the base process has five steps taking a total of 70 minutes. Through a process improvement initiative called a Kaizen event (which will be discussed in the next section, Kaizen), members of the team determined that two steps could be eliminated by allowing all of the screens to be completed at one station, thereby eliminating waiting time and the need for recipients to move to a new location for each test. As seen in Figures 11.3 and 11.4, time has been reduced

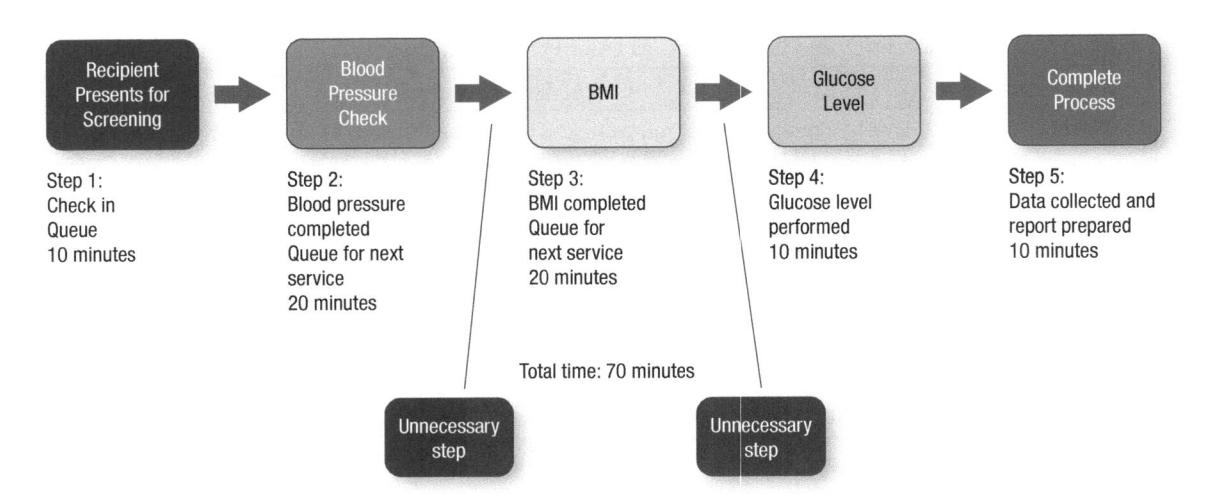

Figure 11.3 Value Stream Mapping: Base Process Example

Step 1: Check in / Queue / 10 minutes
→ **Step 2:** Blood pressure completed / Queue for next service / 20 minutes
→ **Step 3:** BMI completed / Queue for next service / 20 minutes (Unnecessary step)
→ **Step 4:** Glucose level performed / 10 minutes (Unnecessary step)
→ **Step 5:** Data collected and report prepared / 10 minutes

Total time: 70 minutes

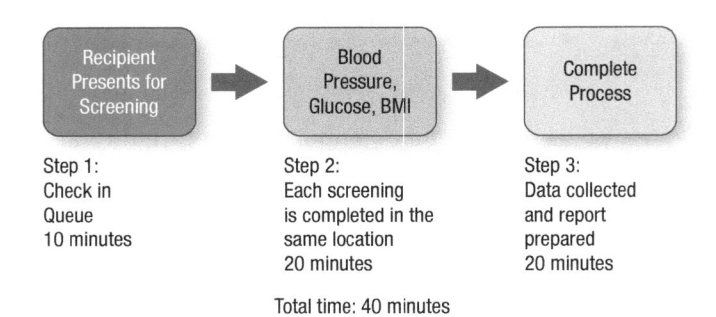

Figure 11.4 Value Stream Mapping: Improved Process Flow

Step 1: Check in / Queue / 10 minutes
→ **Step 2:** Each screening is completed in the same location / 20 minutes
→ **Step 3:** Data collected and report prepared / 20 minutes (Blood Pressure, Glucose, BMI / Complete Process)

Total time: 40 minutes

by 30 minutes. Lean thinking would indicate that there was 30 minutes of wasted time in the process.

The VSM is also valuable to better communicate activities related to the service provided. Visual representations allow all team members to clearly view the process and contribute to potential gaps in delivery.

Kaizen

Kaizen is the Sino-Japanese word for "improvement." The Kaizen is conducted by the team leader organizing participants at every level of the process, especially those providing the service, creating value stream maps, and looking for opportunities for improvement. These are often "bottlenecks" or unnecessary steps in the process. Kaizen events are very appropriate when big impacts are needed on a process. This might include serious dissatisfaction on the part of recipients due to bottlenecks in the process creating delays, inefficiencies, and added costs. The Kaizen event allows all participants to provide input and ideas (Josh Wright, 2020; Voehl, 2014).

DID YOU KNOW?

Sample Kaizen Action Steps

1. **Training and starting the activities.** Everyone participating in a kaizen event needs to be oriented and trained so that they can fully participate in the activities.
2. **Deciding on tools of continuous improvement (e.g., VSM, 5 Whys?).** Various tools will be required in any Kaizen event and selecting those which are most appropriate is important. These should be familiar to the team.
3. **Analysis of current "state."** Review the VSM created by the team and analyze each step (e.g. Exhibit 2)
4. **Select area of concern.** Focus on areas that appear to be of the greatest concern; remember one cannot always fix everything at once.
5. **Create possible solutions.** The team should consider what solutions might be appropriate for the concern that has been identified in the Kaizen.
6. **Select solutions.** Once selected, solution should be implemented in a pilot fashion to determine quickly if they improve the process.

5 Whys

The 5 Whys in Lean methodology is a simple yet elegant root cause analysis technique. By asking a series of questions with each question forming the basis for the next, it is possible to determine the root cause of an issue. Five iterations are used because it has been observed that the root cause is often discovered by the fifth question. This does not necessarily mean that a solution has been found only that the root cause becomes more evident.

An example of the 5 Whys might be as follows:

1. Question: Why did you not take your medication?

   Answer: Because I did not pick it up

2. Question: Why didn't you pick it up at the pharmacy?

   Answer: Because I do not have a car.

3. Question: Why don't you have it delivered? Answer:

   Because I did not ask them too.

4. Question: Why did you ask them to deliver it?

   Answer: Because I did not have the money.

5. Question: Why do you ask for assistance with the cost?

   Answer: Because I really do not want to take the medicine anyway.

Although a rather simple example, it illustrates the fact that we often take superficial responses to questions about actions without ever getting to the root cause of why they actually had occurred which is essential for making any permanent correction to the problem (IHI—Institute for Healthcare Improvement, 2020a). In this simple example, the root cause is going to bed to late, not missing the bus or not hearing the alarm. Maybe suggesting here that this behavior may be exhibited by hundreds of individuals within a population. Getting to the root cause could have a dramatic effect in improving the health outcome of many. This is truly patient engagement.

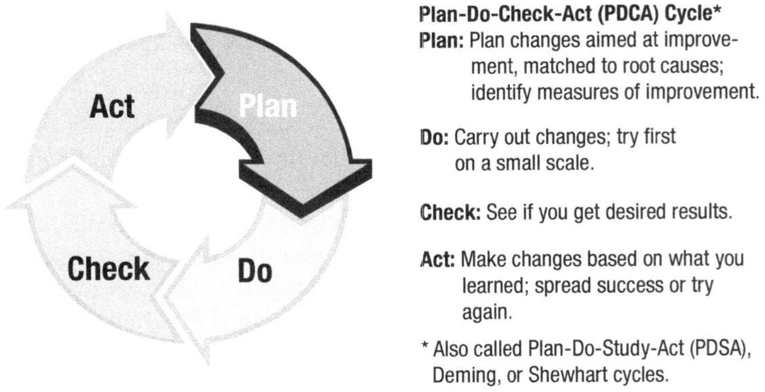

Plan-Do-Check-Act (PDCA) Cycle*

Plan: Plan changes aimed at improvement, matched to root causes; identify measures of improvement.

Do: Carry out changes; try first on a small scale.

Check: See if you get desired results.

Act: Make changes based on what you learned; spread success or try again.

* Also called Plan-Do-Study-Act (PDSA), Deming, or Shewhart cycles.

FIGURE 11.5 Plan-Do-Check-Act Cycle
Source: CDC (2017).

Plan–Do–Study–Act Cycle

The plan–do–study–act (PDSA) Worksheet is a useful tool for documenting and piloting a change in the QI process suggested in a Kaizen or other activity. The PDSA cycle is away to (plan), carrying out the test (do), observing and learning from the consequences (study), and determining what modifications should be made to the test (act). See Figure 11.5.

A worksheet can be found at IHI.org. (IHI—Institute for Healthcare Improvement, 2020c). Readers should reach out for more resources on Kaizen and other lean tools. Lean.org has many resources available as well as the IHI (IHI, 2020b).

Six Sigma Statistical Tools

Six Sigma is much more statistically oriented and uses many statistical tools. Some of the more common ones are as follows:

- *Pareto charts* usesthe Pareto principle. The Pareto principle states that 80% of outcomes result from 20% of the causes. By far charting issues of concern, it is easy to visually see what area or issue is creating the most concern.

- *Histograms* are graphic representations of numeric or continuous data. This tool allows you to quickly identify the spread of variation in the data.

- *Process control charts* help the manager of the process understand the upper and lower boundaries of performance. This demonstrates how well the process delivers expected outcomes and provides another analytical tool for reducing variation.

- Statistical analysis with an *ANOVA* charts allows managers to determine the accuracy of their measurement and when different people are involved in an activity (Seidl & Newhouse, 2012).

Six Sigma requires a significant level of training to properly use this QI technique in practice (Deming et al., 2016; Juran & De Feo, n.d.).

These process QI strategies and techniques offer multiple options for the PH managers to improve health delivery activities and positively impact a large number of individuals. It is also just as important to monitor and evaluate various PHM programs to determine heath status outcomes.

Comparative Effectiveness Research

Comparative effectiveness research (CER) is a technique used to compare various PH programs and assess their viability and effectiveness. Although the term research is included in the name, this assessment tool differs significantly from the standard randomized control trial as population programs are not randomized for study. They are tailored to priority populations, and the focus is on efficacy of the program intervention.

- Assessing the financial impact of healthcare interventions is a critical component to support decision-making for funding and program prioritization. CER, as a part of every PHM effort, can demonstrate the effectiveness of programs, policies, and interventions (Grosse et al., 2007b). Often routine data, which are readily available, can be used to evaluate various PH initiatives and can be used to compare the outcomes of the program with what one would expect, which becomes essential to overcoming barriers to supporting such programs (MacDonald et al., 2016). Many data sources can be found at the National Library of Medicine (Health Data Sources, n.d.). They include the following:

  Surveys
- Medical records
- Claims data

    Vital records

    Surveillance reports

    Peer-reviewed literature

Cost is measured against the effectiveness of two or more treatments and/or program initiatives. The term effectiveness is of critical importance here because we are not only concerned with cost, but how effective the intervention is. This is especially true when it is measuring such things as avoiding future medical cost, the value of quality of life or extra years of productive life which are difficult to evaluate (Feldstein, 2019; Slabaugh et al., 2017a). The timeline and end points, which are measured, may have serious implications for this type of analysis. For example, the effectiveness of diet and exercise on cholesterol levels may take much longer to be determined than a pharmaceutical (proscribed medication), but in the long run, it may be more effective and less costly. If the effects of these treatments on longevity were the end point, rather a simple measurement of cholesterol levels a much longer time frames are needed.

Cost–benefit analysis (CBA) is used less often because of the difficulty in valuing health and life (Neumann & Greenberg, 2009; Pearson, 2019; Phillips, 2009). Quality-adjusted life years (QALYs) and disability-adjusted life years (DALYs) are used in other countries to determine cost–benefit (Neumann & Greenberg, 2009; "WHO |Metrics: Disability-Adjusted Life Year (DALY)," 2014; Zarate, 2007), but the United States has been less engaged in using a strict economic model to determine value (Greenberg & Neumann, 2011; Neumann & Greenberg, 2009). It may be because such measures imply rationing of care or programs, which is often done de facto through resource allocation (Pearl, 2017).

> ### ❓ DID YOU KNOW?
>
> **Cost–Benefit Analysis**
>
> *The Inputs*
> Net cost is the intervention cost minus averted medical and other identifiable cost of outcomes that can be quantified in dollars: changes in health outcomes with the intervention in place minus outcomes without the intervention in place (Grosse et al., 2007a). Examples of health outcomes include heart attacks and deaths from heart disease, childhood obesity prevention and intervention, and tobacco use abatement.
>
> *The Output*
> CBA provides information on health and cost impacts of an intervention compared with an alternative intervention (or the status quo). If the net cost of an intervention is positive (which means a more effective intervention may be more costly), then the results are presented as a cost-effectiveness ratio. A cost-effectiveness ratio is the net cost divided by changes in health outcomes. Examples include cost per case of disease prevented, medical costs attributed to a health condition such as obesity, or cost per death averted. If the net costs are negative (which means a more effective intervention is less costly), the results are reported as net cost savings. The following is the CBA example (intervention is more effective and less costly).
>
> *Example*
> The following example is a comparison between a childhood program focused on reducing obesity and its complications, such as diabetes to the status quo of no program. The cost of implementing the program is much less than the medical costs averted, not to mention the lifelong benefits, which in this simple example are not determined. One of the issues that does arise in doing such evaluation is the lack of available data, so estimates are often necessary and at times very difficult to determine (Owen et al., 2018). It is essential to be as accurate as possible to avoid unwarranted criticism of the validity of the analysis. In this case, the outcome metric for the intervention is cost savings; the results are not presented as a cost-effectiveness ratio. Instead, they are presented as net cost savings (Siegel, 2002).
>
> *Childhood Obesity Program Example*
> *The Three-Step Process*
> Calculate Net Cost
> Costs of implementation (cost of testing, program activities, education, and treatment):
> Cost averted (cost of treating childhood disease related to obesity):
> Net costs (positive value means money spent):
> Identify change in health outcomes:
> Calculate cost-effectiveness ratio:
> Net costs/change in health outcome = 7.5/76.4
>
> *Childhood Obesity Program Results*
> | | |
> |---|---:|
> | Costs of implementation: | $7.5 million |
> | Cost averted (medical costs): | −$76.4 million |
> | Net costs (negative value means cost savings): | − $68.9 million |

Program Evaluation and Certification

Ensuring the quality of any PHM program requires selecting the most appropriate measurement tool to assess both effectiveness and efficacy. For many heath promotion and other types of programs, an alternative strategy can be the integration of population evaluation.

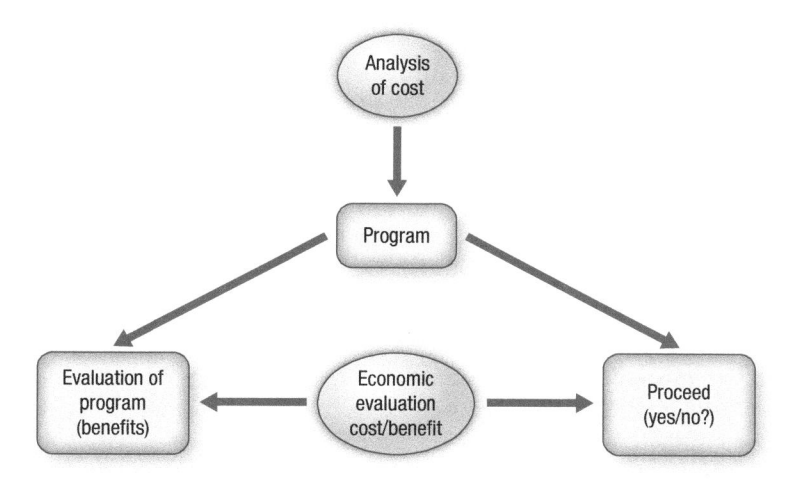

FIGURE 11.6 Cost-Effectiveness Research

In addition to comparative effectiveness research (CER), program evaluation is a systematic way to improve and account for PH programs by involving procedures that are useful, feasible, ethical, and accurate (CDC-PPEO, 2020). Without assessing the health impacts of a program, CBA alone may not provide a complete understanding of the PH program's value.

Figure 11.6 illustrates the use of program evaluation using both cost-effectiveness and program benefits as a criterion.

The National Committee on Quality Assurance

One prominent certification program for PHM is one provided by the NCQA. The NCQA standards are a road map for improvement—organizations use them to perform a gap analysis and align improvement activities with areas that are most important to state and employers, such as network adequacy and consumer protection. Standards evaluate plans on the following:

- Quality management and improvement
- Population health management
- Network management
- Utilization management
- Credentialing and recredentialing
- Members' rights and responsibilities
- Member connections
- Medicaid Benefits and Services (NCQA, 2018, 2020)

NCQA Population Health Program Accreditation helps organizations align their operations with the industry's best PHM practices. Having a solid PH strategy is reassuring to all that programs can monitor and address opportunities and challenges in their populations.

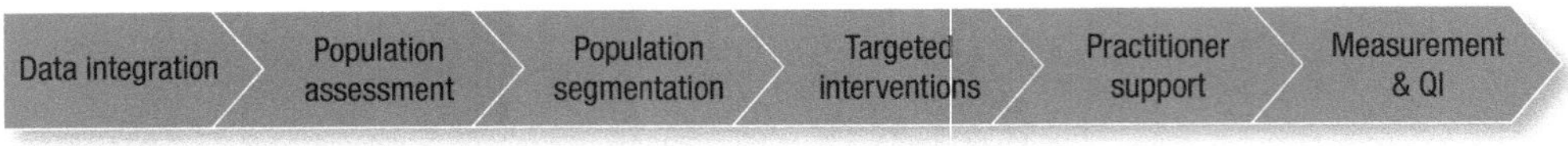

Data integration → Population assessment → Population segmentation → Targeted interventions → Practitioner support → Measurement & QI

FIGURE 11.7 NCQA Population Health Program Assessment Criteria

NCQA, National Committee on Quality Assurance.

The National Committee on Quality Assurance Uses a Quality Improvement Framework

NCQA's standards provide a framework for organizations to standardize care, become more efficient, and manage complex needs better. This helps keep members healthier, reduce risks, and prevent unnecessary costs from poor care management.

The NCQA population health program evaluates organizations in six key areas as presented in Figure 11.7 (NCQA, 2020).

NCQA PH programs help to create a **high-reliablity program (HRP)** similar in character to a HRO.

High-Reliability Programs

Establishing reliability in PH interventions requires valid clear specific measures. It also requires a culture focused on patient safety and quality. One model for improvement suggests the following action steps:

- Identify evidence-based interventions that focus on improved outcomes.
- Select outcomes that covert to behaviors.
- Develop measures to evaluate reliability.
- Measure baseline performance.
- Determine and ensure the targeted population receives evidence-based interventions (Gawande, 2007; Pronovost et al., 2006).

For more in-depth information on HRPs, read references by Weick, Pronovost, White, Morrow, Wilson, and their colleagues (Morrow, n.d.; Pronovost et al., 2006; Weick & Sutcliffe, 2015; White et al., 2016; Wilson et al., 2005).

> **? DID YOU KNOW?**
>
> QI options provide PH managers multiple models for assessment and obtain the status of an HRP. The common characteristics of HRP are presented in Table 11.3.

TABLE 11.3 Common Characteristics of High-Reliability Programs

Characteristic	Description
Preoccupation with failure	Everyone is aware of and thinking about the potential for failure. People understand that new threats emerge regularly from situations that no one imagined could occur, so all personnel actively think about what could go wrong and are alert to small signs of potential problems. The absence of errors or accidents leads not to complacency but to a heightened sense of vigilance for the next possible failure. Near misses are viewed as opportunities to learn about systems issues and potential improvements, rather than as evidence of safety.

Reluctance to simplify	People resist simplifying their understanding of work processes and how and why things succeed or fail in their environment. People in HROs understand that the work is complex and dynamic. They seek underlying rather than surface explanations. While HROs recognize the value of standardization of workflows to reduce variation, they also appreciate the complexity inherent in the number of teams, processes, and relationships involved in conducting daily operations.
Sensitivity to operations	Based on their understanding of operational complexity, people in HROs strive to maintain a high awareness of operational conditions. This sensitivity is often referred to as "big picture understanding" or "situation awareness." It means that people cultivate an understanding of the context of the current state of their work in relation to the unit or organizational state—i.e., what is going on around them—and how the current state might support or threaten safety.
Deference to expertise	People in HROs appreciate that the people closest to the work are the most knowledgeable about the work. Thus, people in HROs know that in a crisis or emergency the person with greatest knowledge of the situation might not be the person with the highest status and seniority. Deference to local and situation expertise results in a spirit of inquiry and de-emphasis on hierarchy in favor of learning as much as possible about potential safety threats. In an HRO, everyone is expected to share concerns with others and the organizational climate is such that all staff members are comfortable speaking up about potential safety problems.
Commitment to resilience	Commitment to resilience is rooted in the fundamental understanding of the frequently unpredictable nature of system failures. People in HROs assume the system is at risk for failure, and they practice performing rapid assessments of and responses to challenging situations. Teams cultivate situation assessment and cross monitoring so they may identify potential safety threats quickly and either respond before safety problems cause harm or mitigate the seriousness of the safety event.

HROs, high-reliability organizations.

Sources: From https://psnet.ahrq.gov/primers/primer/31/high-reliability; Chassin & Loeb, 2013; Hines et al., 2008; Rochlin, 1999; Weick & Sutcliffe, 2015

HRPs serve as attainable examples for the value of QI as an integrated strategy in achieving both positive health outcomes and cost savings.

SUMMARY

As we have seen with the 2020 pandemic of COVID-19, the need for better PHM and epidemiological research is more important than ever before (Rogawski et al., 2016). QI efforts combine these skills and competencies to consistently address challenges and barriers that limit the success of PH processes and programs. Common QI process models include Six Sigma, Lean, and various related strategies. Program evaluation models commonly recognized are the Comparative Effectiveness Research, NCQA program assessment criteria, and the HRO model.

DISCUSSION QUESTIONS

1. PH managers struggle with quality outcomes, accountability, and patient safety. Briefly compare the differences between Lean and Six Sigma, and summarize why each has been so effective for improving healthcare delivery.
2. Have you ever experienced working with any of the following QI tools: VSM, 5 Whys, Kaizen, PDSA, or any of the control charting methods? Which one had the most value for your organization?
3. Why would it be beneficial to receive NCQA certification for your PH program?
4. Discuss why clinical research protocols based on the randomized control model may not be appropriate for PHM programs?
5. Develop a scenario comparing two PH programs and involving the use of a CBA.

Toolkit Competency Application: Mini Scenarios for Quality Improvement

Directions: PH managers constantly focus on attaining positive outcomes for their various and populations. Healthcare service delivery gaps often occur during transitions of care and/or hand-offs to specialized care. Each of the three vignettes suggests a need for a QI initiative. Choose between the diverse QI options covered in this chapter for each one of the vignettes and then briefly outline a rationale for your decisions. Assume you are the PH manager in each of these situations.

#1 Teamwork and coordination between primary care providers and health specialists can be especially difficult to improve. You are responsible for a patient-centered medical home, where providers can receive incentives for attaining various benchmarks. Recent patient comments support operational scheduling data that follow-up visits are not being completed for a particular service (orthopedics/rehab). Which QI initiative would you choose and why?

#2 To prevent the potential of a twindemic[1] occurring, XYZ hospital developed a new social media program tailored to seniors to encourage an increase in flu shots. To date, the program has not increased the number of flu shots provided especially to minority seniors. Which QI initiative would you choose, and why?

1 *Twindemic* refers to the dual threat of a severe flu outbreak on top of the COVID-19 pandemic in the fall and winter of 2020 (https://www.dictionary.com/e/tech-science/twindemic).

#3 A large heathcare system operated 20 mobile (drive-up) COVID testing sites. Data show extreme variation in the number of tests collected among these sites despite a standardized number of personnel involved. Which QI initiative would you choose, and why?

REFERENCES

Arnwine, D. L. (2002). *Effective governance: The roles and responsibilities of board members.* Baylor University of Medical Center Proceedings (BUMC). https://www.ncbi.nlm.nih.gov/pmc/articles/PMC1276331/pdf/bumc0015-0019.pdf

ASQ. (n.d.). *Six sigma definition. What is lean six sigma?* Retrieved June 29, 2020, from https://asq.org/quality-resources/six-sigma

Bahensky, J. A., Roe, J., & Bolton, R. (2005). Lean Sigma—Will it work for healthcare? *Journal of Health Informatics and Management, 19*, 39–44.

Baicker, K., & Levy, H. (2013). Coordination versus competition in health care reform. *New England Journal of Medicine, 369*(9), 789–791. https://doi.org/10.1056/NEJMp1306268

Bielaszka-DuVernay, C. (2011). Innovation profile: Redesigning acute care processes in Wisconsin. *Health Affairs*. https://doi.org/10.1377/hlthaff.2011.0087

Blendon, R. J., Brodie, M., Benson, J. M., Altman, D. E., & Buhr, T. (2006). Americans' views of health care costs, access, and quality. *The Milbank Quarterly, 84*(4), 623–657. https://doi.org/10.1111/j.1468-0009.2006.00463.x

CDC. (2017). *National Public Health Performance Standard Program: User guide*. https://www.cdc.gov/NPHPSP/PDF/UserGuide.pdf

CDC. (2018). *Health and economic costs of chronic disease | CDC*. Health and Economic Costs of Chronic Diseases. https://www.cdc.gov/chronicdisease/about/costs/index.htm

CDC-PPEO. (2020). *Framework for program evaluation*. A Framework for Program Evaluation. https://www.cdc.gov/eval/framework/index.htm

Chassin, M. R., & Loeb, J. M. (2013). High-reliability health care: Getting there from here. *The Milbank Quarterly, 91*(3), 459–490. https://doi.org/10.1111/1468-0009.12023

Coleman, S. Y. (2012). Six sigma in healthcare. In *Statistical methods in healthcare*. https://doi.org/10.1002/9781119940012.ch14

Deloitte Development. (2017). *Deloitte 2017 Survey of US Health System CEOs: Moving forward in an uncertain environment*. Deloitte Development.

Deming, W. E. (1986). *Out of the crisis*. MIT Press.

Deming, W. E., Jackson, T., James, J., Liker, J., Munger, C., Mosadeghrad, A. M., Martin, K., Osterling, M., Shewhart, W., Deming, E., Makary, M., Daniel, M., McGlynn Asch, Steven, Adams, John, Keesey, Joan, Hicks, Jennifer, DeCristofaro, Alison, K., Eve, E., Tent, M. B. W., Drucker, P., Jackson, T., Pyzdek, T., Keller, P., Barry, R., ... Miller, H. D. (2016). The six sigma book for healthcare: Improving outcomes by reducing errors. In B. Quick (Ed.), *http://rube.asq.org/gov/* (Vol. 28, Issue 5). McGraw-Hill Education. https://doi.org/10.1377/hlthaff.28.5.1418

Feldstein, P. J. (2019). *Health policy issues: An economic perspective*. Health Administration Press.

Fillingham, D. (2007). Can lean save lives? *Leadership in Health Services, 20*(4), 231–241. https://doi.org/10.1108/17511870710829346

Gaikwad, R., & Warren, J. (2009). The role of home-based information and communications technology interventions in chronic disease management: A systematic literature review. *Health Informatics Journal, 15*(2), 122–146. https://doi.org/10.1177/1460458209102973

Gawande, A. (2007). The checklist: If something so simple can transform intensive care, what else can it do? *New Yorker*. https://doi.org/10.1097/ACM.0b013e3180556d21

Goitein, L. (2014). The argument against reimbursing physicians for value. *JAMA Internal Medicine, 174*(6), 845. https://doi.org/10.1001/jamainternmed.2014.1063

Greenberg, D., & Neumann, P. J. (2011). Does adjusting for health-related quality of life matter in economic evaluations of cancer-related interventions? *Expert Review of Pharmacoeconomics & Outcomes Research, 11*(1), 113–119. https://doi.org/10.1586/erp.11.1

Grosse, S. D., Teutsch, S. M., & Haddix, A. C. (2007a). Lessons from cost-effectiveness research for United States public health policy. *Annual Review of Public Health, 28*, 365–391. https://doi.org/10.1146/annurev.publhealth.28.021406.144046

Grosse, S. D., Teutsch, S. M., & Haddix, A. C. (2007b). Lessons from cost-effectiveness research for United States public health policy. *Annual Review of Public Health, 28*(1), 365–391. https://doi.org/10.1146/annurev.publhealth.28.021406.144046

Health Data Sources. (n.d.). Retrieved July 2, 2020, from https://www.nlm.nih.gov/nichsr/stats_tutorial/section3/index.html

Health Quality Ontario. (2020). *Quality is... What is health quality*. https://www.hqontario.ca/What-is-Health-Quality/Quality-Is

Hines, S., Luna, K., Lofthus, J., & Marquardt, M. S. D. (2008). *Becoming a high reliability organization: Operational advice for hospital leaders*. https://archive.ahrq.gov/professionals/quality-patient-safety/quality-resources/tools/hroadvice/hroadvice.pdf

IHI – Institute for Healthcare Improvement. (2020a). *5 Whys: Finding the root cause*. Tools. http://www.ihi.org/resources/Pages/Tools/5-Whys-Finding-the-Root-Cause.aspx

IHI – Institute for Healthcare Improvement. (2020b). *Lean and six sigma: A one-two punch*. Lean and Six Sigma: A One-Two Punch. http://www.ihi.org/resources/Pages/Publications/LeanandSixSigma.aspx

IHI – Institute for Healthcare Improvement. (2020c). *Plan-Do-Study-Act (PDSA) worksheet*. Tools. http://www.ihi.org/resources/Pages/Tools/PlanDoStudyActWorksheet.aspx

Institute for Healthcare Improvement. (2005). *Going lean in health care 7 innovation series 2005*. www.ihi.org

Institute of Medicine. (2001). *Crossing the quality chasm: A new health system for the 21th century*. IOM. https://doi.org/10.17226/10027

IOM. (2001). *Crossing the quality chasm*. http://www.nationalacademies.org/hmd/~/media/Files/Report Files/2001/Crossing-the-Quality-Chasm/Quality Chasm 2001 report brief.pdf

Jenni, K., Loewenstein, G. (1997). Explaining the "Identifiable victim effect." *Journal of Risk and Uncertainty, 14*(3 special issue on the value of life), 235–257. https://www.jstor.org/preview-page/10.2307/41760854?seq=1

Joosten, T., Bongers, I., & Janssen, R. (2009). Application of lean thinking to health care: Issues and observations. *International Journal for Quality in Health Care, 21*(5), 341–347. https://doi.org/10.1093/intqhc/mzp036

Josh Wright. (2020). *Kaizen: The complete guide to implementing the smart concept of continuous improvement of all the strategic operations in the development process involving the Lean and Agile startup team*. https://www.amazon.com/Kaizen-Implementing-Continuous-Improvement-Development/dp/B087HF2WR9/ref=sr_1_21?crid=2A8EX65D36FQV&dchild=1&keywords=lean+process+improvement&qid=1593610661&sprefix=lean+improvement%2Caps%2C151&sr=8-21

Juran, J. M., Joseph, M., & De Feo, J. A. (n.d.). *Juran's quality handbook: The complete guide to performance excellence*. http://qpr.buaa.edu.cn/_local/4/D4/C0/81CC8D81E1AE0E0518FBECD1CB2_F5D24D52_50DBCF.pdf?e=.pdf

Kang, J. O., Kim, M. H., Hong, S. E., Jung, J. H., & Song, M. J. (2005). The application of the Six Sigma program for the quality management of the PACS. *American Journal of Roentgenology, 185*, 1361–1365.

Kent, J. (2018). *Addressing chronic disease with population health management strategies*. Health IT Analytics. https://healthitanalytics.com/news/addressing-chronic-disease-with-population-health-management-strategies

Leape, L. L., & Berwick, D. M. (2005). Five years after to err is human: What have we learned? *Journal of the American Medical Association, 293*, 2384–2390. https://doi.org/10.1001/jama.293.19.2384

MacDonald, M., Pauly, B., Wong, G., Schick-Makaroff, K., van Roode, T., Strosher, H. W., Kothari, A., Valaitis, R., Manson, H., O'Briain, W., Carroll, S., Lee, V., Tong, S., Smith, K. D., & Ward, M. (2016). Supporting successful implementation of public health interventions: Protocol for a realist synthesis. *Systematic Reviews, 5*(1), 1–11. https://doi.org/10.1186/s13643-016-0229-1

Mandal, A. K., Tagomori, G. K., Felix, R. V., & Howell, S. C. (2017). Value-based contracting innovated medicare advantage healthcare delivery and improved survival. *American Journal of Managed Care, 23*, e41–e49

Mazzocato, P., Thor, J., Bäckman, U., Brommels, M., Carlsson, J., Jonsson, F., Hagmar, M., & Savage, C. (2014). Complexity complicates lean: Lessons from seven emergency services. *Journal of Health Organization and Management, 28*(2), 266–288. https://doi.org/10.1108/JHOM-03-2013-0060

McConnell, K. J., Chang, A. M., Maddox, T. M., Wholey, D. R., & Lindrooth, R. C. (2014). An exploration of management practices in hospitals. *Healthcare, 2*. https://doi.org/10.1016/j.hjdsi.2013.12.014

Merkley, K., & Bickmore, A. M. (2017). *The Top five recommendations for improving the patient experience*. http://www.healthcatalyst.com/wp-content/uploads/2016/09/Top-Five-Recommendations-for-Improving-Patient-Experience.pdf

Morrow, R. (2016). *Leading high-reliability organizations in healthcare.* Productivity Press. https://doi.org/10.1201/b19529 ISBN 9780367737283

National Academies of Science. (1999). *To err is human: Building a safer health system.* Press Release. http://www8.nationalacademies.org/onpinews/newsitem.aspx?Record ID=9728

NCQA. (2018). *The state of health care quality 2018.* https://www.ncqa.org/report-cards/health-plans/state-of-health-care-quality-report/

NCQA. (2020). *Population Health Program Accreditation – NCQA.* Population Health Program Accreditation. https://www.ncqa.org/programs/health-plans/population-health-program-accreditation/

NEJM Catalyst. (2017). *What is value-based healthcare?* NEJM Catalyst. https://catalyst.nejm.org/what-is-value-based-healthcare/

Neumann, P. J., & Greenberg, D. (2009). Is the United States ready For QALYs? *Health Affairs, 28*(5), 1366–1371. https://doi.org/10.1377/hlthaff.28.5.1366

Owen, L., Pennington, B., Fischer, A., & Jeong, K. (2018). The cost-effectiveness of public health interventions examined by NICE from 2011 to 2016. *Journal of Public Health (United Kingdom), 40*(3), 557–566. https://doi.org/10.1093/pubmed/fdx119

Pearl, R. (2017, February). Why healthcare rationing is a growing reality for Americans. *Forbes Magazine.* https://www.forbes.com/sites/robertpearl/2017/02/02/why-healthcare-rationing-is-a-growing-reality-for-americans/#1c3522e92dba

Pearson, S. D. (2019). Why the coming debate over the QALY and disability will be different. *The Journal of Law, Medicine & Ethics, 47*(2), 304–307. https://doi.org/10.1177/1073110519857286

Phillips, C. (2009). *What is a QALY?* Hayward Medical Communications.

Porter, M. E. (2010). What is value in health care? *New England Journal of Medicine, 363,* 2477–2481. https://doi.org/10.1056/NEJMp1011024

Pronovost, P. J., Berenholtz, S. M., Goeschel, C. A., Needham, D. M., Sexton, J. B., Thompson, D. A., Lubomski, L. H., Marsteller, J. A., Makary, M. A., & Hunt, E. (2006). Creating high reliability in health care organizations. *Health Services Research, 41*(4 Pt 2), 1599–1617. https://doi.org/10.1111/j.1475-6773.2006.00567.x

Quinn, K. (2015). The 8 basic payment methods in health care. *Annals of Internal Medicine, 163,* 300–306. https://doi.org/10.7326/M14-2784

Ramos, L. (2016). 6 Business imperatives for population health management. *Healthcare Executive, 31,* 16–20.

Richardson, A. K. (2012). Investing in public health: Barriers and possible solutions. *Journal of Public Health, 34*(3), 322–327. https://doi.org/10.1093/pubmed/fds039

Rochlin, G. I. (1999). Safe operation as a social construct. *Ergonomics, 42*(11), 1549–1560. https://doi.org/10.1080/001401399184884

Rogawski, E.T., Gray, C.L., Poole, C. (2016). An argument for renewed focus on epidemiology for public health. *Annals of Epidemiology, 26*(10). https://doi.org/10.1016/J.ANNEPIDEM.2016.08.008

Seidl, K. L., & Newhouse, R. P. (2012). The intersection of evidence-based practice with 5 quality improvement methodologies. *The Journal of Nursing Administration, 42*(6), 299–304. https://doi.org/10.1097/NNA.0b013e31824ccdc9

Siegel, M. (2002). The effectiveness of state-level tobacco control interventions: A review of program implementation and behavioral outcomes. *Annual Review of Public Health, 23,* 45–71. https://doi.org/10.1146/annurev.publhealth.23.092601.095916

Slabaugh, S. L., Shah, M., Zack, M., Happe, L., Cordier, T., Havens, E., Davidson, E., Miao, M., Prewitt, T., & Jia, H. (2017a). Leveraging health-related quality of life in population health management: The case for healthy days. *Population Health Management, 20*(1), 13–22. https://doi.org/10.1089/pop.2015.0162

Slabaugh, S. L., Shah, M., Zack, M., Happe, L., Cordier, T., Havens, E., Davidson, E., Miao, M., Prewitt, T., & Jia, H. (2017b). Leveraging health-related quality of life in population health management: The case for healthy days. *Population Health Management, 20*(1), 13–22. https://doi.org/10.1089/pop.2015.0162

Smith, B. (2006). *Lean and six sigma.* Management Services, April, 14–17.

Thompson, C. P. (2011). *What is cost-effectiveness?* Education for Health. https://doi.org/10.1007/s00383-011-3028-8

Toussaint, J. (2009). Writing the new playbook for U.S. health care: Lessons from Wisconsin. *Health Affairs (Project Hope), 28*(5), 1343–1350. https://doi.org/10.1377/hlthaff.28.5.1343

Toussaint, J. S., & Berry, L. L. (2013). The promise of lean in health care. *Mayo Clinic Proceedings, 88*(1), 74–82. https://doi.org/10.1016/j.mayocp.2012.07.025

Vest, J. R., & Gamm, L. D. (2009). A critical review of the research literature on Six Sigma, Lean and StuderGroup's Hardwiring Excellence in the United States: The need to demonstrate and communicate the effectiveness of transformation strategies in healthcare. *Implementation Science, 4*, 35.

Viau, M., & Southern, B. (2007). Six Sigma and Lean concepts, a case study: Patient centered care model for a mammography center. *Radiology Management, 29*, 19–28.

Voehl, F. (2014). *Lean Six Sigma black belt handbook: Tools and methods for process acceleration*. CRC Press (an imprint of Taylor & Francis).

Weick, K. E., & Sutcliffe, K. M. (2015). *Managing the unexpected: Sustained performance in a complex world*. Wiley.

Weil, A. (2008). *Healthy aging: A lifelong guide to your well-being* (Reprint Edition). Random House, LLC. https://www.amazon.com/Healthy-Aging-Lifelong-Guide-Well-Being-ebook/dp/B000SEFKA8/ref=sr_1_4?ie=UTF8&qid=1550928006&sr=8-4&keywords=healthy+aging

Wen, L., Divers, C., Lingohr-Smith, M., & Lin, J. (2016). Overview of national leading organizations involved in quality of care in oncology. *Value in Health, 19*, A38. https://doi.org/10.1016/j.jval.2016.03.397

White, K. R., Kenneth R., & Griffith, J. R. (2016). *The well-managed healthcare organization*. Health Administration Press/AUPHA.

WHO | Metrics. (2014). *Disability-Adjusted Life Year (DALY)*. WHO. https://www.who.int/healthinfo/global_burden_disease/metrics_daly/en/

Wilson, K. A., Burke, C. S., Priest, H. A., & Salas, E. (2005). Promoting health care safety through training high reliability teams. *Quality & Safety in Health Care, 14*(4), 303–309. https://doi.org/10.1136/qshc.2004.010090

Zarate, V. (2007). DALYs And QALYs in developing countries. *Health Affairs, 26*(4), 1197–1198. https://doi.org/10.1377/hlthaff.26.4.1197-a

CHAPTER 12

Collaborations and Coproduction of Health

Stephen L. Wagner and Anne M. Hewitt

KEY TERMS

Collaboration
Convener Model
Coproduction Decision-Making Pathway (CDMP)
Coproduction of Health

Health in All Policies (HIAP)
Integrator
Interlocking Chain for Health Outcomes
Nontraditional Competitors

LEARNING OBJECTIVES

1. Define coproduction of health and identify the major aspects of this collaborative strategic approach.
2. Describe collaboration strategies applicable for population health managers.
3. Apply skills and tool options appropriate for the coproduction of health process that will improve population health (PH) intervention effectiveness.
4. Discuss the importance of culturally competent interventions for the coproduction of health.
5. Apply strategies for cross-sectional intervention in communities.

> Podcasts that exemplify the content of this chapter are available at Springer Publishing Connect™
>
> Podcast 12.1. Isn't Cooperation the Same as Collaboration?
> Podcast 12.2. Collaborators and Not Competitors

Access the podcast online at http://connect.springerpub.com/content/book/978-0-8261-4427-0/part/part04/chapter/ch12

INTRODUCTION

> None of us is as smart as all of us.
>
> Ken Blanchard

Population health management (PHM) continually seeks new ways to deliver better health services to our communities and change the healthcare culture from simply a service provider to one that focuses on the outcome of better health and well-being. We are entering a time when the goals of population healthcare management, other health sector stakeholders, and nonhealth corporations and parties are beginning to merge and focus on a collaborative approach to improved health for all Americans. **Collaboration,** working with others, is not new for PHM as relationship with public and community health organizations is common. The healthcare sector is transforming to include potential and unique partnerships with previous competitors, venture capitalists, nonprofit agencies, and public health.

Exacerbated by events like the COVID-19 crisis, PHmanagers need to recognize that others external to the hospital sector contribute to the well-being and health of a community. In the past, management of institutions, medical practices, state and federal agencies, and public health organizations were separate activities and seen as distinct in many ways with separate missions (Bialek et al., 2020). Previously, collaboration with these and other community resources such as grocery stores and fitness centers like the YMCA was limited or nonexistent. The involvement of the "consumer," the community, and the service recipient (patient) has been limited especially as we develop programs and services to improve the health of our citizens.

The health sector is transforming. As healthcare organizations (HCOs) become larger and payment mechanisms require more accountability from providers of healthcare, changes will become even more apparent as our system of care evolves. Providers of services must be more accountable in a way that delivers value to the patient and society at large (Berwick et al., 2008). The inevitable outcome of this coalescence of purpose is the need to focus on root cause of disease, ailments, and social determinants of health (Ellner & Phillips, 2017; Emanuel et al., 2016).

Coproduction of Health

PHM strategies offer an effective framework for managing the cause of disease as well as the delivery of healthcare in a more efficient and effective way (Deloitte Health, 2020). The Population Health Alliance (PHA) is the only industry organization of its kind that strives to work along the continuum of health and well-being through participation by all stakeholders (PHA, 2020).

Health policymakers have long recognized that many of today's primary causes of health disparities and inequities are beyond the scope of any single organization or even group of health systems to alleviate. The **Health in All Policies** (HIAP) adopted by many communities and municipalities is a universal approach to integrate positive health outcomes across various social and policy sectors.

🅿 DID YOU KNOW?

Health in All Policies

HIAP is a collaborative approach to improving population health by incorporating health considerations into decision-making across various sectors and policy issues (Strategy, 2016). For PH managers, the HIAP approach offers a framework for developing partnerships and programs in four categories: Clinical & Community Preventive Services, Elimination of Health Disparities, Empowered People, and Healthy and Safe Community Environments.

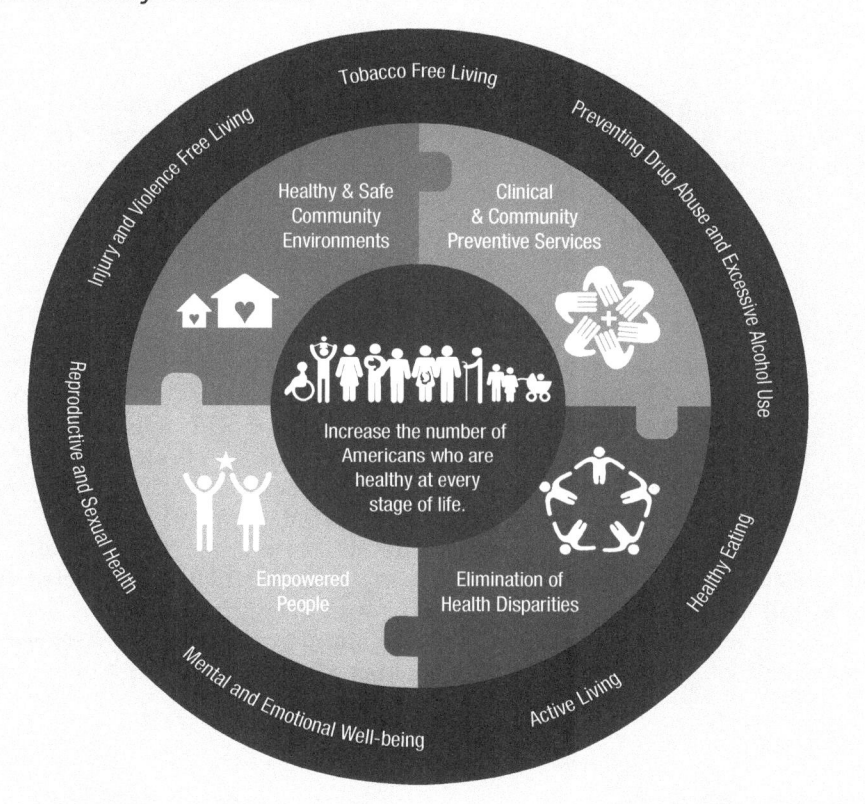

The Centers for Disease Control and Prevention (CDC) sponsors a Health In All Policies website with available resources for all communities and organizations (https://www.cdc.gov/policy/hiap/index.html). The World Health Organization supported this perspective with a clarifying statement in 2013 that emphasized the need for all public policies to adopt an approach that both avoided harmful health impacts and addressed health equity and disparities (Kieny, 2013).

Going forward, healthcare administration, public health, and PHM will be inseparable. Every healthcare administrator and manager will need to become more adept at PHM to be effective and for their organization to survive in this new age. Understanding the overlap of public health, population health, and traditional healthcare administration has implications for the coproduction, coordination, and collaboration of health and has become essential for all manager and leaders if they are to be successful in the future of an evolving healthcare system focused on outcomes and the Triple AIM as its metric.

The coproduction of health is going to become one of the new norms (Bodenheimer & Sinsky, 2014; Ellner & Phillips, 2017; Genuino, 2018; IOM, 2001; Katz, 2001; McGinnis et al., 2002).

Coproduction of health can be summed up in a beautiful poem by John Donne (1839):

> *No man is an island, entire of itself; every man is a piece of the continent, a part of the main; if a clod be washed away by the sea, Europe is the less, as well as if a promontory were, as well as if a manor of thy friend's or of thine own were; any man's death diminishes me, because I am involved in mankind, and therefore never send to know for whom the bell tolls; it tolls for thee.*

Although the aforementioned quote refers to a single individual, this thought should include all people. The idea that we are connected and have accountability for one another cannot be lost. The alignment with health and nonhealth sector collaborators is primary for PHM. That is the essence of coproduction of health.

Coproduction of Health Strategies

A single modern definition has not been established for coproduction of health. The idea of coproduction of a service or product did not originate from the healthcare industry as so often is the case with new innovation, but from other industries (Grönroos, 2011) where consumers became highly engaged in the development of products and services and they are offered together for convenience and to increase access (Bettencourt et al., 2002; Realpe & Wallace, 2010). The consumer or, in the case of PH, the recipients of service and the community are the focus and must be engaged for there to be a credible coproduction of health effort as seen in Figure 12.1.

The coproduction of health is inclusive and has a basis in the civil rights movement of the 1960s as well. Consider that the involvement in your

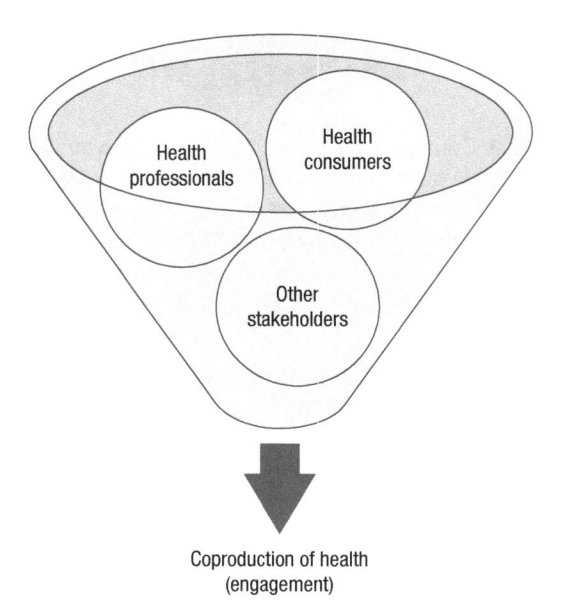

FIGURE 12.1 Engaging All Stakeholders for Inclusive Coproduction of Health

personal healthcare decision-making would certainly qualify as a human right, not to mention the inequality health and healthcare has seen in our population with many groups seeing large disparities in health outcomes (Office of Disease Prevention and Health Promotion [ODPHP], 2019; Rosa Dias & O'Donnell, 2013).

From a PH perspective, **coproduction of health** requires a close collaboration between clinicians, social services, government agencies, community organizations, and all parties focused on the well-being of the population (Turakhia & Combs, 2017b).

Figure 12.2 provides a visual image of how the coproduction of health can be optimized in a community. Public health organizations, government resources, medical practices and providers, and health facilities such as hospitals all combined with community resources and the patients to produce the desired outcome for a targeted population. It should be emphasized that the priority population be involved from the beginning of any coproduction effort (Janamian et al., 2016). Hippocrates once said, "The Physician must not only be prepared to do what is right [himself,] but also make the patient…cooperate" (Hippocrates, 1886, p. 113, volume 2). It is necessary for each individual and all involved in a coproduction effort to help bring about change in behavior.

Maximizing PH programs, hospitals, and other healthcare institutions cannot occur in a vacuum without community collaboration as illustrated in Figure 12.3. Without the engagement of all stakeholders, any coproduction initiative will be less effective at achieving the desired outcome (Enthoven,

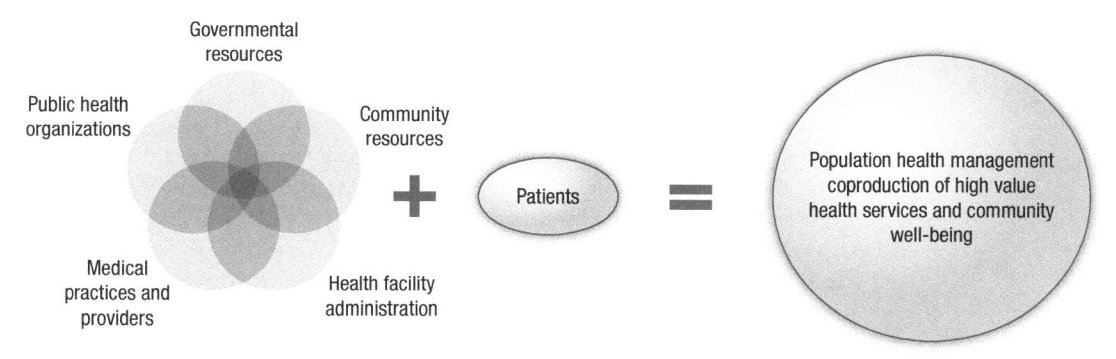

FIGURE 12.2 Aligning Coproduction of Health Stakeholders and Organizations

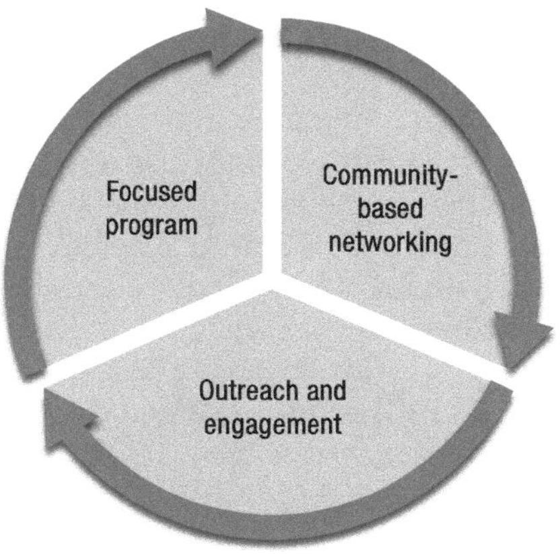

FIGURE 12.3 Input Requirements for Inclusive Community Collaborations

2009; Sultz & Young, 2011). Service recipients (patients) may be in the best position to lead coproduction efforts with the support of other coalitions of groups and providers, which provides the resources and expertise and allows for an inclusive and culturally competent process (McNally, 2016; Realpe & Wallace, 2010).

Barriers to aligning these three sectors and strategies will exist and must be overcome by those in leadership. Common challenges include the following:

- Lack of knowledge, expertise, and information
- Lack of resources and commitment
- Poor communication
- Lack of stakeholder empowerment and self-efficacy

Many of these barriers can be surmounted by creating partnerships with community groups, demonstrating success and positive experiences of inclusion with stakeholders, and careful planning and structuring of the program or initiative (Batalden et al., 2016; Holland-Hart et al., 2019).

Advancing Collaboration and Integrating Coproduction Models into Population Health Management

The healthcare delivery system previously included various types of inter sector collaborations with local communitiy nonprofit agencies. Formalized collaborations occurred on a regular basis with local public health departments and municipalities via disaster preparedness and emergency management planning (Hewitt et al., 2015). The significant challenges for co production of health strategy implementation today are the scale, complexity, diversity of partnerships, and financial arrangements.

The starting point for a coproduction of health program should be a community health needs assessment to determine what interventions or programs would have the greatest impact on improving the health and well-being of the targeted population (Hibbard & Greene, 2013). Community health needs assessments as well as other data sources which are widely available from hospitals. Not-for-profit hospitals are required to conduct these assessment under the Affordable Care Act of 2010 (HHS.gov, 2018; U.S Government Internal Revenue Service, 2018). Other data sources are widely available from government sources (DHHS, 2020) and other organzations, for example, the Darmouth Atlas (Darmouth College, 2018).

The **Interlocking Chain Model of Outcomes** illustrates the codependency of various health sectors.

Figure 12.4 illustrates types of organizations, programs, and services that combine in an interlocking chain to produce the desired targeted health outcomes along with the members of the target population. The organization of co production of health can present significant challenges simply because of the potential number of people, organizations, and agencies involved but also establishing ownership proper roles and relationships and ensuring that the targeted population is equitably represented in designing and implementing the program.

A PH manager might follow the **coproduction decision-making pathway** (CDMP), which consists of a sequential checklist framework for PH managers as outlined in Table 12.1.

With these steps functioning as a checklist, the PH manager can effectively align with the appropriate health sector partners to product a quality health outcome.

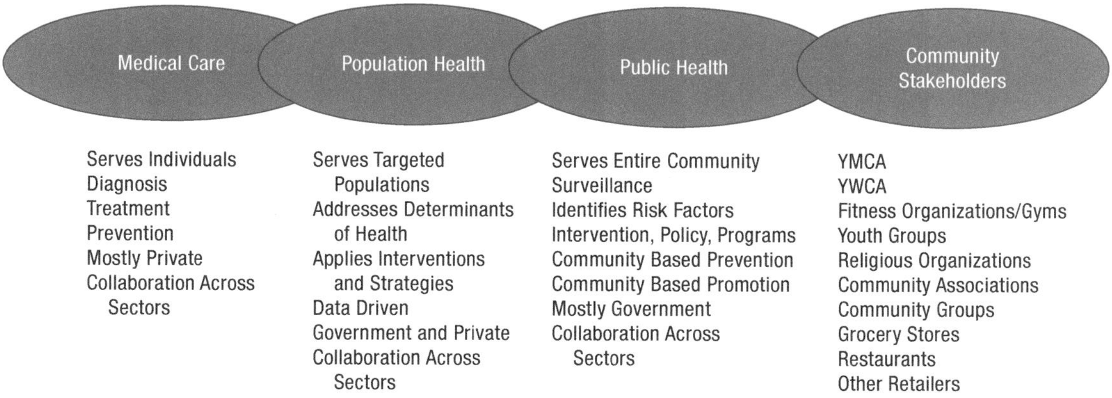

The Interlocking Chain for Health Outcomes

Medical Care
- Serves Individuals
- Diagnosis
- Treatment
- Prevention
- Mostly Private
- Collaboration Across Sectors

Population Health
- Serves Targeted Populations
- Addresses Determinants of Health
- Applies Interventions and Strategies
- Data Driven
- Government and Private
- Collaboration Across Sectors

Public Health
- Serves Entire Community
- Surveillance
- Identifies Risk Factors
- Intervention, Policy, Programs
- Community Based Prevention
- Community Based Promotion
- Mostly Government
- Collaboration Across Sectors

Community Stakeholders
- YMCA
- YWCA
- Fitness Organizations/Gyms
- Youth Groups
- Religious Organizations
- Community Associations
- Community Groups
- Grocery Stores
- Restaurants
- Other Retailers

FIGURE 12.4 The Interlocking Chain for Health Outcomes
Adapted from Wagner, 2020

TABLE 12.1 Coproduction Decision-Making Pathway

Step	Description
Step 1	**Determine Need(s).** The identified need(s) for intervention often obtained by community health surveys, interviewing residents, community health assessments, health statistics, and other available data. Questions: "What are the needs?" and "What is the focus of the activity?"
Step 2	**Input.** The resources, such as people, facilities, and equipment, needed to implement the program. Questions: "What resources will be required to carry out the intervention and what are our funding sources?"
Step 3	**Activities.** The events or actions done by the program and its people. Question: "What activities are required to complete the plan?"
Step 4	**Decision-Making.** Identification, prioritization, and selection of best option to meet the need. Question: "Who is the most effective and offers the best cost to deliver the service?"
Step 5	**Outputs.** The direct results of program activities measured in accountable and subjective terms. Question: "How do we determine success?"
Step 6	**Tools and resources.** These are the models and processes required to carry out the program and activities. Question: "What models are best suited for our program?"
Step 7	**Outcomes.** These are the changes that result from the program's activities and outputs. In population health programs, outcomes are often expressed as short-term, intermediate, and long-term outcomes. Question: "How do we define short-term intermediate and long-term outcomes?"
Step 8	**Impact.** These are the measurable achievements of the program's goals. Questions: "Did our program have a significant impact in improving the health and well-being of our targeted population?" and "What are the metrics?"

Aligning Health Sector Relationships: Population Health Options

In the previous discussion, relationships involved a hospital or health system entity and either a nonprofit, community organization or public entity. Community relationships often refer to generic connections between organizations and groups of individuals that share a common health goal and are physically located within a defined geographic area (Hewitt et al., 2015) Recent events clearly indicate that coproduction of health is transforming to include relationships with private and for-profit entities. As depicted in Figure 12.5, these arrangements offer an additional opportunity to meet the needs of vulnerable populations through nontraditional partnerships or other alignment options.

Examples of these new and diverse nontraditional entrants into the PH sector include drug stores (CVS, Walgreens), retail (Walmart), venture capitalists, e-commerce businesses (Amazon), third-party vendors offering PHM patient-engagement solutions, and fortune 500 companies. PHM managers may need to view these organizations as potential partners whether their previous relationship has been a collaborator or competitor.

Figure 12.6 introduces both a traditional business model and a collaborative version that highlights the different types of relationships and the potential forms of alignment between participants.

The differences between the two perspectives highlight both legal and operational characteristics that require different management skills and accountability. As nontraditional private, nonprofit entities continue to enter the market, PH managers will need to expand their skill base in designing

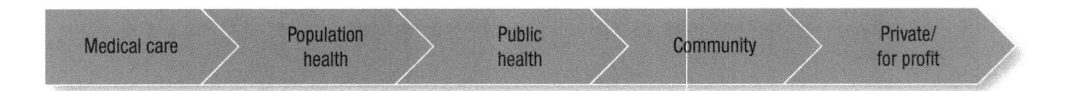

FIGURE 12.5 Aligning Atypical Stakeholder Relationships

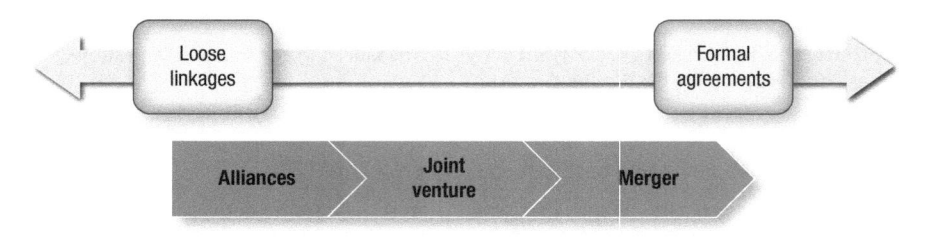

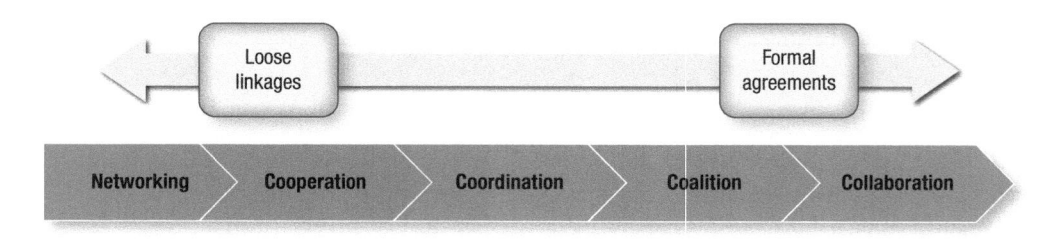

FIGURE 12.6 Relationship Continuums for Business and Community Collaborative Perspectives
Adapted from Hewitt et al., 2015

PH delivery options that may include alternative financial options such as capitated payments to for-profit entities.

Coproduction Models for Population Health Managers

With the introduction of new models of collaboration and an emphasis on the coproduction of health to ensure safe and positive PH outcomes, PH managers can adopt the leadership role of integrator. An **integrator** can be described as a facilitator capable of convening all necessary health stakeholders across diverse sectors to achieve positive outcomes in health and well-being for a defined population. (Nemours, 2012)

The integrator's role includes at least five components:

- **Partnership** with individuals and families in the community to build trust and obtain insight to the needs and concerns of the targeted population. Families are important because they are often the bridge to better outcomes for any individual member. We are often better able to address issue as a group rather than by ourselves.
- **Redesign of primary care.** Patient-centered medical homes, for example, as the name implies, offer a place of the patient to begin any health journey [National Committee for Quality Assurance (NCQA), 2018].
- **Population health management.** The management of any program is essential to success. The nature of coproduction requires active involvement of management because of the dynamic nature of the many people and entities engaged in the process.
- **Financial management.** Managing for accountability of financial resources is essential. Often PH programs must compete with other priorities for funding; demonstrating the efficacious use of resources is important and expected in value over volume contracts.
- **Macrosystem integration.** The operations involving necessary resources for any coproduction of health initiative including information technology, medical records, resources management programs, equipment, and staffing require intensive integration especially when multiple partners are involved.

Another emerging model seeks to directly link healthcare providers with social care providers to help with social determinants of care. The **convener model** involves a third party so healthcare providers do not make direct investments in social needs services or forge direct partnerships with community-based organizations (CBOs). The purpose of the convener organization is to be a "trusted broker" and establish a network of social service providers that takes electronic referrals from healthcare providers (Cheney, 2020). A successful example of this model in New York involved a state-funded organization that served in the role of intermediary between healthcare providers, payers, and CBOs.

These new coproduction models for PHM represent several reasons that a healthcare organization would be interested in effective PH strategies including, better service to their community, reduction in the burden of disease, better outcomes overall, and reducing hospital readmissions and the overall cost of care (Gray, 2017). Financial obligations that are increasingly being shared by large healthcare organizations and through various alternative payment models are becoming more predominant (Berwick &

Hackbarth, 2012; McHugh et al., 2017). These organizations have a pressing need to develop new strategies that demonstrate better outcomes and reduce the cost of care and improve outcomes (Emanuel et al., 2016; Pham et al., 2007; Sharfstein et al., 2017).

Example of Coproduction

Two successful and recent coproduction of health examples are a direct result of the COVID-19 pandemic and can illustrate how healthcare organizations can actively work with government to promote healthy behaviors. CBOs can serve as essential safety net providers beyond what health providers and systems can deliver (Kosel & Nash, 2020).

> **DID YOU KNOW?**
>
> **COVID-19 as a catalyst for the Coproduction of Health**
>
> The CDC and other health experts recommended mass testing for the COVID-19 virus to help reduce the spread of the disease (Centers For Disease Control and Prevention, 2020). One of the major obstacles to increase testing was access especially as populations in low-income areas had limited access to testing. The major health systems in Charlotte developed multiple mobile testing sites in these underserved communities in order to increase testing of its residents (Atrium Health, 2020).
>
> On June 26, 2020, Governor Roy Cooper issued a statewide mandate in North Carolina for all citizens to wear face coverings (masks) when in public and unable to properly social distance. Immediate concerns were raised because underserved communities had limited access to masks. Atrium Health organized effort with other large employers in Charlotte to donate 1 million masks that would be targeted toward vulnerable and underserved communities. The partnership represents a large cross section of health and nonhealthcare organizations including the Carolina Panthers (a sports team) Bank of America, Honeywell, Lowe's, Blue Cross Blue Shield, and Red Ventures in addition to Atrium Health. Other businesses also joined in the effort to supply masks to the community (Kuznitz & Smoot, 2020).
>
> In the first example, a major healthcare system partnered directly with communities. In the second example, the healthcare system partnered with industry leaders who normally would not be actively involved in solving healthcare problems to supply masks and meet the community's needs. In this case, the collaboration included public, health sector, and nonhealthcare organizations to ensure the health of the entire population. Recent studies suggest that Connected Communities of Care (CCC) can offer a tremendous strategic and tactical advantage over nonconnected peers when a major disaster occurs (Kosel & Nash, 2020).

National health policy and funding organizations, such as the Commonwealth Fund, strongly support these types of partnership as opportunities for quality improvement initiatives (Hostetter & Klein, 2021). The positive impact is the capability of prioritizing health needs and streamlining resources to address them within the community.

Nontraditional Health Partnership Model for the Coproduction of Health

In 2018, the healthcare and corporate sector were amazed at a formal announcement by Amazon, Berkshire Hathaway, and J.P. Morgan to form a healthcare company (HAVEN) with Atul Gawande, M.D., at the helm. This alliance had the potential to be a health sector game changer. Dr. Gawande is considered one of the premier thought leaders in healthcare today, and this may be a signal of things to come in the healthcare industry. In the past, consolidation was often limited by several factors, which included the following:

- The lack of capital
- The lack of expertise
- The lack of organizational structure and governance

These three giants, all Fortune 100 companies, brought significant resources to each of these areas and together, and they covered 1.25 million lives making the investment in exploring better ways to deliver healthcare feasible. Each partner had significant capital to invest; Amazon has tremendous logistical and information services support, Berkshire Hathaway with great business acumen and significant resources in the insurance industry, and J.P. Morgan as a successful bank with significant financial expertise (Gawande, 2019; Tozzi, 2019). Most importantly, there seemed to be the will to innovate and provide better care for their employees and family through a coproduction concept that engages the consumer in their care (Dyrda, 2020; Haven, 2020). But during the first week 2021, the three corporate founds announced that HAVEN was closing with an official explanation that much had been accomplished including progress exploring a wide range of healthcare solutions (LaMonica, 2021). Speculators suggested that the healthcare delivery conundrum presented too much of a challenge for companies with other primary interests.

Despite this outcome, the HAVEN example spurred other nonprofit companies to expand as well as healthcare systems. In 2020, there were seven hospital and health system mergers involving two companies with more than $1 billion in annual revenue, and of the 79 deals announced in 2020, 37% of them involved a for-profit partner representing almost a 60% increase from the previous year (Paavola, 2021). The era of collaboration and coproduction of health appears to be a primary focus for the healthcare sector, and the implications for PH managers suggest continuing transformations.

Additional Nontraditional Competitors: CVS, Walmart, and Walgreen

Other segments of the care delivery system have been quick to focus new services for priority populations. In recent years, other large companies have entered the healthcare delivery space. Although Walgreen, CVS, and Walmart have traditionally provided some healthcare-related products and services such as pharmaceuticals and durable medical equipment, they have effectively expanded their scope and included more of the healthcare continuum. Using many retailing concepts and focusing on many of the areas where consumers have expressed the most dissatisfaction with the traditional healthcare delivery system, these organizations are providing more traditional clinical healthcare services such as primary care, dental, consulting, lab and x-ray services, immunizations, hearing testing and employment physicals in more innovative ways.

The advantages of **nontraditional health organizations** in the health market are important. Unlike more traditional healthcare delivery organizations, they can respond to consumer needs for lower cost and better access because they have limited the services that they provide to more basic primary care needs and colocate these serves in existing stores. These existing business attributes offer serious challenges to traditional PH delivery systems. Many of them are beginning to expand into the chronic disease management, another area that is particularly suited to the coproduction of healthcare in a retail setting (Sanborn, 2018; Tyler, 2012).

The integration of care might have the potential to improve. For example, if a patient is taking a medication they receive from the pharmacy and receive their chronic care at the same location, compliance might be easier to confirm. As we know from example such as the cases highlighted by Atul Gawande in the article the Hot Spotters, failure to take medication properly contributes to poor healthcare outcomes (Gawande, 2011).

In addition, these organization have also demonstrated that doing good and achieving business goals are not mutually exclusive. CVS, for example, has made a strong commitment to social responsibility by providing community support through financial contributions, community grants, and partnerships with national organizations through both their foundation and the Aetna foundation. They also provide a resource library and focus on stakeholder engagement by working with such organizations as the American Academy of pediatrics, the American Cancer Society, Campaign for Tobacco-Free Kids, Doing Something.org, Scholastic Corporation, and Truth Initiative (CVS, 2020). They were one of the first Fortune 100 companies to stop retailing tobacco, and as stated by the CEO, "We are a healthcare company" (Melo, 2014). The roll of the traditional drug store chain continues to transform rapidly as both CVS and Walgreens were selected to provide COVID-19 vaccinations to America's seniors (Repko, 2020).

By working with other organizations and providing additional segments of the care continuum, these organizations are effective competitors for traditional medical providers in the service areas which they target (Walgreen, 2020; Walmart, 2020).

Consumers as Central to the Coproduction of Health

As highlighted in the Population Health Alliance Framework, the patient/consumer is the central consideration in PHM. The consumer aspect of a patient relationship is key to improving PH outcomes. Without patient engagement, any coproduction of health initiative will face the common barriers identified earlier. The consumerism influence on healthcare delivery requires health interventions to meet the expectations of the patient, and often, only a collaboration of organizations can fulfill those needs in a manner that satisfies and enhances patient engagement. The coproduction of health requires patient involvement to create value (Turakhia & Combs, 2017a).

SUMMARY

The healthcare sector, as it continues to address the continuing intractable challenges to providing access and quality of care, now recognizes the emerging opportunities available through the coproduction of health. Aligning relevant stakeholders, whether public, private, for-profit or not-for-profit, in not just identifying or delivering healthcare but also becoming part of production process of healthcare, has emerged as a viable option for healthcare organizations. Partnering with nontraditional, former competitors, and nonprofit entities not previously aligned with healthcare offers a transformational solution. Both the integrator and convener models provide frameworks for population health managers. Challenges going forward will include resolving management, governance, legal, ethical, and financial parameters and developing implementation plans that are feasible. The overarching goal remains providing convenient quality care and at a lower cost.

DISCUSSION QUESTIONS

1. The coproduction of health is considered transformational for the health sector. Provide several reasons for this conclusion.
2. Compare the integrator and convener model of coproduction organization.
3. Develop a rationale for why a nontraditional, for-profit company would be interested in expanding into the health sector.
4. Identify operational challenges that may occur in aligning traditional and nontraditional organizations for coproducing health.
5. Search the Internet for examples of each of the following and clearly identify the product or process that required their aligned partnership. Please provide the url.
    a. Two not-for-profit health organizations working together
    b. A hospital/health system collaborating with a public agency or department
    c. Two hospitals/health systems currently competitors collaborating on a project
    d. A non-for-profit health organization and a for-profit nonhealth company.

Toolkit Competency Application: Mini Case Study

Community and Healthcare Organizations Joining Forces

Healthy Families, Healthy Communities is a coalition of organization and community groups in Charlotte, North Carolina, which engaged in coproduction of health. In the following example, it was a part of the CDC's REACH 2010 initiative (Plescia et al., 2008). REACH is a national program administered by the CDC to reduce racial and ethnic health disparities (CDC Division of Nutrition, Physical Activity, 2020). The coproduction team was a collaboration of 45 neighborhoods and 25 agencies, a large medical practice, a healthcare system, and the local and state health departments. The CDC provided funding and guidance as part of the REACH program. It should be noted that this coalition existed long before it sought grant funding and was actively pursuing the community's health needs; however, the CDC grant funding allowed the collaborative to coalesce into a more organized effort. This demonstrates the importance of funding to achieve important coproduction health goals.

The targeted population was several underserved communities in West Charlotte. Heart disease and diabetes were the specific ailments targeted

The Role Of Physician Group Practices in the Health Communities Movement

Healthy Families, Healthy Communities
A collabortive effort of more than 45 neighborhoods and 25 agencies to help improve the physical and mental health of underserved communities

General Strategy
- Increase awareness of health care issues
- Increase community leadership and goodwill
- Position the medical group as a active and contributing member of the community

Benefits
Effects such as *Healthy Families, Healthy Communities* cannot be measured entirely by financial statements or traditional measure of success. We must also consider the intrinsic value to ourselves and the communities we serve, including:
- Better, stronger, healthier communities
- Personal and professional fulfillment by medical staff
- Placing medical staff communities as leaders and builders for the future

Serving The Entire Community
With 50 staff physicians specializing in cardiovascular medicine and thoracic and cardiovascular surgery, we combined our individual efforts into community success. An Outreach Clinics was established at a local health center, we participated in sponsorship of health fairs, Heart Walks, a speakers bureau and the distribution of Heart/Health Assessment literature in underserved communities.

Results
To date, approximately 5,000 people have been provided information, initial and /or follow-up treatment through this collaborative effort. The Outreach Clinic has treated 41 seriously ill patient thus far. These people would not have had traditional access to a health care system, or would have done so only on an emergency basis.

Your Turn
"Why are you here, and what do you bring to the table?"
If you have questions, or would like information on starting a program in your community, contact:

Dr. Stephen Wagner. Ph.D.,FACMPE
Administrator
Sanger Clinic
J00J Rlythe Blvd
Suite 300
Caarlotte, NC 28203
(704) 373-0212 ■ Fax (704) 372-1-88

Not Just Meeting Health Care Needs, Exceeding Them.

THE SANGER CLINIC

EXHIBIT 12.1 Coproduction of Health: Physician Practices and Communities

due to their high prevalence in this population. As shown in Exhibit 12.1, a large cardiovascular practice as well as the Carolinas Medical Center participated in a far-reaching strategy, which included providing information, outreach clinics, health fairs, dietary instruction, and the development of a community health workforce, which serve to communicate and encourage community members to participate in the process (The American Hospital Association, 2018; Plescia et al., 2008). Over the past 15 years, thousands of people have received a wide variety of services to combat heart disease and diabetes. Other benefits included building trust between the partners and increasing awareness of the important issues that each of the participants faces in improving healthcare in these underserved communities in addition to providing services.

CASE STUDY QUESTIONS

1. Identify all the various stakeholders in this coproduction of health example.
2. What was the impetus for this collaboration?
3. Describe the impact of this partnership.
4. List the specific benefits to the physician practice.
5. If this initiative occurred today, what other innovations could you consider?

REFERENCES

The American Hospital Association. (2018). *Community Health Initiatives at the American Hospital Association.* http://www.aha.org/about/pathforward.shtml

Atrium Health. (2020). *Mobile coronavirus testing | Atrium health.* Mobile Corona Virus Testing. https://atriumhealth.org/about-us/coronavirus/mobile-unit

Batalden, M., Batalden, P., Margolis, P., Seid, M., Armstrong, G., Opipari-Arrigan, L., & Hartung, H. (2016). Co-production of healthcare service. *BMJ Quality & Safety, 25*(7), 509–517. https://doi.org/10.1136/bmjqs-2015-004315

Berwick, D. M., & Hackbarth, A. D. (2012). Eliminating waste in US health care. *JAMA – Journal of the American Medical Association, 307*(14), 1513–1516. https://doi.org/10.1001/jama.2012.362

Berwick, D. M., Nolan, T. W., & Whittington, J. (2008). The triple aim: Care, health, and cost. *Health Affairs, 27*(3), 759–769. https://doi.org/10.1377/hlthaff.27.3.759

Bettencourt, L. A., Ostrom, A. L., Brown, S. W., & Roundtree, R. I. (2002). Client Co-Production in knowledge-intensive business services. *California Management Review, 44*(4), 100–128. https://doi.org/10.2307/41166145

Bialek, R., Moran, J., Amos, K., Lamers, L. (2020). *Cross-sector collaboration: Making partnerships work for your community public health foundation* (p. 36). Public Health Foundation. http://www.phf.org/events/Pages/Cross_Sector_Collaboration_Making_Partnerships_Work_for_Your_Community.aspx#:~:text=Cross-sector collaboration is a,to a community they serve.&text=Resources to help you address common community health challenges

Bodenheimer, T., & Sinsky, C. (2014). From triple to quadruple aim: Care of the patient requires care of the provider. *Annals of Family Medicine.* https://doi.org/10.1370/afm.1713

CDC Division of Nutrition, Physical Activity, and O. (2020). *Racial and ethnic approaches to community health.* Racial and Ethnic Approaches to Community Health. https://www.cdc.gov/nccdphp/dnpao/state-local-programs/reach/index.htm

Center For Disease Control and Prevention. (2020). *Testing for COVID-19 | CDC.* Coronavirus Disease 2019 (Covid-19). https://www.cdc.gov/coronavirus/2019-ncov/symptoms-testing/testing.html

Cheney, C. (2020). *Convener model helps healthcare providers address social determinants of health.* HealthLeaders Media. https://www.healthleadersmedia.com/clinical-care/convener-model-helps-healthcare-providers-address-social-determinants-health

CVS. (2020). *Homepage | CVS Health.* https://cvshealth.com/

Darmouth College. (2018). *Centers & Institutes | Dartmouth College.* Centers & Institutes. https://home.dartmouth.edu/centers-institutes-02-12-15

Deloitte Health. (2020). *Chapter 2: Population health and value-based care.* Deloitte US. https://www2.deloitte.com/us/en/pages/life-sciences-and-health-care/articles/population-health-based-model.html

DHHS. (2020). *Health data.* HealthData.gov. https://healthdata.gov/

Donne, J. (1839). *The works of John Donne.* In H. Alford (Ed.). John W. Parker.

Dyrda, L. (2020). *Haven has been quiet for the past 2 years—What does that mean for healthcare?* Becker's Health IT and CIO Report. https://www.beckershospitalreview.com/healthcare-information-technology/haven-has-been-quiet-for-the-past-2-years-what-does-that-mean-for-healthcare.html

Ellner, A. L., & Phillips, R. S. (2017). The coming primary care revolution. *Journal of General Internal Medicine, 32*(4), 380. https://doi.org/10.1007/s11606-016-3944-3

Emanuel, E. J., Ubel, P. A., Kessler, J. B., Meyer, G., Muller, R. W., Navathe, A. S., Patel, P., Pearl, R., Rosenthal, M. B., Sacks, L., Sen, A. P., Sherman, P., & Volpp, K. G. (2016). Using behavioral economics to design physician incentives that deliver high-value care. *Annals of Internal Medicine, 164*(2), 144. https://doi.org/10.7326/M15-1330

Enthoven, A. C. (2009). Integrated delivery systems: The cure for fragmentation. *The American Journal of Managed Care, 15*(10 Suppl), S284–S290. http://www.ncbi.nlm.nih.gov/pubmed/20088632

Gawande, A. (2019). *Haven.* Haven Healthcare. https://havenhealthcare.com/

Gawande, A. (2011). The hot spotters. *The New Yorker.*

Genuino, M. J. (2018). Effects of simulation-based educational program in improving the nurses' self-efficacy in caring for patients' with COPD and CHF in a post-acute care (PACU) setting. *Applied Nursing Research, 39*, 53–57. https://doi.org/10.1016/j.apnr.2017.10.012

Gray, M. (2017). Value based healthcare. *BMJ (Online)*. https://doi.org/10.1136/bmj.j437

Grönroos, C. (2011). Value co-creation in service logic: A critical analysis. *Marketing Theory, 11*(3), 279–301. https://doi.org/10.1177/1470593111408177

Haven. (2020). *Vision | Haven Healthcare*. Vision Statement. https://havenhealthcare.com/vision

Hewitt, A., Wagner, S., Twal, R. & Gourley, D. (2015). Community Hospitals with Local Pubic Health Departments: Collaborative emergency management. In S. B. Hamner, S. Stovall, & D. Taha (Eds.), *Emergency management and disaster reponse utilizing public-private partnerships* (pp. 218–239). IGI Global.

HHS.gov. (2018). *About the ACA*. About the Affordable Care Act. https://www.hhs.gov/healthcare/about-the-aca/index.html

Hibbard, J. H., & Greene, J. (2013). What the evidence shows about patient activation: Better health outcomes and care experiences; fewer data on costs. *Health Affairs, 32*(2), 207–214. https://doi.org/10.1377/hlthaff.2012.1061

Hippocrates. (1886). The genuine works of hippocrates: Hippocrates: Free download, borrow, and streaming: Internet archive. In F. Adams & W. Wood (Eds.), *Sydenham Society*. https://archive.org/details/genuineworkship02hippgoog/mode/2up

Holland-Hart, D. M., Addis, S. M., Edwards, A., Kenkre, J. E., & Wood, F. (2019). Co-production and health: Public and clinicians' perceptions of the barriers and facilitators. *Health Expectations, 22*(1), 93–101. https://doi.org/10.1111/hex.12834

Hostetter, M., & Klein, S. (2021). *Improving population health through community-wide partnerships commonwealth fund*. What's Trending-The Commonwealth Fund. https://www.commonwealthfund.org/publications/newsletter-article/improving-population-health-through-communitywide-partnerships

IOM. (2001). *Crossing the quality chasm*. http://www.nationalacademies.org/hmd/~/media/Files/Report Files/2001/Crossing-the-Quality-Chasm/Quality Chasm 2001 report brief.pdf

Janamian, T., Crossland, L., & Wells, L. (2016). On the road to value co-creation in health care: The role of consumers in defining the destination, planning the journey and sharing the drive. *Medical Journal of Australia, 204*(S7). https://doi.org/10.5694/mja16.00123

Katz, D. L. (2001). *Clinical epidemiology & evidence-based medicine: Fundamental principles of clinical reasoning & research*. Sage Publications.

Kieny, M.-P. (2013). *Closing the health equity gap policy options and opportunities for action*. WHO.

Kosel, K., & Nash, D. (2020). Connected communities of care in times of crisis | Catalyst non-issue content. *NEJM Catalyst*. https://catalyst.nejm.org/doi/full/10.1056/CAT.20.0361

Kuznitz, A., & Smoot, H. (2020). COVID-19 in NC: Donated masks with new mandate from Cooper. *Charlotte Observer*. https://www.charlotteobserver.com/news/coronavirus/article243766737.html

LaMonica, P. (2021). *Haven—The joint health care venture by Amazon, Berkshire and JPMorgan—is shutting down*. CNN Business. https://www.cnn.com/2021/01/04/investing/haven-shutting-down-amazon-jpmorgan-berkshire/index.html

McGinnis, J. M., Williams-Russo, P., & Knickman, J. R. (2002). The case for more active policy attention to health promotion. *Health Affairs, 21*(2), 78–93. https://doi.org/10.1377/hlthaff.21.2.78

McHugh, J. P., Foster, A., Mor, V., Shield, R. R., Trivedi, A. N., Wetle, T., Zinn, J. S., & Tyler, D. A. (2017). Reducing hospital readmissions through preferred networks of skilled nursing facilities. *Health Affairs, 36*(9). https://doi.org/10.1377/hlthaff.2017.0211

McNally, D. (2016). *Joining up 'co-production' and 'patient leadership' for a new relationship with people who use services*. NHS Blog. https://www.england.nhs.uk/blog/david-mcnally/

Melo, L. (2014). *CVS stops selling tobacco—Message from Larry Merlo | CVS Health*. CVS Website. https://cvshealth.com/thought-leadership/message-from-larry-merlo-president-and-ceo

National Committee for Quality Assurance (NCQA). (2018). *Patient-Centered Medical Home (PCMH)—NCQA*. NCQA Website. https://www.ncqa.org/programs/health-care-providers-practices/patient-centered-medical-home-pcmh/

Nemours. (2012). *Integrator role and functions in population health improvement initiativese*. https://www.improvingpopulationhealth.org/Integratorrole and functions _FINAL.pdf

Office of Disease Prevention and Health Promotion (ODPHP). (2019). *Disparties*. Healthy People 2020. https://www.healthypeople.gov/2020/about/foundation-health-measures/Disparities

Paavola, A. (2021). *7 healthcare transactions were megamergers in 2020*. Becker's Hospital Review. https://www.beckershospitalreview.com/hospital-transactions-and-valuation/7-healthcare-transactions-were-megamergers-in-2020.html?origin=SupplyE&utm_source=SupplyE&utm_medium=email&utm_content=newsletter&oly_enc_id=1450I5993723C6U

PHA. (2020). *About PHA*. PHA. https://populationhealthalliance.org/about/

Pham, H. H., Ginsburg, P. B., McKenzie, K., & Milstein, A. (2007). Redesigning care delivery in response to a high-performance network: The Virginia Mason Medical Center. *Health Affairs, 26*(4), W532–W544. https://doi.org/10.1377/hlthaff.26.4.w532

Plescia, M., Groblewski, M., & Chavis, L. (2008). A lay health advisor program to promote community capacity and change among change agents. *Health Promotion Practice, 9*(4), 434–439. https://doi.org/10.1177/1524839906289670

Realpe, A., & Wallace, L. M. (2010). *What is co-production?* (p. 19). The Health Foundation.

Repko, M. (2020). *CVS Health has 10,000 staffers ready to vaccinate seniors at nursing homes*. CNBC. https://www.cnbc.com/2020/12/10/cvs-health-has-10000-staffers-ready-to-vaccinate-seniors-at-nursing-homes.html

Rosa Dias, P., & O'Donnell, O. (2013). *Health and inequality*. Emerald.

Sanborn, B. J. (2018). *Here's what Walmart says about non-traditional companies moving into healthcare*. Health Finance. https://www.healthcarefinancenews.com/news/heres-what-walmart-says-about-non-traditional-companies-moving-healthcare

Sharfstein, J., Moriarty, E., Chin, D., & Gerovich, S. (2017). *An emerging approach to payment reform: All-Payer global budgets for large safety-net hospital systems Sule Gerovich Senior Researcher Mathematica policy research an emerging approach to payment reform: All-payer global budgets for large safety-net hospital systems an emerging approach to payment reform: All-Payer global budgets for large safety-net hospital systems 3*. https://www.commonwealthfund.org/sites/default/files/documents/___media_files_publications_fund_report_2017_aug_sharfstein_all_payer_global_budgets_safety_net_hospitals.pdf

Strategy, O. of the A. D. for P. and. (2016). *Health in All Policies | AD for Policy and Strategy | CDC*. Health in All Policies. https://www.cdc.gov/policy/hiap/index.html

Sultz, H. A., & Young, K. M. (2011). *Health care USA: Understanding its organization and delivery* (7th ed.). Jones and Bartlett.

Tozzi, J. (2019). Amazon-JPMorgan-Berkshire health-care venture to be called haven. *Bloomberg*. https://www.bloomberg.com/news/articles/2019-03-06/amazon-jpmorgan-berkshire-health-care-venture-to-be-called-haven

Turakhia, P., & Combs, B. (2017a). Using principles of co-production to improve patient care and enhance value. *AMA Journal of Ethics, 19*(11), 1125–1131. https://doi.org/10.1001/journalofethics.2017.19.11.pfor1-1711

Turakhia, P., & Combs, B. (2017b). Using principles of co-production to improve patient care and enhance value. *AMA Journal of Ethics, 19*(11), 1125–1131. https://doi.org/10.1001/journalofethics.2017.19.11.pfor1-1711

Tyler, V. (2012). *Top 10 non-traditional hospital competitors to consider*. Becker's Hospital Review. https://www.beckershospitalreview.com/hospital-management-administration/top-10-non-traditional-hospital-competitors-to-consider.html

U.S Government Internal Revenue Service. (2018). *Requirements for 501(c)(3) Hospitals Under the Affordable Care Act – Section 501(r) | Internal Revenue Service*. Charitable

Organizations. https://www.irs.gov/charities-non-profits/charitable-organizations/requirements-for-501c3-hospitals-under-the-affordable-care-act-section-501r

Wagner, S. L. (2020). *The United States Healthcare System, overview, driving forces and outlook for the future* (first). Health Administration Press/AUPHA.

Walgreen. (2020). *Find care | Services | Walgreens*. Walgreen Website. https://www.walgreens.com/findcare/services

Walmart. (2020). *Care clinic—Walmart.com*. Walmart Website. https://www.walmart.com/cp/care-clinics/1224932

CHAPTER 13

Leadership for the Future Health Sector: Transformation, Innovation, and Change for Population Health Managers

Stephen L. Wagner, Patrick D. Shay, and Edward J. Schumacher

KEY TERMS

Bridges Model of Change
Change Management
Design Thinking
Divergent Thinking
Drexler/Sibbet High-Performing Teams Model
Empathy Map
Innovation
PAST Change Model
Radical Collaboration
Salerno and Brock's Cycle of Change
Wicked Problem

LEARNING OBJECTIVES

1. Articulate the Factors underlying a need for health sector transformation.
2. Discuss current population health management challenges.
3. Describe design thinking and apply the three-part innovation model.
4. Identify the common barriers to innovation and offer potential solutions.
5. Analyze change model examples and applications.
6. Apply the team building model to change transformations.

> Podcasts that exemplify the content of this chapter are available at Springer Publishing Connect™
>
> Podcast 13.1. Understanding Design Thinking
> Podcast 13.2. From Transactions to Transformations: Innovation at Work

Access the podcast online at http://connect.springerpub.com/content/book/978-0-8261-4427-0/part/part04/chapter/ch13

INTRODUCTION

Looking into the future, tomorrow's healthcare leaders can expect to be confronted not only by the challenges they experience in providing services to the patients that walk through their facilities' doors in person or virtually, but more broadly by the enormity of changes disrupting the health sector. Major challenges include diverse and evolving workforces and worksites, new digital and clinical technologies, healthcare payment reform with increased emphasis on assuming risk for positive patient/consumer outcomes, and the entry of for-profit companies as both competitors and collaborators. To truly transform healthcare and provide services that are deeply meaningful, leaders must effectively

(a) connect to their communities,

(b) understand their populations' experiences, needs, and challenges, and then

(c) utilize that knowledge to develop creative and desirable solutions.

This chapter addresses how population health managers can be become prepared leaders for the future health sector.

The Role of Healthcare Leaders: Caring for Populations and Communities

Today's healthcare industry faces considerable change, with unique key issues that demand population health (PH) managers consider which strategies and approaches will enable them to effectively lead their healthcare organizations. Change can be categorized as either a transition—the process of incremental change, or transformation—inspired and motivated change. The type of change selected reflects both external and internal environments. The health crisis stemming from the COVID-19 pandemic provides a powerful illustration of ways these issues intersect and demand effective leadership.

DID YOU KNOW?

The COVID-19 challenge for Population Health Managers

As communities throughout the United States witnessed the emergence and spread of COVID-19, all health managers and leaders were challenged by this century's unexpected and unprecedented pandemic to pivot immediately and navigate different policies and regulations that directly impacted their populations. These policies included, among others, government assistance in acquiring personal protective equipment, ventilators, and other resources required to effectively treat patients; the need for financial relief to support healthcare organizations in the midst of significant losses in elective procedures; the expansion of scope of practice for nonphysician providers to enable increased access to needed care; the broadened reimbursement for telehealth services to enable safe and effective care that maintained access in a socially distant environment; and policies placing public health restrictions and guidelines on local populations to mitigate the spread of COVID-19 and the demand for intensive care resources. They also served as content experts to provide critical information surrounding the impact of such policies and regulations on the frontlines of care.

PH managers soon recognized that social determinants of health greatly influenced their populations' risk of exposure, probable outcomes, and postacute transitions of care options. Community capabilities and assets became an essential resource for most health systems and helped introduce the coproduction of the health among multiple and diverse organizations. Health sector leaders witnessed varying demands from key stakeholders, such as community officials looking to them to provide critical information and guidance during the pandemic. They also struggled to address the tremendous physical and psychological burden on their own workforce.

Industry observers now recognize that COVID-19 serves as an illustration of a **wicked problem,** which consists of challenges that have no easy solutions "because they involve many interdependent, changing, and difficult to define factors" (Nembhard et al., 2020). And just as COVID-19 presented healthcare leaders with wicked problems relating to excess patient demand, mortality, care management, supply chains, testing, staffing, and other factors, healthcare leaders can anticipate the continued demands of wicked problems that require systems thinking and a sense of creative confidence, "adopting a learning rather than performance mindset and embracing the…quick implementation of iterative changes to respond to new problems that arise" (Nembhard et al., 2020).

Transformation of the Health Sector

Moving forward, these transformative types of changes will confront leaders from myriad directions, not only from the continued advancement of health technology, including the progression of personalized medicine and the widespread embrace of mobile health technology that enables individuals to be more connected and empowered in their own health, but also from the integration of healthcare analytics and enhanced abilities to pursue predictive care and artificial intelligence methodologies to unlock new PHM approaches and strategies. The ongoing expansion and adoption of telehealth throughout society and the continued progression of useful electronic health records continue the emphasis on interoperability across the health sector and not just limited to the primary hospital or health system (see Figure 13.1).

Similarly, healthcare leaders can expect challenges relating to healthcare financing, including efforts to address concerns with the continued rise of health spending, continual attempts to shift away from fee-for-service medicine and experiment with alternative payment models, increased consumerism, and a retail mind-set that has gradually permeated the healthcare industry. Conversations about the future of health insurance at both the private and public health insurance program levels may yield additional policy transformations.

Also highlighted by the recent COVID-19 pandemic, PH managers recognize the need to overcome continuing burnout and fatigue among clinicians and healthcare professionals. Problems with ensuring the healthcare workers' safety from heightened risks of injury and violence, clinician maldistribution and shortages in specific parts of the healthcare delivery system, and questions surrounding scope of practice and the appropriate limits of varied roles within healthcare delivery remain major obstacles to delivering quality healthcare.

External issues and additional disruptors include the increase in consumerism and the rapid ascent of ambulatory and alternative care sites, such as those provided by retail entities, which support the continued shift toward

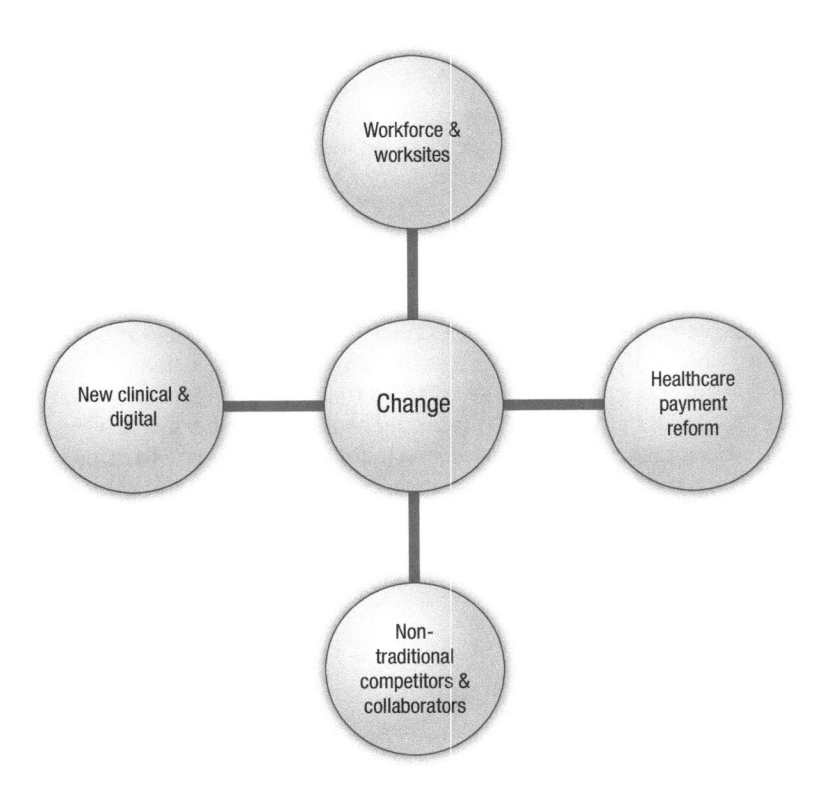

FIGURE 13.1 Future Challenges: Drivers of Change

TABLE 13.1 Transformative Health Sector Challenges

Patient/ Consumer	Technology	Financial Issues	Delivery
Personalized medicine Connected and empowered patients	Decision-making with artificial intelligence Expanding continuum of care via Telehealth	Alternative payment models and risk integration	Coproduction of health and interoperability among health sectors Closing gaps in health coverage and disparities

outpatient services. Innovative efforts, (m-health wellness programs) surrounding primary and preventive care, and the growth of convenient care models suggest additional transitions for PH managers. Geographical coverage and viability issues include threats to the viability of facilities in rural and inner-city areas, questions surrounding hospital consolidation, and the importance of trust and transparency in hospital systems' relations with the populations they serve. The COVID-19 pandemic's impact also exposed the growing needs of the behavioral health sector and accompanying efforts to integrate mental health services and continued demand for postacute care services especially surrounding long-term care. See Table 13.1.

The common task for PH managers and leaders, who now are at the intersection of their populations' demands and health needs, is to solve these complex challenges. Fortunately, the framework of population health management represents a catalyst for improving health policy and processes and reimagining current paradigms of delivering healthcare.

Leading and Innovating: Designing the Future

Innovation can be understood as executing an idea, which addresses a specific challenge and achieves value for both company and customer (Skillicorn, 2016). Today's healthcare delivery system demands innovative solutions across many levels to create meaningful change and improvement, beyond the sustaining efforts that prolong the status quo. Yet such demands are not new; for nearly 20 years, the healthcare industry has faced criticisms regarding its lack of creativity, with industry experts pointing to a variety of problems across healthcare that plead for innovative solutions (Herzlinger, 2006). If a paradigm shift is a major change in the way the world views and acts accordingly (Wagner, 2017), then PHM needs to embrace innovation.

The Call for Innovation

Innovation has captured widespread attention throughout the healthcare industry. Recent health reform efforts, stemming from the Patient Protection and Affordable Care Act of 2010, have placed considerable emphasis on the funding, promotion, and development of innovative healthcare delivery and financing models. At the state and local market levels, policymakers continually encourage experimentation to identify what innovative efforts might be effective and translate to dissemination in other markets across the country. Beyond the public sector, private entities are also promoting and fueling innovation, as illustrated in the considerable growth of healthcare start-ups, incubators, and innovation centers. These efforts to fuel innovation come from both entrepreneurial efforts to disrupt and transform healthcare, as well as *intrapreneurial* efforts to adapt and reimagine the status quo from the perspective of incumbent healthcare organizations.

Yet, in all these efforts, some suggest that innovation has become a trendy buzzword throughout the healthcare industry, leading to a lack of true meaning. Concerns of a "bandwagon effect," in which innovative practices and symbols are embraced to maintain legitimacy and fit in with what will eventually become a passing fad, can be used to dismiss the value and opportunity of innovative efforts. Healthcare leaders who remain tethered to innovation as part of their leadership principles recognize the indelible value of innovation in exercising leadership, and this stems from a foundational understanding of innovation's definition.

Although varying interpretations exist, a common perspective views innovation as something new (e.g., a new idea, a new way of thinking, or a new application of an approach or practice), Other individuals may lack even a clear definition of what innovation means to them, but a helpful definition of innovation states "executing an idea which addresses a specific challenge and achieves value for both the company and customer" (Skillicorn, 2016). This definition recognizes the importance of not only developing an idea to solve a specific problem or issue but also executing that idea in a way that ultimately is valued by those experiencing that problem or issue. As previously noted in the considerations of the role of healthcare leaders, empathy and creative problem-solving are once again integral to the leader's success, as highlighted in the path to exercising leadership through innovation.

As industry leaders, experts, and observers have recognized the need for innovation in healthcare, there have been attempts to pinpoint the source of this challenge. In short, why do our complex problems continue to persist in healthcare, and why have we not been able to meaningfully solve them? Some believe that the difficulty experienced in developing innovative solutions does not stem from "a lack of vision, passion, or resources," instead it is due to "a chronic lack of creativity...to understand problems and their solutions differently" (Roberts, 2017). This then leads us to consider what barriers may be limiting the creative potential of healthcare leaders in pursuing innovative solutions to persistent healthcare problems (see Figure 13.2).

Barriers to innovation are abundant, existing at the individual, organizational, and system levels.

Note the similarities between the individual and organizational level barriers, but at the system level, the barriers become more complex (see Table 13.2).

Health sector leaders can confront and overcome innovation barriers using critical mind-sets and approaches. The cofounder of Pixar Animation Studios, Ed Catmull (2014), highlighted important elements that characterized Pixar's famed "Braintrust," which worked to create a powerful culture of innovation. These included not fearing failure, but instead viewing failure

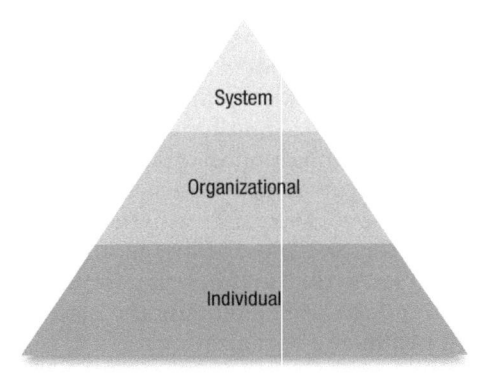

FIGURE 13.2 Levels of Innovation Barriers

TABLE 13.2 Individual-, Organizational-, and System-Level Barriers to Innovation

Individual Barriers	Organizational Barriers	System Level Barriers
• The assumption that innovative abilities are innate, limiting one's recognition of their own capabilities in innovative thinking. • A limited attention span or capacity to find a problem that would benefit from meaningful innovation. • A sense of doubt regarding the potential of one's innovative concept that ultimately leads to the quiet dismissal of that idea before it is shared with others. • A concern that one's innovative idea may be stolen or face failure. • A resistance to constructive criticism or opportunities to advance and improve the idea (Weisberg et al., 2014).	• The assumption that innovative efforts must be tied to one's title or job description. • A limited attention span to address a problem with meaningful innovation due to a strict focus on immediate concerns. • A sense of doubt regarding the potential of an innovative concept considering the potential risks or time it would take to realize the solution's benefit. • A concern that innovative efforts lead to straying from organizational practices and culture. • A lack of organizational support for innovative efforts. • A resistance to change and adaptation that views innovative efforts as potential threats (Weisberg et al., 2014).	• Myriad stakeholders and competitors that may distract or impede innovation. • Limited access to funding resources. • Regulations that inhibit efforts to advance innovative solutions. • Customers that are challenged to imagine solutions beyond the status quo. • Technology that may complicate, confuse, and drive-up expenses. • A lack of accountability (Herzlinger, 2006).

as a necessary by-product of innovation and, ultimately, success. By embracing failure in this sense, innovators aim to "fail fast," working to quickly detect and analyze opportunities for improvement, and then experiment until a breakthrough solution is identified. Related to this, candid feedback is prioritized, as it is viewed to gain the criticism that can highlight where current failures exist. Similarly, other lauded experts in design thinking emphasize the importance of overcoming one's fear of failure, which is a common barrier to innovation, and instead viewing failure as a part of the learning process. To do this, they suggest that one must give themselves permission to fail, allowing them to approach ideas as experiments, and they should practice "urgent optimism" that is motivated in a belief that an innovative breakthrough is just around the corner if one persists in moving quickly toward finding a solution.

In these efforts, population health managers are challenged to not be limited to the status quo—the "way things are"—but to instead create organizational cultures that perpetually consider how healthcare *ought* to be and how they can get there. To ensure innovative capabilities are promoted in their organizations, leaders must also create cultures and organizational structures that actively support new ideas and new approaches when good ideas emerge, rather than ceremonially embracing innovation through an annual offsite event or one-off creativity exercise. Leaders can frame the search for new, innovative ideas by considering their competencies, customers, and environment (see Table 13.3).

In the past decade, significant attention has been drawn toward the application of a human-centered approach to problem-solving, also referred to as design thinking. Advocates suggest that to fuel innovation and transformation in healthcare, leaders would greatly benefit from a human-centered approach, which ultimately uncovers problems and solutions that are truly valued.

The Value of Design Thinking

Design thinking is an approach to problem-solving that emphasizes empathy, innovation, collaboration, and continual experimentation. Population health managers can use design thinking to help them resolve health processes and develop novel models rather than follow an incremental pathway of change that may not produce the desired health outcomes at the desired level.

Design thinking dates to the mid-20th century, with the work of IDEO—a global design and innovation company famous for designing environments and products such as the first usable computer mouse, the first notebook-style computer, and the Palm PDA handheld organizer, and Stanford University's design school, or d.school. This unique way of thinking has recently gained

TABLE 13.3 Framing the Search for Innovative Ideas

Competency Level	How personal capabilities and strengths provide an opportunity for new endeavors?
Customers	What needs they experience as well as *how* those needs get experienced?
Environment	What broader trends or environmental shifts might create future opportunities to pursue in the present? (Parmar et al., 2014)

interest among healthcare leaders, and it has been applied in renowned organizations such as Mayo Clinic, Johns Hopkins Hospital, and Kaiser Permanente. There has been a growing consensus that design thinking is useful for healthcare and can be a tool for its transformation, and major corporations that have embraced design thinking—such as Microsoft—suggest that it is an essential skill for future leaders.

Design thinking leads problem-solvers on a journey to identify and solve the right problems. It requires individuals to deeply understand problems by first gaining empathy for those who experience the pain of that problem, and from that empathy to generate critical insights that more effectively define the problem. Design thinking then challenges individuals to engage in ideation and continual experimentation, embracing an iterative creative process that stays tethered to a foundational understanding of the problem and those who experience that problem. With this approach, design thinkers pursue ideas or concepts that are truly and meaningfully innovative, with innovation suggested to be found at the intersection of ideas that are technically feasible, financially viable, and—perhaps most importantly—deeply desirable among those who experience the pain of the problem. In healthcare, advocates of design thinking have recognized that this approach fuels creative confidence, and it "helps us avoid doing what we do so well in health care: elegantly solve the wrong problems" (Roberts, 2017). See Figure 13.3.

Part 1: Understanding Problems

Design thinking suggests that to understand a problem, one must strive to embrace empathy and see the problem from the perspective of those who feel the pain of that problem. Through empathy, meaningful insights to the problem can be identified, helping to define the problem more clearly and effectively.

DID YOU KNOW?

Understanding the Problem

A popular quote that is often attributed to Albert Einstein conveys the sentiment that if someone had only an hour to solve a problem on which their life depended, they should spend the first 55 minutes defining and understanding the problem, rather than thinking through a potential solution. In other words, most of the effort in meaningful problem-solving requires determining what proper questions to ask to deeply understand and gain insights regarding the problem, and only then can the problem be meaningfully resolved.

Design thinking suggests that to understand the problem, we must discover insights by *empathizing with others*. This means exploring a problem by working to understand what the experiences and perspectives are of those who feel

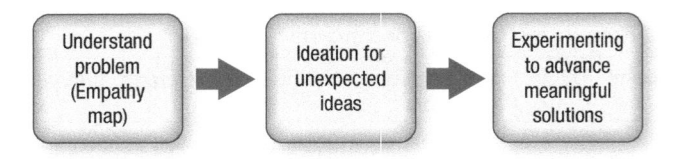

FIGURE 13.3 Three-Step Design Thinking: Innovation Process

the pain of the problem, or of those who are immersed in the problem and letting go of assumptions about what that experience may be like, or what the root of the problem is, and instead adopting a beginner's mindset to listen, seek to understand why, and observe. Through this mindset, one continuously strives to grasp what lies beneath the surface of what is visible or initially presumed, and instead to identify patterns that can point to critical needs or insights that may not be initially appreciated or recognized. Curiosity is essential throughout the effort to understand the problem. In doing this work and uncovering such key insights, leaders can engage in the process and are able to define the problem more effectively at its core—the true problem.

DID YOU KNOW?

Power of Observing

A popular design thinking exercise that illustrates the power of observing—even in just examining objects—has individuals reveal to someone who is "observing" what is in their wallet or their bag or perhaps their backpack. The person observing is then challenged to begin to understand more about the individual by considering what the contents in their wallet or bag tell them about that individual, and it fosters an experience in which the observer asks questions about what they notice. These observations also point the observer to actively listen, for both what they hear and what they *do not* hear in the individual's responses. What patterns or even inconsistencies emerge? Such areas merit further exploration and can point to value. These patterns and inconsistencies can often be a path to gaining key underlying insights to the problem. And ultimately, the observer is tasked with designing a new wallet or bag for the individual based upon insights they have gained regarding what that individual values.

In addition to observing and listening, design thinking also encourages empathy through *feeling* the experiences of those who suffer from the problem or experience at hand. There are a variety of creative ways in which design thinkers embrace this approach to gaining empathy, often referred to as empathy exercises that include various scenarios of imaging things as others experience them. A common exercise is imaging yourself much taller or shorter. In their book, *Value Proposition Design*, Osterwalder and colleagues (2014) share helpful questions to help identify potential pain points as well as obtaining clear consumer insights into the problem (see Table 13.4).

Throughout efforts to embrace empathy in the design thinking journey, a helpful tool that has been widely embraced is the empathy map (Gray et al., 2010; Osterwalder et al., 2014) The **empathy map** offers varied considerations to be aware of during the work of observing, listening, and feeling (see Figure 13.4). These considerations include the consumers perceptions of what they see, hear, think, feel, say, feel, and want in their environment. With this information, the design thinker begins to make sense of all that was gained in understanding the experience of those who feel the pain of the problem.

The insights become the foundation of the solutions because these deep glimpse into the experiences of others—their thoughts and feelings—and they take us beyond what is immediately expected or imagined.

TABLE 13.4 Understanding the Problem-Probing Questions

Identification of Consumer Pain Points	Consumer Insights of the Problem
• What makes your target audience feel bad? • What frustrates, annoys, or gives them a headache? • How are current solutions underperforming? What is missing? • In what ways are alternatives annoying or inadequate? • What are the main difficulties and challenges encountered? • Does the target audience understand how things work? • Do they have difficulties getting certain things done? • Do they resist tasks for specific reasons? • What common mistakes do they make? • Are they using a potential solution the wrong way?	• What need are they trying to satisfy? • What problem are they trying to solve? • What task are they trying to complete? • What is their perspective? • What is the context in which the task or problem occurs? • Are there any constraints or limitations imposed by the situation or environment? • How important is this task or problem to the target audience? • What were the patterns or themes that emerged, or the moments of interest that were particularly noticeable?

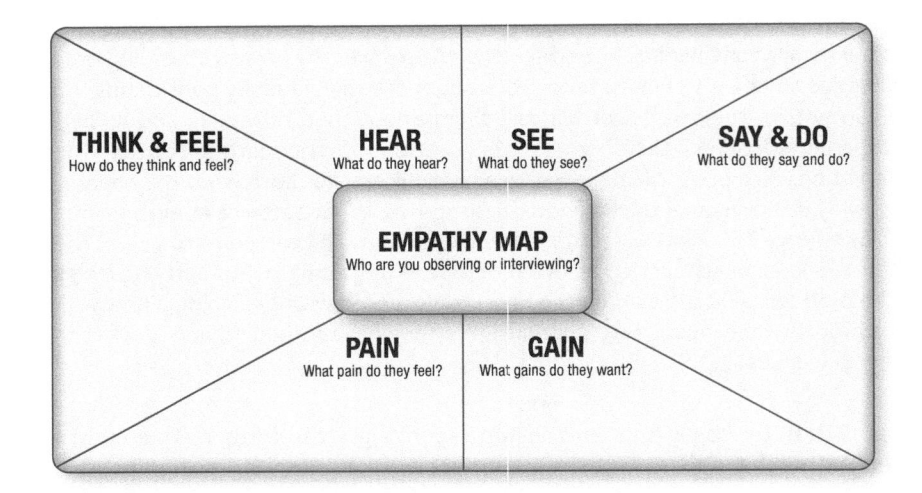

THINK & FEEL — How do they think and feel?
HEAR — What do they hear?
SEE — What do they see?
SAY & DO — What do they say and do?
EMPATHY MAP — Who are you observing or interviewing?
PAIN — What pain do they feel?
GAIN — What gains do they want?

FIGURE 13.4 Sample Empathy Map

Part 2: Ideating to Generate Unexpected Ideas

Once a deep understanding of the problem has been gained and insights have emerged that inform the creative problem-solving process, design thinkers are equipped to engage in the process of ideation, generating many unique ideas and concepts that may ultimately be explored as a potential solution. Ideating allows us to reframe our challenges by pushing us to continuously explore and pursue new perspectives while also continually maintaining focused on the problem. It asks us to look for new opportunities from all different angles and perspectives.

? DID YOU KNOW?

Innovation Does Not Always Lead to Success

A brief example illustrates the importance of staying tethered to the problem, and how losing that focus can lead to results that are lauded for their creativity but ultimately fail for their lack of desirability. In the late 2010s, a Silicon Valley startup named Juicero captured significant attention and interest for its potentially disruptive juicer machine. This expensive, high-tech, Wi-Fi-enabled juicing machine was promised to allow customers to easily cold-press their own fresh fruit and vegetable juice, if customers also purchased and used the packets of fruits and vegetables that were to be plugged into the Juicero machine. Juicero gained widespread attention and millions of dollars in investments due to its creativity and innovative concept, but when curious reporters discovered that the juice customers enjoyed did not even need the machine—the Juicero juice packets could effectively be squeezed simply by hand rather than requiring the expensive Juicero machine—the company suffered tremendous embarrassment and ultimately shut down, becoming a widely used example of a solution to a problem that did not really exist. To avoid this trap, ideating requires us to be willing to courageously explore new ideas, but to always stay tethered to the problem that we are working to solve.

In the process of ideation, as we work to stay connected to our problem while also continuously engaging in a cycle of exploration, it is necessary to continuously ask questions and be aware of human values—utilizing the **beginner's mindset**, a keen sense of curiosity, and an emphasis on empathy that design thinking promotes. In ideation, we must ask questions continuously: How might we…? What if…? Could we…? Why? We must also be willing to call into question our common assumptions, and this often requires altering our point of view and seeing the situation in new ways that uncover critical insights and lead to possibilities for breakthrough ideas.

Ideation also requires us to intentionally stretch our thinking and push ourselves to develop multiple ideas. This prevents us from becoming possessive of the few ideas that exist so that when there is an abundance of ideas to work with, there is less temptation to become territorial (Kelley & Kelley, 2013).

During the ideation process, the goal is to produce as many ideas as possible, which is also referred to as **divergent thinking.** As divergent thinking describes the process during ideation of developing multiple ideas, it is paired with convergent thinking, which shifts through those ideas to explore concepts of merit and leads to iteration and experimentation.

Part 3: Experimenting to Advance Meaningful Solutions

As the design thinking journey progresses, an iterative process takes shape in which potential solutions are prototyped and tested to gain feedback that can identify where the solution falls short as well as what additional insights can be captured to further understand the problem. Design thinkers use their insights, their judgment, and their intuition to explore a select group of concepts and then explore those concepts through the development of **prototypes.** These prototypes allow for meaningful feedback, judgment, and iteration to occur, enabling concepts to be further developed and advanced, and a "fail fast" mentality is embraced to identify opportunities for improvement in an expedited fashion. This is often referred to as a "bias toward action," and it challenges design thinkers to find their concept's faults quickly, and without significant investment of resources in a prototype, so that the solution is more quickly developed. It also requires participants to resist becoming defensive, protective, or territorial with their concept, and instead to be fully open to feedback and constructive criticism from others. The process of experimentation and iteration is one that can become a perpetual loop, and it can also send design thinkers back to either better understand their problem in a new perspective or, alternatively, to further ideate on new insights gained from the exercise of iterating.

Throughout the design thinking journey, leaders must embrace radical collaboration. **Radical collaboration** suggests an organizational strategy of working with nontraditional or unexpected organizations or entities. This value recognizes that our best ideas often come from being able to share and build upon ideas with others. Design thinking thrives with the incorporation of diverse perspectives that may surprise and lead us in unexpected directions or may challenge our assumptions or path dependence. It emphasizes that the process of design thinking—and creative problem solving—is a team sport, requiring a sense of humility that resists the idea we can do it all on our own. Instead, radical collaboration fosters a sense of community and camaraderie that can be a powerful antidote to the fear of failure that is often such a powerful barrier to innovation.

Ultimately, as healthcare leaders embrace the design thinking process, they gain from an approach to problem-solving that emphasizes empathy and creative confidence. However, once a leader effectively develops a meaningful solution to the problem they have identified, validated, and explored, their work as a leader is not done. Rather, the solutions they have identified can often require change, and leaders must then embrace the role of managing change to successfully implement the solution and navigate the changes that are required. This leads us to consider more closely change management.

Change Management: Essential Leadership Skills for the Future

Managing change is an essential skill for leaders regardless of the endeavor; however, it may be more important in population health management because of the diversity of the people, groups, organizations, and stakeholders impacted by any initiative. Behavior is often seen as "contagious," and to get true change, behavior must change. Consider that it is nearly impossible to know what one thinks or to know what another person truly feels, but one can know another's behavior because it can be seen and assessed. A quote attributed to Leonardo da Vinci sums this idea up well: "I have been impressed with the urgency of doing. Knowing is not enough; we must apply. Being willing is not enough; we must do."

Change management and the related tools can be used to help people understand, accept, move forward, and appreciate change, and then act. Just as design thinking highlights the importance of empathy and observing the behaviors and emotions of others, much of change management is about addressing behaviors and emotions, which is a critical part of many population health strategies.

An essential competency is to understand the neurobiology of change. Our modern society is moving faster than the evolution of our neural biological system, and we often experience negative emotional responses to change because, in the past, change meant danger. Patterns of behavior were essential to survival, and any alteration of that pattern could mean death or serious negative consequences. That may explain why the first response to or feeling about a change is often an emphatic "no," and why such resistance to change can be so strong (Greene, 2014; Phan et al., 2002; Sebastian & Ahmed,

2018). Although this may not be true in modern society, our brains will often have a similar emotional threat response to change—even though it may not be life-threatening or have the adverse consequences that one might have experienced in earlier human history—and make this reaction to change a programmed response.

Models to Understand and Manage Change

Over the years, models have been developed to manage diverse change transitions. Today, PHM can refer to these diverse change models as useful tools and a framework for leading change and transforming healthcare.

The Bridges Model

The **Bridges Model of Change** helps us understand the change process in a straightforward way. The model is composed of three important segments of the process of change:

1. The first segment of change according to Bridges is *Ending, Losing, Letting Go*. In this stage, people are analyzing and trying to understand the nature of change, and they require time to let go of what they perceive as being lost.
2. This is then followed by *the Neutral Zone*. This represents a time when our feelings regarding the change are somewhat ambiguous, and it is during this time that we can accept or reject change.
3. The Neutral Zone is followed by the *New Beginnings Phase*. During this time, we are further understanding the change and beginning to accept change as a new reality (Bridges, 2020).

Not all change models, either for the individual or for groups of people, necessarily move smoothly and sequentially through these stages. People will often vacillate between one aspect of change and another, feeling positive at some points and more negative at other times. The key then is perseverance to continue to inform, support, and encourage people toward constructive change.

The PAST Change Model

The **PAST Change Model** developed by Wagner (2017) has four principal parts or action steps as illustrated in Exhibit 13.1.

The first activity is *Preparation*. What is your case for change or for the intervention? It is important to incorporate sensitivity around the emotions of change and help people understand that a sense of loss is a natural response to change. By acknowledging doubts and ushering people through the stages of discomfort, helping them discover new realities to understand the change, they can then begin to integrate it into their daily lives. One must also assess their gap in readiness. Is it possible to engage in the project or intervention that is needed by the participants? This can often be accomplished through discussions and awareness of the project or intervention. A formal assessment of attitudes about the potential intervention may also be useful.

Next, one must *Act*. This is best done by assessing the current state of the situation: do we understand what we are attempting to do, and are we sure that the design and development of the intervention is a suitable match for its intended purpose? Effective implementation and measurement are needed to determine program status.

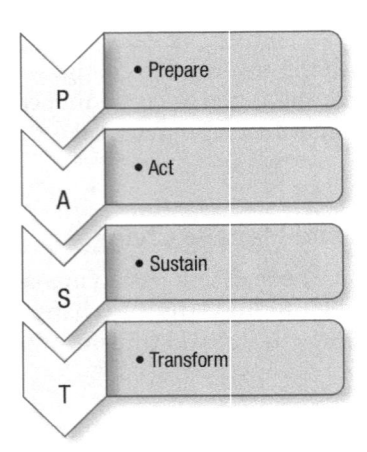

EXHIBIT 13.1 The PAST Change Model

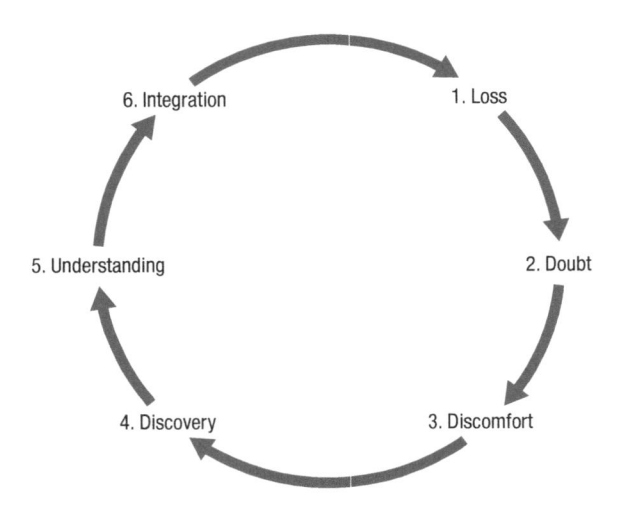

FIGURE 13.5 The Six Stage Change Cycle

Sustaining Change is often a challenge. There is a natural tendency for things to regress to their previous status, and less vigorous action is taken to reinforce the change, to continually monitor and improve the change, and to put new work standards in place to ensure that the program is implemented true to its intention.

Transformation then occurs. Such transformation requires defining the standards of the program, not just the rules. Expectations must be set, and there must be feedback and accountability to see that those standards and expectations are adhered to. As George Bernard Shaw once said, "Those who cannot change their minds cannot change anything" (Wagner, 2017).

Salerno and Brock's Cycle Change

Figure 13.5 is an illustration of the six stages of change developed by Salerno and Brock (2008). The **Salerno and Brock's cycle of change model** focuses heavily on the emotions of the individual experiencing change. Each stage contains certain feelings, thoughts, and behaviors. This model suggests that we focus on the observation of individuals' behaviors as opposed to supposition about their feelings or thoughts.

The stages are as follows:

1. *Loss*. In this stage, a person feels fear and has thoughts of cautiousness, and their behavior is quite paralyzed because they do not know what to do.
2. *Doubt*. In this stage, feelings are likely to be those of resentment and thoughts of skepticism, and we typically see resistance to change emerging in this stage.
3. *Discomfort*. During this stage, feelings of anxiety, confusion, and unproductive behaviors are likely to occur. During this time, a person is not sure what to think about the change, and they are still making up their mind. Because of this, they often enter a danger zone where—when less effectively managed—they may revert to earlier, more dangerous stages of loss and doubt.
4. *Discovery*. At this stage of the change cycle, things become decidedly more positive. The individual may experience feelings of anticipation, thoughts of resourcefulness, and more energized behavior. During this period, the individual has begun to accept the change and is beginning to think about how they will fit into the new way of doing things.
5. *Understanding*. At this stage, positive change has begun to occur with feelings of confidence, pragmatic thoughts, and productive behaviors.
6. *Integration*. At this point, the individual is putting it all together with feelings of satisfaction. Thoughts become more focused, and behaviors become more generous, meaning they can effectively interact with others to support the change and help others through it.

Once a person has completed the six stages of the cycle, true change can occur and can be lasting. It is also important to note that people do not necessarily spend any length of time at any single stage; however, they must go through all the stages, and they can revisit stages based upon the resolution of the issues involved. This often depends heavily on the effectiveness of management (Salerno & Brock, 2008).

The change cycle provides a good opportunity to discuss injured individual feelings about a change that individuals are experiencing or being asked to make. It is appropriate for the manager or leader to ask people where they are in the change cycle and what they can do to help them move forward. There are several exercises that can assist in helping people progress. These include the following:

- A reframing exercise that allows the project manager to help people through change by asking them the following question: "What questions can I answer that would help you understand and clarify the change?"
- Another exercise is to develop a "Resistance to Change" worksheet, asking the individual to examine their understanding of the change, why it is happening, whether they support the change, if they need further education (implying that they may need additional skill training or education on a topic important to the project or intervention), and what support they need.

The Influencer Model

The Influencer Model for Change is one that can be effectively utilized in implementing new interventions and programs in population health management

(Grenny et al., 2005a). Fundamentally, the model is built on the research that demonstrated that people would change if they were motivated and able to make the change (Grenny et al., 2005b), and it focuses on two issues: motivation and ability. To start, one must identify the sources of influence—which can be personal, social, and structural—and find the vital new behavior that will produce change (see Figure 13.6).

As true of all the domains, *Personal* sources of influence can be broken down into motivation to change and the ability to carry out the desired change. In the case of personal sources of influence, making an undesirable change desirable is an effective strategy. One should ask, Do I enjoy it? Is a person able to do it? For example, a person may wish to quit smoking cigarettes; however, they first must desire to do so, because they likely either enjoy smoking or have an addiction to nicotine. They must change their perspective to enjoy better health as a motivation and use new change vital behaviors to increase their personal mastery and ability to make the change. This might include not having cigarettes in their home or workplace, which would be a source of temptation.

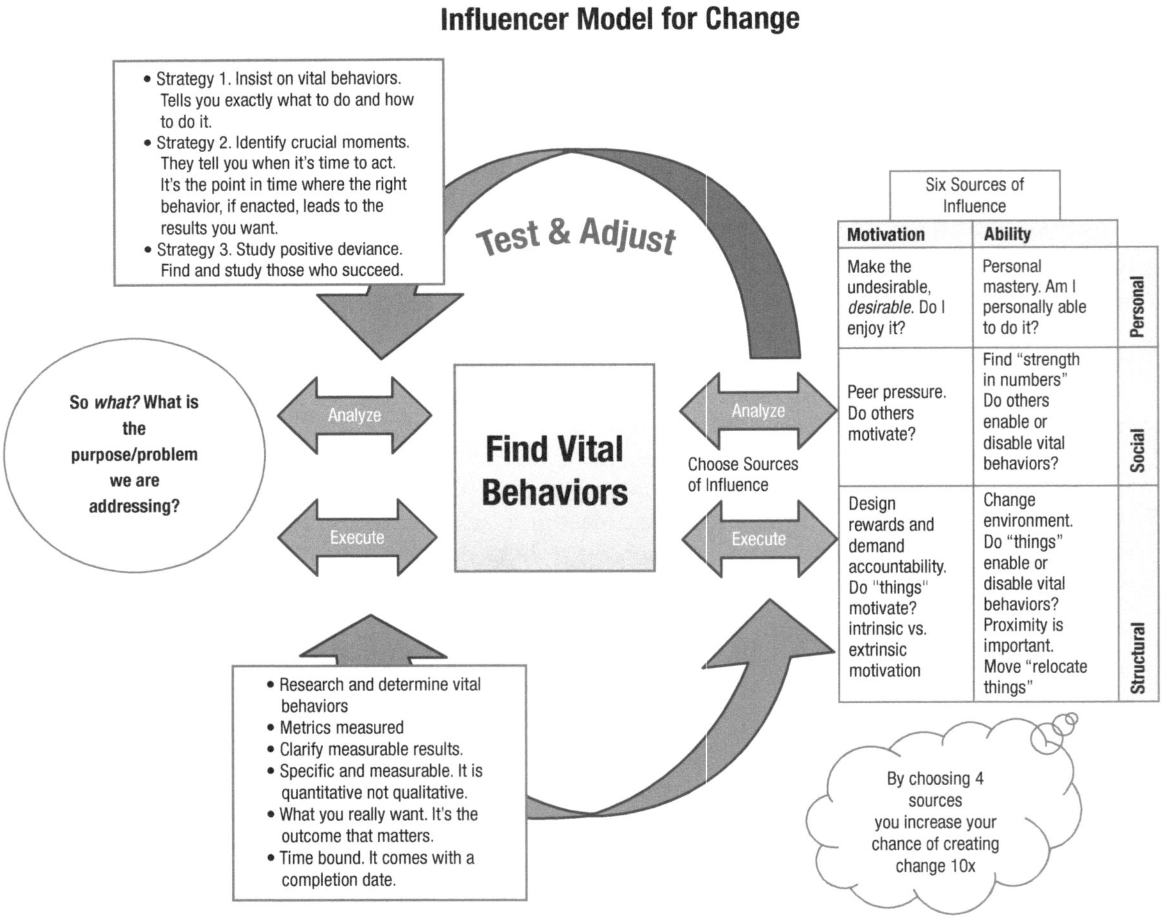

Influencer Model for Change

- Strategy 1. Insist on vital behaviors. Tells you exactly what to do and how to do it.
- Strategy 2. Identify crucial moments. They tell you when it's time to act. It's the point in time where the right behavior, if enacted, leads to the results you want.
- Strategy 3. Study positive deviance. Find and study those who succeed.

So *what?* What is the purpose/problem we are addressing?

Test & Adjust

Analyze — **Find Vital Behaviors** — Analyze
Execute — — Execute
Choose Sources of Influence

- Research and determine vital behaviors
- Metrics measured
- Clarify measurable results.
- Specific and measurable. It is quantitative not qualitative.
- What you really want. It's the outcome that matters.
- Time bound. It comes with a completion date.

Six Sources of Influence

	Motivation	Ability	
	Make the undesirable, *desirable*. Do I enjoy it?	Personal mastery. Am I personally able to do it?	Personal
	Peer pressure. Do others motivate?	Find "strength in numbers" Do others enable or disable vital behaviors?	Social
	Design rewards and demand accountability. Do "things" motivate? intrinsic vs. extrinsic motivation	Change environment. Do "things" enable or disable vital behaviors? Proximity is important. Move "relocate things"	Structural

By choosing 4 sources you increase your chance of creating change 10x

FIGURE 13.6 The Influencer Model of Change
Reprinted by permission from Wagner, 2017

Motivation and ability regarding *social factors* would include such things as peer pressure and finding strength in numbers, which often allows us to persevere toward a change. A vital behavior might be walking groups, which are often more effective than people simply attempting to exercise alone. The walking group offers an element of camaraderie and a little peer pressure to consistently engage in exercise.

Structural sources of influence include designing reward and developing mechanisms that intrinsically and extrinsically motivate the individual or group. Changing the environment, for example, with the vital behavior is the insistence on the availability of healthier foods such as fresh fruits and vegetables. A community garden may be another vital behavior, which would offer not only exercise but also fresh produce. Notice that the vital behavior is both group- and individual-based, because a community garden would likely be done by a group, while changing what a person eats is an individual vital behavior. As the model indicates, the greater the number of influence factors employed, the greater the level of success (Grenny et al., 2005b).

Change Management Skills for Population Health Managers

When managing change, it is important to consider the potential responses that individuals may show. The four primary responses can be categorized as get on board, accept, and thrive on the change. Individuals can also push back, which can be positive if the pushback is used to obtain more information or a better understanding of the change. A person can refuse to accept the change and essentially remove themselves from participating in the intervention. Or they can remain as a participant in the intervention, while at the same time they serve as a consistent naysayer and detractor, providing a disruptive influence on those who are more engaged.

Why is change management so difficult? Population health managers need to understand what people want to know regarding any change or new activity. Without appropriate communication, delivered by a skilled manager at the right time and the right place, essential organizational changes and workflows risk not being fully implemented leading to potential negative outcomes for consumers, patients, employees, and the organization.

People typically want to know four things, and it is important to note the nature of this information and how people perceive these things. Table 13.5 aligns these types of concerns with the questions that the manager needs to answer and provides the appropriate response.

Once individual employees are comfortable with change, building successful teams will be easier.

Team Building: The Drexler/Sibbet High-Performing Teams Model

Healthcare is not a team sport—but a team enterprise. The **Drexler/Sibbet High-Performing Teams Model** is an excellent way to organize population health management teams for implementing new strategies. The model consists of a seven-stage process: three of which are creating the team, three of which are sustaining the team, and a pivotal stage that is the point of commitment. Each stage represents a question essential to team-building. The

TABLE 13.5 Team's Concerns, Questions, and Leadership Responses

Team Concern	Underlying Question	Leadership Response
People often want to know the vision on a grand scale, and they are satisfied with this macro view of the change intervention.	Where are we going?	Articulate and explain the vision for the organization and the importance of this change.
Others want more detail and are looking for a sense of purpose, and they focus on the question: Why are we doing this?	Why are we going there?	Discuss the purpose and focus and outcome of the change.
Then, there are those who want to know more specifics and are interested in the actual plan.	How do we get there?	Provide the plan of action.

model further requires the assessment of the consequences of resolved and unresolved issues during each stage.

The stages, questions, and the diagnostics for resolved and unresolved issues are presented in Table 13.6.

As with the creating phases of the teambuilding process, if we do not resolve the issues within implementation, high performance, and renewal, we must return to the unresolved stage for further action and resolution.

DID YOU KNOW?

Leading change also requires belief in yourself.

Leading change required belief in what one is doing and a passion for change. Each day, we must ask ourselves three questions:

1. Who am I?
2. Why am I here?
3. What do I bring to the table?

The author learned this lesson years ago when challenged by a community leader to do more than just show up (Wagner, 2003).

SUMMARY

The challenges we confront in healthcare today are complex and daunting, and they do not promise to easily fade or grow tempered as time progresses. Instead, tomorrow's healthcare leaders must rise to the challenge, anticipating and meeting the demands of the future health sector. In the next decade, healthcare leaders will likely navigate their organizations through the continued effects of the COVID-19 pandemic, the continued rise of chronic care needs in an aging population, potential significant changes to health reform (whether the overturning of the Affordable Care Act, the progression toward a public option or single-payer system, or something else), potential disruption in health coverage among many in the U.S. population, the continued rise of consumerism, the continued advance of health technology including personalized medicine and analytics, continued pressures surrounding health spending, and many other challenges, including those not currently anticipated or imagined. This chapter emphasized the importance for leaders to embrace such future challenges by considering their role in addressing

TABLE 13.6 The Drexler/Sibbet High-Performing Teams Model

Team Stages	Team Characteristics
Orientation: why am I here?	If this stage is resolved, one could expect a clear understanding of purpose, team identity, and membership. If this stage remains unresolved, one can expect disorientation, uncertainty, and fear.
Trust building: who are you?	If this stage is resolved, one can expect mutual respect, forthrightness, and reliability. If this stage remains unresolved, one can expect caution, mistrust, and a façade.
Goal clarification: what are we doing?	If this stage is resolved, one can expect explicit assumptions, clear and integrated goals, and a shared vision. If this stage is unresolved, one can expect apathy, skepticism, and irrelevant competition.
Commitment: how will we do it?	If the first three stages are resolved, one can expect commitment on the part of the team. At this point, we can assign roles, allocate resources, and make decisions. Our team is now formed and functioning, and now we must sustain it. If unresolved, we must return to the point where resolution has been lost.
Implementation: who, does what, when, where	If this stage is resolved, one can expect clear processes, alignment, and disciplined execution. If left unresolved, one can expect conflict and confusion, nonalignment, and missed deadlines.
High performance: wow!	If this stage is resolved, one can expect spontaneous interaction, synergy, and surpassing expectations for results. If unresolved, we will see overload and disharmony.
Renewal: why continue?	If this stage is resolved, we can expect recognition and celebration, change mastery, and sustaining/staying power. If unresolved, we will have boredom and burnout.

the health needs of the populations they serve, leading with empathy and creative confidence to solve the challenging problems they confront, and navigate the difficulties that can accompany change to lead their healthcare organizations into a brighter future.

DISCUSSION QUESTIONS

1. Identify five major management challenges for population health managers.
2. Which factors were instrumental in creating the healthcare sector's demand for innovation?
3. Which barriers to innovation would be the easiest to overcome? Which would be the most difficult.
4. Briefly explain the three-part innovation model and use an example.
5. Why are change management skills so crucial for population health managers?
6. Select one of the change management models and apply it to a current situation in your experiences.
7. Team-building has been described as both an art and a science. How would you respond?

Toolkit Competency Application: Mini Scenarios

Part A. The Empathy Map

An accountable care organization with over 50 primary care physicians has begun a design thinking process to develop a better pathway for patient engagement in the hopes of positively impacting regular medication routine use. One of their primary steps is to complete an empathy map. Outline the steps and activities that would need to be completed to construct a useful empathy map.

Part B: Change Management Strategy

As Vice President of Population Health for your health organization, you just completed a meeting with six of your regional directors. In the last year, strong clinical and financial evidence suggested that the targeted population health management interventions were still not effectively "reaching" many of the high acuity/ high-cost chronic disease patients in your population.

Based on a recommendation provided by the VP of strategic planning, you decided to implement a remote patient monitoring initiative over an alternative Community Health Worker care coordination approach. The regional directors report that many care coordination teams seem reluctant to adopt this new strategy and are either "dragging their feet" or seriously trying to undermine the success of the initiative via failure to follow protocols and processes. How would you manage this organization change? What would be your response?

REFERENCES

Bridges, W. (2020). *William bridges—Change transitions and how to navigate them.* http://www.strategies-for-managing-change.com/william-bridges.html

Catmull, E. (2014, March 12). *Inside the Pixar braintrust.* Fast Company. https://www.fastcompany.com/3027135/inside-the-pixar-braintrust

Gray, D., Brown, S., & Macanufo, J. (2010). *Gamestorming: A playbook for innovators, rulebreakers, and changemakers.* O'Reilly Media.

Greene, J. D. (2014). *Moral tribes: Emotion, reason, and the gap between us and them* (Reprint ed). Penguin Books.

Grenny, J., Patterson, K., Maxfield, D., McMillan, R., & Switzler, A. (2005a). *Influencer: The new science of leading change.* McGraw-Hill Education.

Grenny, J., Patterson, K., Maxfield, D., McMillan, R., & Switzler, A. (2005b). *Influencer: The new science of leading change.* McGraw-Hill Education.

Herzlinger, R. E. (2006). Why innovation in health care is so hard. *Harvard Business Review, 84*(5), 58–66.

Kelley, T., & Kelley, D. (2013). *Creative confidence: Unleashing the creative potential within us all.* Crown Publishing.

Nembhard, I. M., Burns, L. R., & Shortell, S. M. (2020, April 17). Responding to COVID-19: Lessons from management research. *NEJM Catalyst.* https://doi.org/10.1056/CAT.20.0111

Osterwalder, A., Pigneur, Y., Bernarda, G., & Smith, A. (2014). *Value proposition design.* John Wiley & Sons.

Parmar, R., Mackenzie, I., Cohn, D., & Gann, D. (2014). The new patterns of innovation: How to use data to drive growth. *Harvard Business Review, 92*(1–2), 86–95.

Phan, K. L., Wager, T., Taylor, S. F., & Liberzon, I. (2002). Functional neuroanatomy of emotion: A meta-analysis of emotion activation studies in PET and fMRI. *NeuroImage, 16*(2), 331–348. https://doi.org/10.1006/NIMG.2002.1087

Roberts, J. (2017). Design thinking gains converts in health care after finding success in other fields. *H&HN Magazine.* www.hhnmag.com/articles/7812-how-design-thinking-could-transform-a-health-care-organization

Salerno, A., & Brock, L. (2008). *The change cycle: How people can survive and thrive in organizational change*. Berrett-Koehler Publishers.

Sebastian, C. L., & Ahmed, S. P. (2018). The neurobiology of emotion regulation. *The Wiley Blackwell Handbook of Forensic Neuroscience, 1–2*, 125–143. https://doi.org/10.1002/9781118650868.ch6

Skillicorn, N. (2016, March 18). What is innovation? 15 experts share their innovation definition. *Idea to Value*. https://www.ideatovalue.com/inno/nickskillicorn/2016/03/innovation-15-experts-share-innovation-definition/

Wagner, S. L. (2003). Defining the ACMPE Fellow. *College View, Fall*, 28–31.

Wagner, S. L. (2017). *Fundamentals of medical practice management*. Health Administration Press.

Weisberg, R. W., Speck, R. M., & Fleisher, L. A. (2014). Fostering innovation in medicine: A conceptual framework for medical centers. *Healthcare, 2*, 90–93. https://doi.org/10.1016/j.hjdsi.2013.09.007

PART V

Population Health Management Cases

CHAPTER 14

Case Studies

This chapter includes four original and unique case studies that offer students the opportunity to test their decision-making and critical thinking abilities when faced with typical population management health problems and scenarios. Each example requires the student to apply a related theory, model, strategy, or tool and produce an innovative synthesis and solution that meets the real-world challenge.

CASE STUDY 1. COPRODUCTION OF HEALTH: *BABY'S FIRST* BY ANNE M. HEWITT

Virtual care and telehealth have become a mainstream population health management intervention option especially for populations at risk that require significant social support and reinforcement. This case study also introduces students to a coproduction of health example involving three diverse stakeholders. Although located in a midwestern state, this particular health problem is pervasive nationwide.
   Chapter Alignment: 6, 9, 10, 12

CASE STUDY 2. IMPLEMENTING A POPULATION HEALTH DATA ANALYTICS PLATFORM: A MULTISPECIALTY GROUP CASE STUDY BY ASHISH PARIKH, JAMIE L. REEDY, AND NALIN JOHRI

Combining the diverse and sometimes complex aspects of population health management to develop and implement an integral operation such as a Data Analytics Platform requires an application of multiple tools and frameworks. Not only will the student need to assess the types of data sources and identified data analyses but also explain the complex contract negotiation variables to align with the desired outcome.
   Chapter Alignment: 5, 6, 7, 8, 11, 13

CASE STUDY 3. A CASE STUDY ON POPULATION HEALTH ADDRESSING HEALTH EQUITY DURING A CRISIS: FLATTENING THE CURVE OF HISPANICS WITH COVID-19 IN SOMERSET COUNTY, NEW JERSEY
BY PAULA A. GUTIERREZ AND SERENA COLLADO

Reducing health disparities and inequities remains a major goal for Healthy People 2020 and a continuing initiative for all health sector organizations. Based on the impact of the recent COVID-19 pandemic, this case study uses managerial epidemiological data to risk segment an underserved population at risk. Students should understand not only the impact of various social determinants of health but strategies for community involvement and engagement.

Chapter Alignment: 1, 2, 3, 4, 6, 9, 10, 12

CASE STUDY 4. COPRODUCTION LEADERSHIP FOR THE FUTURE HEALTH SECTOR
BY PATRICK D. SHAY AND EDWARD J. SCHUMACHER

Population health management continues to transform the entire healthcare sector. Aspects of how, where, when, and why care is delivered change rapidly as technological advances now enable workflows, products, and processes unknown even a few years ago. Students' competencies need to integrate both the creativity and commitment of innovation and the organizational management skills to help facilitate the coming changes and transitions. This case study provides students with opportunities to engage in both skill-building processes.

Chapter Alignment: 1, 10, 11, 12, 13

Case Study 1. Coproduction of Health: *Baby's First*

Anne M. Hewitt

Disclaimer: This case study does not offer an endorsement of any company or products discussed.

INTRODUCTION

Due to the predominant rural nature of Nebraska (approximately 1.9 million people located over 77,258 square miles), quick and easy access to care and appropriate social support is not always feasible for parents and families (Populationu, 2021). This can lead to negative health risk factors such as isolation, exhaustion, and in severe cases, infant abuse, and neglect. Abusive head trauma (AHT), formerly referred to as shaken baby syndrome, is a severe form of child abuse causing devastating health and social outcomes for children and families. In 2014, Nebraska diagnosed shaken baby abuse more often than any other state in the country (NBC, 2014).

WellCare of Nebraska, now known as HealthyBlue, a managed care organization (MCO) that serves Medicaid eligible individuals, conducted a detailed medical claims review process as one component of a population assessment (HealthyBlue, 2020). For a comparison perspective, a Canadian study estimated that costs associated with fatal, severe, and least severe AHT averaged $7,147,548, $6,057,761, and $1,675,099, respectively (Beaulieu et al., 2019). However, an investment of $5 per newborn using a health promotion program (PURPLE) resulted in a $273.52 and $14.49 per child cost avoidance by society and by the healthcare system (Beaulieu et al., 2019). The PURPLE Crying Intervention developed by the National Center on Shaken Baby Syndrome is an evidence-based intervention protocol (National Center on Shaken Baby Syndrome, n.d.). Evidence-based interventions rely on established health behavior theories and models as well as scientific study validations.

Population-at-Risk Intervention Analysis

Further population data analysis also identified the need to educate parents on attending infant well visits, the importance of attending mom's postpartum visits, receiving immunizations, and ER diversion for nonemergent illnesses. In addition to decreasing infant abuse and neglect, and specifically abusive head trauma, the healthcare organization wanted to support Nebraska parents through the critical first 15 months of a baby's life.

Evidence from a study in North Carolina had found a health promotion intervention that included nurse-provided education (advice line phone calls), a DVD, a booklet, and reinforcement by primary care practices and a media campaign and showed no significant changes in outcome metrics of AHT hospital admissions, although the proportion of calls concerning crying babies were reduced suggesting that the additional health education may be a positive factor (Zolotor et al., 2015). Given rural health challenges such as logistical challenges with face-to-face visits, the organization recognized that a population health approach was needed that offered convenient, consumer friendly support and real-time interaction if needed. Recent smartphone technology enhancements coupled with the development of tailored digital therapeutics and evidence-based health behavior designed programs suggested selecting an interactive virtual care intervention. Telehealth interventions can expand access to services and improve quality of care at a lower cost (RHIHub, 2019).

Proposed Solution

Although the primary goal was the reduction of infant abuse and neglect, specifically abusive head trauma, it was decided that rather than solely focusing on the connection between infant crying and shaken baby syndrome, the best approach was to increase resiliency in parents by educating and preparing them for typical infant development and behaviors. To meet the population-at-risk needs, WellCare selected a third-party digital therapeutic provider to collaboratively create *Baby's First* * to deliver the intervention. The remote care delivery 15-month postpartum, digital therapeutic education and support program addresses specific needs of each parent through an initial onboarding survey (GoMoHealth, 2020). Parents were stratified by their identified risk level, which enables the program to deliver individualized content and resources to support parents how and when they need it most. Available in multiple languages, the program not only offered mobile support and educational videos, but also at-risk parents received up to six messages per week until the baby became 6-months-old when the number of messages tapered to two to three care messages per week for the duration of the program. Program content focuses on healthy child-rearing, postpartum and pediatric provider visits and vaccination reminders, breastfeeding, how to deal with a crying baby, calming and coping techniques, development milestones, educational play activities, healthy-parenting motivation, local support resources, answers from parent surveys, and more.

Process for Intervention Planning and Implementation

Baby's First was the first member facing mobile resource delivery program for the MCO; thus, systems needed to be conceptualized, created, and implemented prior to launch. As with any organization, such system changes take time and resources. Additionally, as WellCare of Nebraska was contracted as an MCO within the state of Nebraska, state reviews and approvals were required.

As Figure 14.1 and Table 14.1 indicate, the planning and implementation processes are intricate, carefully planned, and executed. Program escalations are utilized for members who indicate that they are in need of social services

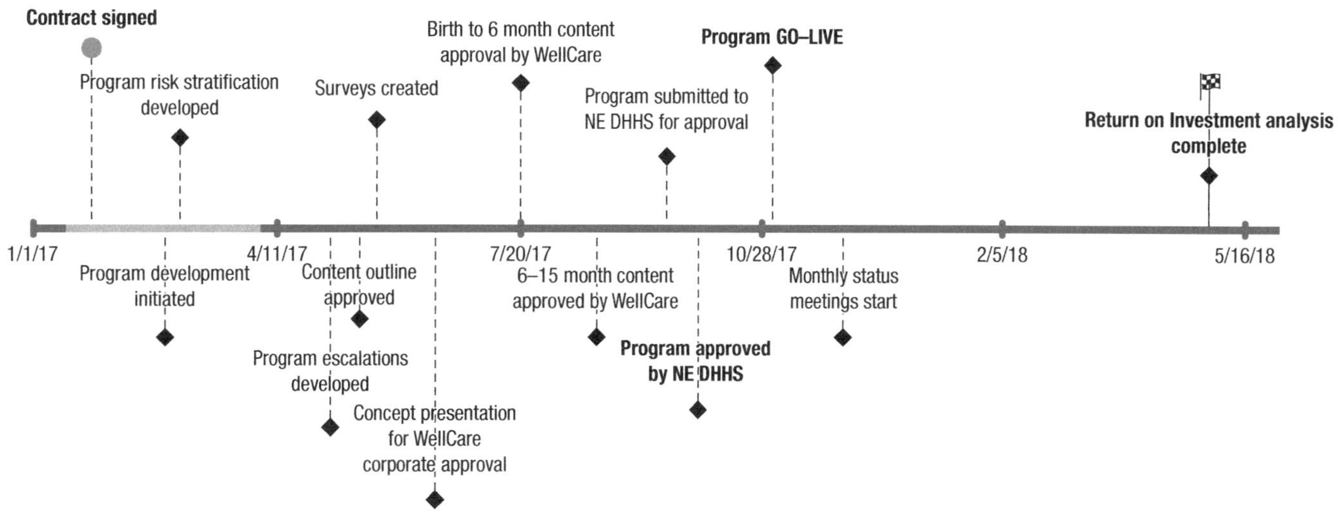

FIGURE 14.1 Baby's First Program Timeline

TABLE 14.1 Milestone Accomplishment Dates

Date	Milestone
1/25/17	Contract signed
2/24/17	Program development initiated
3/2/17	Program risk stratification developed
5/3/17	Program escalations developed
5/1/17	15-month program analysis
5/15/17	Content outline approved
5/22/17	Surveys created
6/15/17	Concept presentation for WellCare corporate approval
7/20/17	Birth to 6-month content approval by WellCare
8/20/17	6- to 15-month content approved by WellCare
9/18/17	Program submitted to NE DHHS for approval*
10/1/17	Program approved by NE DHHS
11/1/17	Program GO–LIVE
12/1/17	Monthly status meetings start
5/1/18	Return-on-investment analysis complete

*Nebraska Department of Health and Human Services

(food, housing, utilities), the baby was in the NICU after birth, potentially at risk for postpartum depression per the Edinburgh and PHQ-2 screenings, or report feeling like they themselves or someone else may hurt themselves or their child (in which case the immediate program response is to call 911 if they are in imminent danger). In addition to this, an escalation to the WellCare crisis line was sent as well as an escalation to the care management team as defined within the program.

Program Components

Stakeholders

Throughout the development, planning, and implementation stages, a team of Nebraska stakeholders were involved to provide an interdisciplinary and global perspective to address the needs of Nebraska parents. The stakeholder team was comprised of the following:

- Physicians: OBGYN, pediatricians, psychiatrists
- WellCare of Nebraska: nurses, social workers, case managers

Budget

$3/per member per month

Care Messages

The program utilizes tailored care messages (sent via text) to deliver content to the parent in their "lived environment" along with valuable information and resource links to additional information from trusted resources such as the American Academy of Pediatrics (AAP) and the Centers for Disease Control and Prevention (CDC). The intent of these messages is to support the family while reinforcing the information covered by pediatricians during most well visits. Figure 14.2 is an example of a program care message.

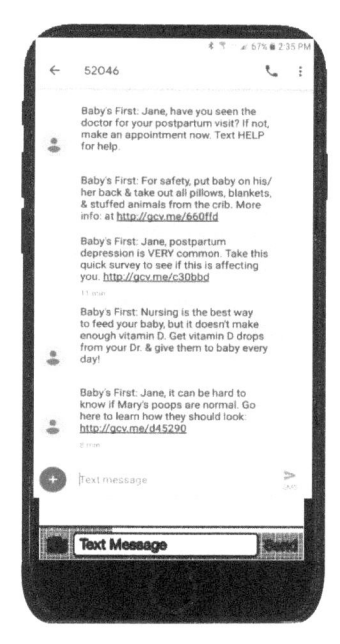

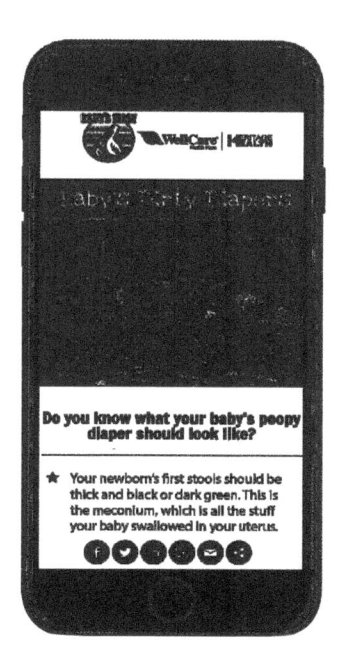

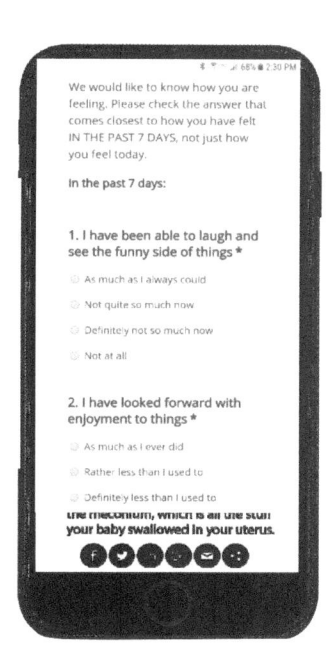

FIGURE 14.2 Baby's First Program Mobile Images

MOBILE SUPPORT

Care messages within the program also include a hyperlink that directs the reader to a mobile web page for additional information. Figure 14.3 is an example of a mobile page snapshot.

Surveys

Parents are encouraged to complete the program surveys.
- Onboarding
- Edinburgh Postnatal Depression Scale (EPDS)
- Patient Health Questionnaire-2 (PHQ-2)
- 6-month, 12-month, and 15-month/program conclusion

Data from surveys are reviewed quarterly by the WellCare stakeholder group. Through the review of program surveys and additional quantitative results, a plan–do–study–act (PDSA) approach to program modifications can be applied.

Outcomes – Qualitative, Quantitative, and Anecdotal = Triangulation of Data

In the spring of 2018, WellCare conducted a retrospective analysis to identify the return on investment (ROI) for *participating* members within their first year of life. The aggregated medical cost savings per participant was $202 month, less the $3 per person per month for the program, netted a $198 month savings, or approximately $2400 for the year.

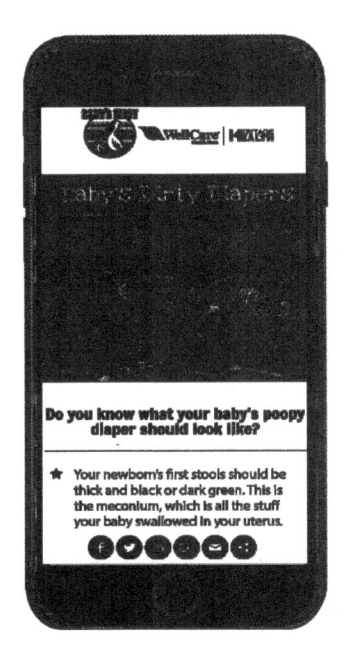

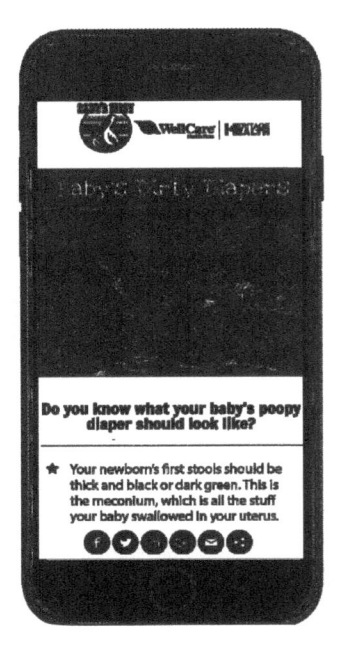

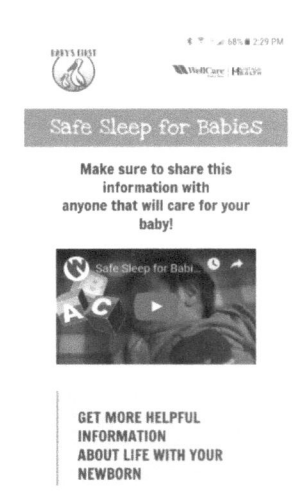

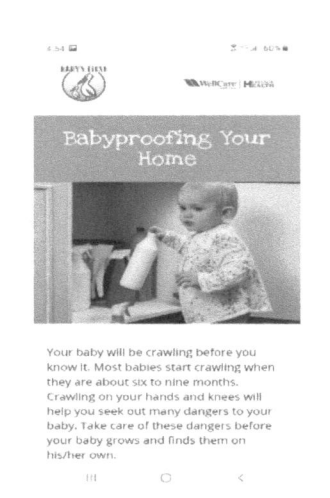

FIGURE 14.3 Mobile Images: Messages With Hyperlinks to CarePages™

WellCare members that participated in the program had
- 75% less inpatient/readmission costs and
- 64% less in emergency room visit costs.

60% reduction in total medical costs
  Additional benefits included the following impacts:
- 86% retention rate of users
- 21 adverse events have been avoided through real-time escalations tied to the postpartum depression screening
- On December 14, 2017, Nebraska Governor Pete Ricketts declared the day "Pelican Day" in recognition of the *Baby's First* Program

In addition to the positive financial and utilization results, using a third-party digital multicomponent initiative had a positive impact on the parenting journey of its users. One hundred percent of surveyed members report that they would recommend the program to others.

The following are anecdotal comments from mothers that responded to program surveys:

- "The information was very good, thank you."
- "The information really helped me."
- "I am a primary care physician, and it was great to see this resource for myself, but also, to recommend it to my patients (I do OB and Peds). Thank you for this service!"
- "I really enjoy the program and getting messages."
- "Very helpful for my boyfriend as he's a first-time parent."

Lessons Learned: Challenges and Successes

One of the biggest challenges the project team encountered during the program was the fairly typical reluctance and "learning curves" when it comes to utilizing new technologies. As the healthcare industry continues to advance, this reluctance to utilize innovations to improve care may result in poor outcomes perpetuating unnecessarily. Healthcare needs to evolve in parallel to the technology and devices that patients have at their fingertips.

Due to the overwhelming ROI, in 2019, the *Baby's First* digital therapeutic was expanded into 11 states across the country.

Additional Material: https://gomohealth.com/2020/measurable-roi-from-babys-first-program/

CASE STUDY QUESTIONS

1. Identify the particular population at risk in this case study by describing the healthcare need, circumstances, and other contextual factors. How was this population identified and selected?
2. Why would an MCO choose to partner with a third-party, for-profit vendor and not deliver the care personally to meet their own population's needs?
3. With the rise of telehealth and m-health, hundreds of population health management companies are now available and offer services similar to GOMOHEALTH. Which five factors would you consider most important to be included in the criteria?
4. Outline the unique features of the Baby's First program.
5. Which metrics were selected and reported to determine success of the program?
6. Why was the cost outlined as per person per month?

REFERENCES

Beaulieu, E., Rajabal, F., Zhang, A., & Pike, I. (2019). The lifetime costs of pediatric abusive head trauma and a cost-effectiveness analysis of the Period of Purple crying program in British Columbia, Canada. *Child Abuse Neglect, 97*, 104133. https://

doi.org/10.1016/j.chiabu.2019.104133. Epub 2019 Aug 29. https://pubmed.ncbi.nlm.nih.gov/31473380/#:~:text=The%20costs%20associated%20with%20fatal,and%20by%20the%20healthcare%20system

GoMoHealth. (2020). *The measurable ROI and improved outcomes from the WellCare of Nebraska Baby's first program.* https://gomohealth.com/2020/measurable-roi-from-babys-first-program/

HealthyBlue. (2020). *Welcome to HealthyBlue.* https://www.healthybluene.com/nebraska/home.html

National Center on Shaken Baby Syndrome. (n.d.). *Believe all babies can be safe from harm…we do.* National Center on Shaken Baby Syndrome. Retrieved May 19, 2021, from https://www.dontshake.org/

NBC News. (2014, May 4). Wrongly accused of shake baby abuse: Case puts focus on legal debate. *NBC News.* https://www.nbcnews.com/news/us-news/wrongly-accused-shaken-baby-abuse-case-puts-focus-legal-debate-n94136

Populationu.com. (2021). *Nebraska population.* World Population. http://www.populationu.com/us/nebraska-population

Rural Health Information Hub. (2019, March 26). *Telehealth use in rural healthcare.* https://www.ruralhealthinfo.org/topics/telehealth

Zolotor, A., Runyan, D., Shanahan, M., Durrance C., Nocera, M., Sullivan K., Klevens, J., Murphy, R., Barr, M., & Barr, R. G. (2015). Effectiveness of a Statewide abusive head trauma prevention program in North Carolina. *JAMA Pediatrics, 169*(12), 1126–1131. https://doi.org/10.1001/jamapediatrics.2015.2690. https://pubmed.ncbi.nlm.nih.gov/26501945/

Case Study 2. Implementing a Population Health Data Analytics Platform: A Multispecialty Group Case Study

Ashish Parikh, Jamie L. Reedy, and Nalin Johri

INTRODUCTION: WHY DOES A PRIVATE MEDICAL PRACTICE NEED DATA ANALYTICS?

As U.S. healthcare costs have risen rapidly over the past several decades, payment reform has emerged as a viable solution for bending the cost curve. There has been a movement away from fee-for-service toward alternative payment models that reimburse healthcare providers for value rather than volume of care delivered. In the face of these changes, providers need to have a comprehensive data analytics strategy to succeed in value-based care.

Data analytics is necessary to inform:

- The overall value-based contracting strategy from choosing which payers to partner with to negotiating risk contract terms
- Development of and investment in a comprehensive clinical model that supports value-based care
- Development of an operational strategy for population health management that includes risk stratification and patient engagement and
- Driving better outcomes and continuous quality improvement
- Converting provider and clinical team into value-based care believers

Background: Summit Health

Summit Health came into existence in 2019 through the merger of Summit Medical Group (SMG) and City MD. SMG is a large multispecialty, outpatient medical practice serving Northern New Jersey for over 100 years. City MD offers efficient walk-in care in the Metro New York area at over 120 urgent care centers. Together the combined entity offers comprehensive, coordinated care across all the care continua (see Table 14.2).

TABLE 14.2 Comprehensive Care Across the Care Continua

Comprehensive Care Across the Care Continua	
The age continuum	Birth to childhood to adulthood to end-of-life
The wellness continuum	Prevention to urgent care to chronic condition management
The care setting continuum	Ambulatory care Virtual care Home care Hospital and postacute care Long-term care

When the movement toward fee-for-value emerged, Summit Health initially partnered with some of the pioneering commercial health plans to develop payment models that would measure and reward high-quality care at a lower cost. This required investment in population health management infrastructure to support operations, quality improvement, and patient management.

It was abundantly clear from the beginning that entering into value-based agreements and successfully managing a population of patients would require strong data analytics. Data analytics is necessary to inform value-based contracting strategy.

Insights, Skills, and Strategies for Negotiating Risk Contracts

As value-based payment models continue to evolve, government payers such as Medicare and Medicaid generally offer providers standard value-based contracts with minimal room for negotiation. In contrast, commercial payers may be willing to innovate and customize agreements with provider groups to drive greater value. In either case, providers must have deep understanding of the contract specifics. With this uncertainty and variability, analytics are the key for preparing, negotiating, and implementing risk contracts.

Key areas where data analytics can help groups analyze and negotiate value-based agreement include the following:

- Data needed prior to contract negotiations
- Attribution of the appropriate population
- Choosing meaningful outcome measures and appropriate benchmarks

Even prior to engagement with payers, providers can use internal data to evaluate their preparedness for value-based agreements that may place a portion of their revenue at risk. In addition, they seek data from their payer partners as well as other external data sets to inform decisions. Exhibit 14.1 describes the sources and types of data that can be used to be well prepared for value-based agreement negotiations.

Attribution of the Appropriate Population

To understand the variables that can impact the attribution of patients, which is very important, a group will be held accountable for their health status. If the population the group truly cares for are not used for measuring outcomes, the chances for success are limited. Figure 14.4 describes factors that are important when negotiating the attribution methodology.

PREPARING TO NEGOTIATE

Going into contract negotiations, you will need to prepare **data about your organization** and make sure your team has a clear, well-aligned understanding of your **organizational priorities**.

Checklist of Data to Prepare

INTERNAL DATA	EXTERNAL DATA—HEALTH PLAN	EXTERNAL DATA SETS/BENCHMARKS
• Financial and revenue cycle data for fee schedule negotiations • EHR quality performance, calculated reliably and accurately for full population and specific health plans • Organizational and services information about clinical programs designed to achieve outcomes • Population demographics including disease burden, adherence, whether specialty care is managed, what mix of patients from that plan you currently care for, etc. • Risk adjustment performance (if you have a PHM platform that can support this) and coding program insights	If you don't already have claims data, ask plan for: • **Standard reporting of utilization across KPIs** to support starting point • **Risk scores of patients** compared to market • **Total medical expense and cost categories** • **Distribution of high-utilizers/high-cost patients** for stop-loss analysis • **IN/OON distribution**	If you have access: • CMS-qualified entities can use PUF to run a comparison MARKET RESEARCH While the health plan will have more insight here, know as much as you can about your services and fees versus the market.

EXHIBIT 14.1 Preparing to Negotiate
CMS, Centers for Medicare and Medicaid Services; EHR, electronic health record; KPI, key performance indicator; PUF, public use files.

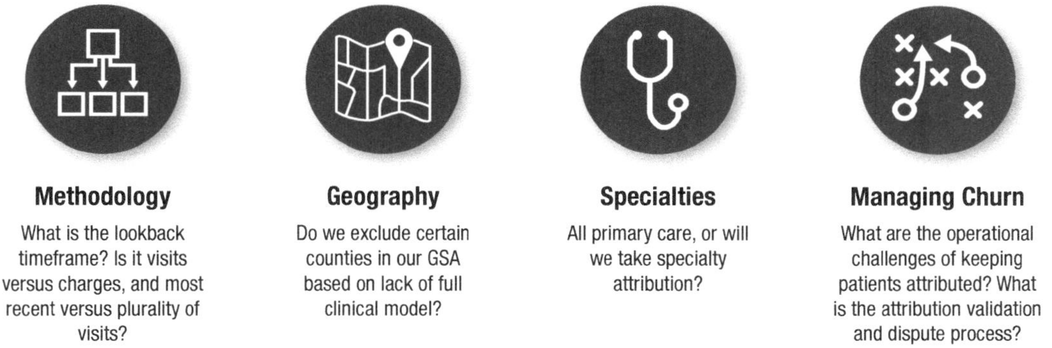

Methodology
What is the lookback timeframe? Is it visits versus charges, and most recent versus plurality of visits?

Geography
Do we exclude certain counties in our GSA based on lack of full clinical model?

Specialties
All primary care, or will we take specialty attribution?

Managing Churn
What are the operational challenges of keeping patients attributed? What is the attribution validation and dispute process?

FIGURE 14.4 Understanding Attribution of Priority Population

Choosing Meaningful Outcomes Measures and Appropriate Benchmarks

Perhaps, most important to success in negotiating risk contracts are the metrics chosen to measure success. Therefore, it is paramount that the agreement includes metrics that providers can truly control and impact outcomes. The benchmarks against which performance is measured should be feasible and meaningful. This applies to measurement of performance of cost as well as quality and utilization.

If a group has the option to choose quality measures, consider the following choices:

- Align metrics across payer contracts and make sure baseline performance is known in order to select measures where there is greater chance for meeting or exceeding benchmarks
- Choose metrics that are clinically relevant and make sense. For example, instead of a cost-cutting metric such as the number of scripts/1,000 patients, consider a more meaningful measure of cost-effectiveness such as generic dispensation rates.

- Equally important is the benchmark against which performance will be compared. Negotiate benchmarks that are fair and achievable. If there is room for improvement from baseline. a good option may be to suggest an X% of improvement rather than a static target. If baseline performance is already high, the measure of success should be maintenance and not further unrealistic improvement.

Consider what will the impact of quality and utilization measures be on overall contract performance? For example, does meeting quality threshold earn the provider a bonus payment or will the quality score be used as a multiplier for any shared savings. Figure 14.5. describes elements to consider when negotiating quality and utilization measures.

A final component is measuring and assessing cost performance, and the details of how and which factors can significantly impact whether a group is financially successful in their risk agreements. Exhibit 14.2. outlines important factors that should be considered when developing cost measures and benchmarks.

UNDERSTANDING QUALITY AND UTILIZATION MEASURES

1 SELECTING MEASURES
Which measures will be used, and how will they be chosen?
- Are the proposed measures **aligned with your other payer contracts?**
- Do you know your **baseline** for these measures?
- Do you have the ability to drive success? Can you **operationalize** performance initiatives?
- Are the measures **clinically relevant** and important to the attributed patient population?

2 DEVELOPING BENCHMARKS
How will you assess your performance?
- Will you use **national, regional, or payer-specific** benchmarks?
- Are the benchmarks **relevant** to your population and organization?
- Are these benchmarks **reasonable and attainable?**
- Can you show your improvement from a baseline, e.g. improve 5% per year until we reach particular benchmark (**glide path**)?
- If you are already doing well, can you maintain performance?

3 UNDERSTANDING CONTRACT IMPACT
How will your quality/utilization measure performance impact your contract performance?

FIGURE 14.5 Understanding Quality and Utilization Measures

UNDERSTANDING COST PERFORMANCE MEASURES AND BENCHMARKS

- **Stop-loss and catastrophic caps**: What is included or excluded? Consider pharmacy stop-loss and caps as well!
- **Comparison group/methodology**: Matched cohort vs. market vs. budget target vs. comparison to self YOY
- **Starting targets**: How is the health plan setting the target at which you will be compared? PMPM targets (budget) or market cohort?
- **Final reconciliation of cost**: What is time frame for final claims run out? Ideal is at least 6 months.

- **Impact of current performance on success**: Will you be hurt if you are already highly efficient? And if you are not, how much work will be required?
- **Cost inclusion/exclusion**: Are there carveouts (ESRD, hospice)? Do you have room to negotiate, or will the plan evaluate TME without carveouts?
- **Are you at risk for pharma?** How much control will you have over spend if taking on that risk? Does your population have rich pharmacy benefits?

EXHIBIT 14.2 Understanding Cost Performance—Measures and Benchmarks
ESRD, end-stage renal disease; TME, total medical expenses; YOY, year-over-year.

Development of and Investment in a Comprehensive Clinical Model That Supports Value-Based Care

The shift to fee-for-value has meant the emergence of alternative payment models and value-based contracts. Success in value requires not only strong population health management including engagement of all stakeholders including patients, providers, clinical and nonclinical teams, and administration.

Summit Health has developed a value formula that has become our call to action for optimal population health management. We must give good care, but we must also prove that we are doing this:

- Deliver high-quality care with experience that drives great outcomes. But equally important is proving this by satisfying quality measures through claims or electronic health records so that the data can be captured and reported.
- Capture the disease burden of the patient population to prove the complexity of care and decision-making. Medical risk must be captured through coding so that payers can set appropriate cost benchmarks for our population.
- Manage costs by offering the right care at the right time to the right person in the right setting. We ensure all people receive their required and recommended high-value care (e.g., preventive services) while avoiding low-value care (e.g., unnecessary tests or medications).

Figure 14.6 illustrates the Summit Health Value Formula that is used to educate and engage providers, staff, and leadership teams and offer them a call to action for high-value care delivery.

$$\left(Value = \frac{Quality + Disease\ Burden}{Cost}\right)$$

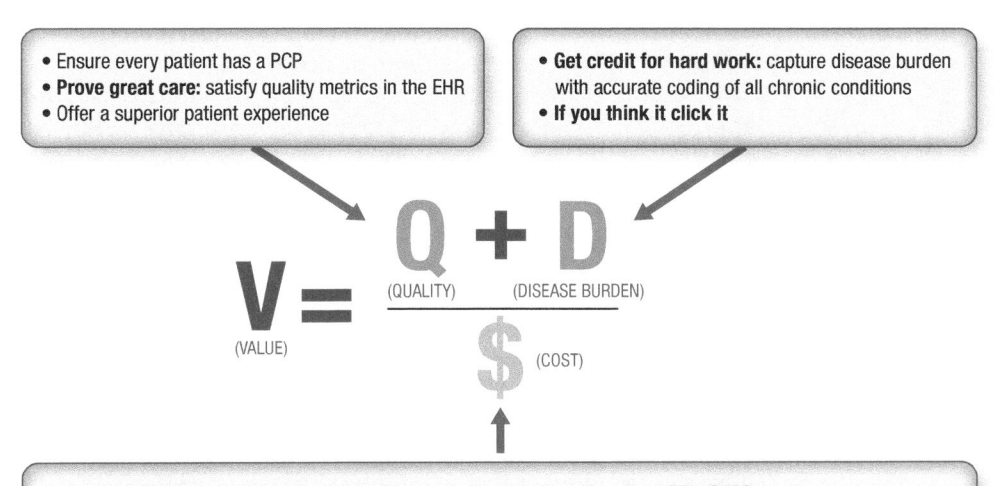

- Ensure every patient has a PCP
- **Prove great care:** satisfy quality metrics in the EHR
- Offer a superior patient experience

- **Get credit for hard work:** capture disease burden with accurate coding of all chronic conditions
- **If you think it click it**

$$V = \frac{Q + D}{\$}$$
(VALUE) = (QUALITY) + (DISEASE BURDEN) / (COST)

- **No place like home:** keep patients out of expensive settings (e.g., hospitals, EDs, SNFS)
- **Choose wisely:** reduce avoidable utilization
- **Keep it in the family:** Use SMG consultants and services

FIGURE 14.6 Summit Health Value Formula

Each component of the value formula requires easily accessible data to drive improvement and ever better outcomes

- Quality: The data analytics platform combines clinical and claims data to report true performance on quality measures. These reports are made easily accessible to care teams so they can reinforce successful workflows and identify areas of opportunity. Drill-down capability allows teams to get to patient level data for direct engagement and closure of care gaps.
- Disease-burden accuracy: For payers to appropriately set cost benchmarks in a value-based agreement, the true disease burden of the population needs to be captured through clinical information systems and submitted claims. Data analytics can identify chronic conditions that have not been captured during care delivery. In addition, artificial intelligence and natural language processing can discover additional potential conditions that need to be addressed by care givers.
- Cost: Analytics are essential to identify areas where care is delivered inefficiently and adversely impacting cost. Examples include the following:
  - Risk stratification to identify populations that require differing types of engagement from high-touch care management for high-risk patients, to identifying patients at end-of-life that may benefit from advance care planning and palliative care, to healthy patient overdue for preventive services.
  - Detecting providers who are outliers and require further education.
  - Identification of inappropriate utilization of inpatient services, labs and radiology, specialty medications, and out-of-network providers.

Data Analytics to Inform Operations and Operational Strategy

Once a provider group has embarked on the value journey, it is important to have in place an operation strategy to evaluate and continually improve on performance in the value-based agreements. This is where technology plays an essential role. Figure 14.7 describes the core functions of a technology strategy used at Summit Health to drive success in risk contracts.

It is important for groups to partner with their payer counterparts to ensure there is appropriate exchange of accurate and timely manner that supports successful PHM. Figure 14.8 describes elements of a successful data exchange strategy.

Process for Intervention Planning and Implementation

The most important factor in implementing a successful PHM data analytics strategy is acceptance of its importance from all stakeholders:

- Leadership needs to accept that financial success in risk contract requires investment in a comprehensive and robust analytics platform and the appropriate analytics team needed to leverage the technology
- Clinical teams and providers must embrace value-based care as the path to optimal outcomes for their patients. And, in turn, they must embrace reporting that helps them manage their patient populations
- Operations and data teams must fully utilize data analytics capabilities to support clinical teams, identify areas of strength and opportunities for improved outcomes, and be transparent, nimble, and innovative.

OUR TECHNOLOGY STRATEGY

6 CORE FUNCTIONS

We needed an information architecture that supports key constituencies and functions for value-based care success under our commercial and other risk-based contracts.

✓ **ACO OPERATIONS**
Contract performance dashboards, ad hoc reporting, payer contract monitoring, PCP scorecards, and ACO performance reports; workflows for attribution management and other focus areas.

✓ **QUALITY IMPROVEMENT**
Quality measure reporting on internal objectives and contract requirements; analysis of performance and workflow tools for improvement efforts.

✓ **DATA ANALYTICS & REPORTS**
Capabilities to generate reports on an ongoing and as-needed basis and conduct analysis to support and enhance performance across all constituencies, e.g., OON leakage.

✓ **CODING COMPLIANCE**
Workflow for coders for using the risk coding model to perform HCC chart prep for targeted patient populations. Monitoring and analysis of provider condition documentation accuracy. Special projects.

✓ **PATIENT MANAGEMENT**
Workflow management and oversight for transitional care management, SNF utilization, high risk patient management, social work, and pharmacy programs.

✓ **PRIMARY CARE CLINICAL SERVICES**
Workflows for clinical office staff for pre-visit planning, chart prep, point-of-care gap identification, registries
Reporting to monitor and manage provider performance

FIGURE 14.7 Technology Strategy at Summit Health

CLAIMS DATA: CRITICAL FOR MUTUAL SUCCESS

Success under risk requires access to claims-based data; it holds **insights about utilization outside your organization** that are not available in your own clinical systems.

How do you convince the plan it is **critical** that you have the data you need...

Use examples of how claims data can help promote high-value care delivery:
- Claims data is necessary to hold physicians accountable for **generic Rx rates** by therapeutic class.
- Reporting on ambulatory procedures allows us to determine the **right sites of care** (ASC, hospital, owned v. not-owned) based on cost, outcomes, and provider block time.

...and then how do you go about **getting** it?

- In **less advanced markets**, plans are not accustomed to providing data.
- Take the time to **educate the plan** about the data you need.
- Set **expectations up front** re: type of data, frequency, quality—and then **monitor and audit!**
- Consider implementing **standard language** about data provision in all your contracts.

FIGURE 14.8 Claims Data: Crucial for Mutual Success

Regardless of where a group is in their value journey, it is never too early to begin using data analytics to inform strategy and operations. Figure 14.9 shows a suggested timeline for building and implementing a PHM data analytics platform for value-based success.

A universal fact in healthcare is that data are stored in various disparate tools, platforms, and databases. The key role of a population health management platform is to aggregate all these data and convert it into meaningful information. Figure 14.10 describes how Summit CityMD leverages its PHM analytics platform to derive actionable reports from clinical and nonclinical data received from various sources.

The following are several examples of how Summit Medical Group-City MD has leveraged analytics in pursuit of its PHM strategy.

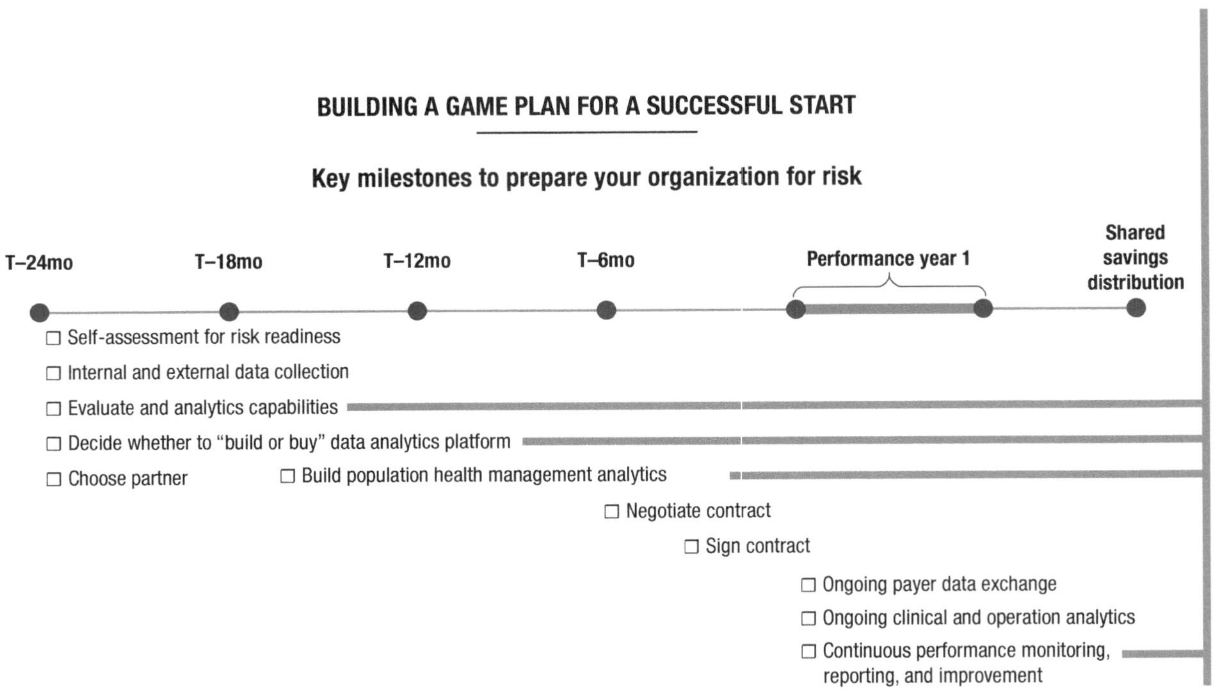

BUILDING A GAME PLAN FOR A SUCCESSFUL START

Key milestones to prepare your organization for risk

T–24mo · T–18mo · T–12mo · T–6mo · Performance year 1 · Shared savings distribution

- ☐ Self-assessment for risk readiness
- ☐ Internal and external data collection
- ☐ Evaluate and analytics capabilities
- ☐ Decide whether to "build or buy" data analytics platform
- ☐ Choose partner
- ☐ Build population health management analytics
- ☐ Negotiate contract
- ☐ Sign contract
- ☐ Ongoing payer data exchange
- ☐ Ongoing clinical and operation analytics
- ☐ Continuous performance monitoring, reporting, and improvement

FIGURE 14.9 Timeframe for Building Data Analytics Platform

- HIE Data (x2)
- Clinical data from EMRs (x3)
- Plan data (x5) — Commercial, Medicare Advantage, Medicare ACO
- ACO
  - Provider hierarchy
  - Care management history, content
  - MPI override
  - Post-acute care registry

→ CNX → Population health management platform (DW) →

- Self-service analytics
- Care management
- Contract analytics
- Medical economics
- Quality performance
- Risk stratification and adjustment

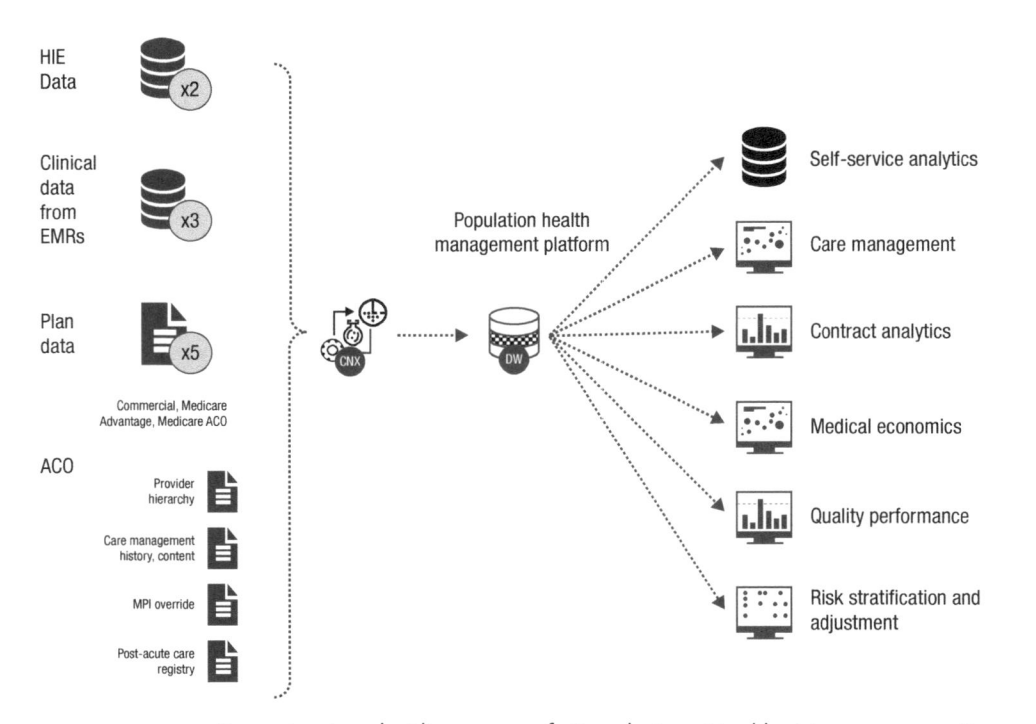

FIGURE 14.10 Organizational Alignment of Population Health Management Data Components

Examples of using data analytics to measure performance and inform strategy:

- What is the impact of Annual Wellness Visits (AWVs) on value-based contact performance and patient outcomes?
    - AWVs are a specific type of visit covered by Medicare. They are an opportunity for providers to perform a comprehensive health risk assessment and develop a personalized prevention plan in collaboration with the patient.
    - Claims and clinical data were used to evaluate whether AWVs improved quality and reduced cost of care.
    - Results:
        - Patients with AWVs have 1.6 more office visits in a 6-month time period when compared with control.
        - While AWVs did not decrease the total cost of care in the year following the visits, they did positively impact quality measures significantly and increase office follow-up, which led to greater patient retention rate of 88% in the following year compared with 67% for patients without AWV.
- Do transitional care management visits (TCMs) impact outcomes?
    - TCMs are outpatient follow-up visits within 1 to 2 weeks of discharge from a hospital or skilled nursing facility. These visits focus on helping patients follow their postdischarge plan and avoid rehospitalization.
    - Using claims data, we measured whether TCMs increased outpatient visits, reduced rehospitalization, and reduced cost of care in period following discharge.
    - Results:
        - High-risk patients with TCM visit had 0- to 30-day readmission rate of 8% compared to 28% for patients without TCM visit.
        - When compared with discharged patients who did not receive a TCM visit, those that did had more outpatient visits and lower cost of care in the following 90 days.

Once a PHM analytics platform has been implemented, it can offer valuable information that continually improves outcomes. Appropriate integration of internal and external data is central to a comprehensive data analytics strategy to support decision-making across the age, wellness, and care-setting continuum to setup for success in managing value-based contracts and their attendant risk (see Figure 14.11). With data touchpoints throughout these continua—including, clinical, pharmacy, ambulatory, and emergency —results are monitored, and immediate feedback provided based on these touchpoints to analyze performance leading to decisions and engaging providers.

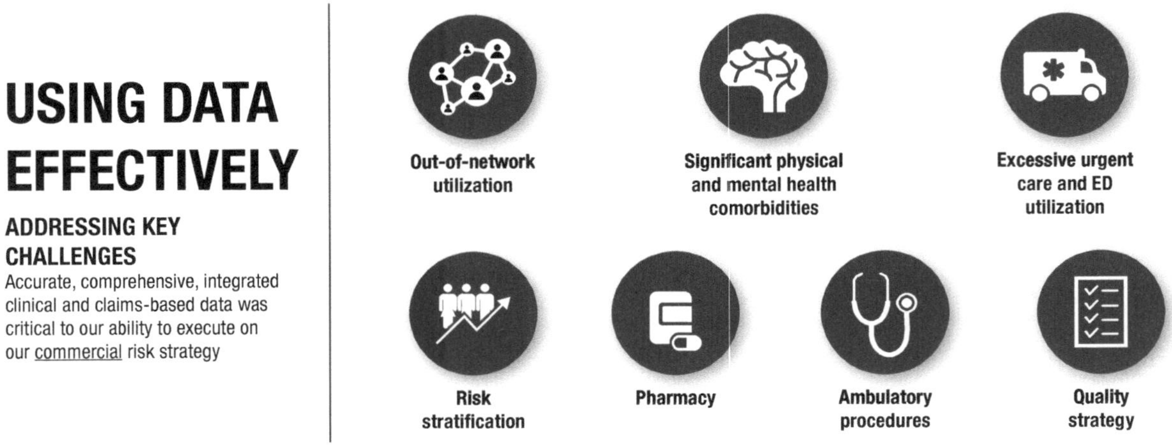

USING DATA EFFECTIVELY

ADDRESSING KEY CHALLENGES

Accurate, comprehensive, integrated clinical and claims-based data was critical to our ability to execute on our commercial risk strategy

- Out-of-network utilization
- Significant physical and mental health comorbidities
- Excessive urgent care and ED utilization
- Risk stratification
- Pharmacy
- Ambulatory procedures
- Quality strategy

FIGURE 14.11 Addressing Key Challenges Through Effective Data Use

DISCUSSION QUESTIONS

1. This case study highlights the use of PHM data analytics to support risk-based contracting. What would be other scenarios that PHM data analytics could potentially be successfully used?
2. In Exhibit 14.1, a general idea of internal and external data is provided. What would be specific internal and external data for a successful PHM strategy and where would these be sourced from.

    What would you consider to be important consideration(s) in a hospital or healthcare system being held accountable for the outcomes of the population that it serves?
3. Discuss how you would identify quality metrics and benchmarks for chosen PH outcomes.
4. In Figure 14.5, Summit Health identifies a value formula as a call to action. Discuss how this could be operationalized for a hospital.
5. Of the six core functions of its technology strategy (Figure 14.6), which is the most indispensable? Why?
6. Discuss how best to provide clinical and operations team with data analytics capabilities.

Case Study 3. A Case Study on Population Health Addressing Health Equity During a Crisis: Flattening the Curve of Hispanics with COVID-19 in Somerset County, New Jersey

Paula A. Gutierrez and Serena Collado

INTRODUCTION

The COVID-19 pandemic has disproportionately affected racial and ethnic minorities across the United States. According to the U.S. Census Bureau, New Jersey is home to 1.8 million Hispanics, which accounts for about 21% of the state's total population. The pandemic has shed light on the health inequities and barriers that have made the Hispanic community especially vulnerable to COVID-19. RWJBarnabas Health (RWJBH)—as the leading academic health system in New Jersey—is advancing innovative strategies in high-quality patient care, education and research to address both the clinical and social determinants of health to ensure health equity for the diverse communities they serve. As New Jersey's largest, most comprehensive healthcare system serving over 5 million people, RWJBH's dedication to patients extends far beyond the care provided within the hospital walls.

Somerset County is at the hub of Central New Jersey. It has over 330,000 residents across 21 municipalities and is equidistant to New York City and Philadelphia. It is also home to about 50,000 Hispanics, which account for 15% of its population. In this case study, we examine how Robert Wood Johnson University Hospital Somerset (RWJUH Somerset), an affiliate of RWJBarnabas Health, responded in a crisis during the first wave of the pandemic to address the health inequity of COVID-19 infections in Somerset County New Jersey's Hispanic population.

Case Problem Statement and Description

According to the Centers for Disease Control and Prevention (CDC), Hispanics are hospitalized from COVID-19 at four times the rate of white Americans. In addition, 26% of people who have died from COVID-19 in the United States are Hispanic. In the weekend of April 10, 2020, approximately 40% of RWJUH Somerset's COVID-19-positive admissions identified as Hispanic. This indicated a severe surge of COVID-19 in Somerset County New Jersey's Hispanic community. While certain preexisting health conditions increase the risk for COVID-19, it is also important to understand the systemic and racial inequities that exist in the Hispanic population to address the disproportionate rate of infection (see Box 14.1).

BOX 14.1 SYSTEMIC HEALTH BARRIERS IN THE U.S. HISPANIC POPULATION

- Limited English Proficiency (LEP)
- High number of essential workers who are unable to work from home or stay home when sick
- Multigenerational families living together in small homes infecting each other
- Lower rates of health insurance due to a segment of the population being undocumented
- Fear of deportation
- Lack of trust in government and large institutions including hospitals
- Food insecurity and lack of resources

RWJBH's Diversity & Inclusion and Social Impact & Community Investment team's missions are rooted in addressing social determinants of health and decreasing health inequities in diverse populations. RWJUH Somerset's leadership and its Community Health and Diversity & Inclusion departments recognized the need to go beyond the hospital walls, into the Hispanic community, and address this disparity in a time of crisis. Through grassroots outreach, education and distribution of resources, they sought to decrease the number of COVID-19 positivity spread among Hispanics in Somerset County, New Jersey.

Case Elements, Context, Supporting Materials

Community Health (CH) and Diversity & Inclusion formed an outreach and educational initiative with CH Spanish speaking staff and the hospital's SALUD (Service and Advocacy for Latinos United for Development) BRG (Business Resource Group). BRGs are comprised of individual employees that come together on a shared characteristic, quality, or life experience. The hospital's SALUD BRG includes staff from various departments, both clinical and nonclinical, who either speak Spanish and/or identify as Hispanic. This resource group sought to educate the Hispanic community on COVID-19, masking, social distancing, and hand hygiene along with providing resources to the community.

Over a 6-week period, the group conducted phone calls in Spanish, sent out culturally and linguistically appropriate mailings, and went out into the community during the peak of the pandemic. Box 14.2 presents the diverse outreach methods and strategies.

14. CASE STUDY 3. A CASE STUDY ON POPULATION HEALTH ADDRESSING HEALTH EQUITY   275

BOX 14.2 OUTREACH METHODS TO REACH PRIORITY HISPANIC POPULATION

Phone Calls:

- Identified Hispanic patients through Community Health and the hospital's databases of previous admissions and community events
- Recruited Spanish speaking staff across hospital including Community Health and Diversity & Inclusion's SALUD BRG that made 4,153 calls to educate Hispanic patients

Mailing:

- Developed and mailed over 3,200 letters in Spanish along with a local resource directory and Spanish RWJBH marketing collateral on prevention of COVID-19, hand hygiene and proper masking

Outreach:

- Partnered with community organizations including Salvation Army, churches, and food pantries to host 16 in-person mask distribution and educational events
- Hospital's Foundation obtained donated masks from community organizations
- Provided a total of 14,132 masks, 3,760 hand sanitizers, and 3,576 soaps

Figure 14.12 presents images and shows RWJUH Somerset staff during various outreach events. This photo also shows RWJUH Somerset masks that CH purchased to supplement donated ones. At height of the pandemic, more supplies need than were donated. Table 14.3 indicates the organizations who donated masks for the outreach.

Table 14.3 indicates the organizations who donated masks for the outreach.

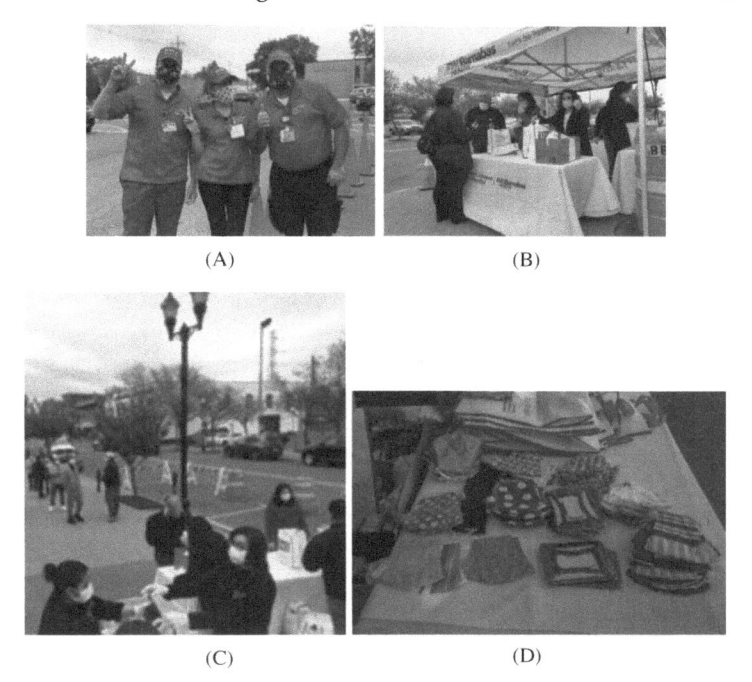

FIGURE 14.12 RWJUH Somerset Outreach Participants and Events. (A, B, and C) Community Health and SALUD BRG Members. (D) Donated and purchased masks

TABLE 14.3 Local Organizations Donating Masks (2020)

Organization	Masks Donated
Bound Brook, NJ	1,000
Community Members	2,439
Empower the Mind	78
Fanatics	1,728
Knit Crochet With Love	485
Liquid Church	1,580
Menlo Park Lions Club	400
Mission Mask Team	70
RWJBarnabas Health	2,670
RWJUH Somerset	1,301
Sewa International	301
Somerset County Library	700
Somerset County OEM	510
The Mask Squad	775
The Sew Strong Project	300
United Against COVID-19	100
Total:	14,437

Guiding Conceptual Models

The disparity of COVID-19 positivity in the Hispanic community became apparent in Week 3. Community Health and Diversity & Inclusion, however, first learned about the surge in week 6 when the departments immediately launched an education and outreach intervention. The hospital collected the necessary patient data, assembled a team of bilingual staff, and collected enough resources to distribute to the entire community. After 6-weeks of outreach, Figure 14.13 shows the number of COVID-19 cases steadily begins to decline in the Hispanic community resulting in an 85% reduction in COVID-19 cases. This chart also illustrates the glaring contrast between the rates of infection in the Hispanic community and the rest of the population. In all other populations, the rate of infection reaches a plateau and then declines. However, in the Hispanic community, the infection does not plateau and continues to increase before it declines. The significance of this outreach is that Hispanics account for only 15% of the county's population yet they had the highest rate of infection. Based on the research and outreach, systemic barriers are likely the leading cause of the disproportionate number of Hispanics impacted by the pandemic.

Figure 14.14 focuses on the borough of Bound Brook, New Jersey, which has the largest Hispanic population in the county and had the highest number of Hispanics infected with COVID-19 in Somerset County. The chart shows that the number of positive cases dropped as personal protective equipment (PPE) donations increased. When COVID-19 positivity peaked in mid-April, the team began mask and hand sanitizer distribution. By early May—the next distribution event in Bound Brook—the number of infections started to decline. When the team conducted its third outreach in mid-June, the positivity rate dropped significantly. As a result, the rate of COVID-19 infection decreased by 87% in Bound Brook, New Jersey at the end of 6 weeks after the hospital distributed over 5,340 masks.

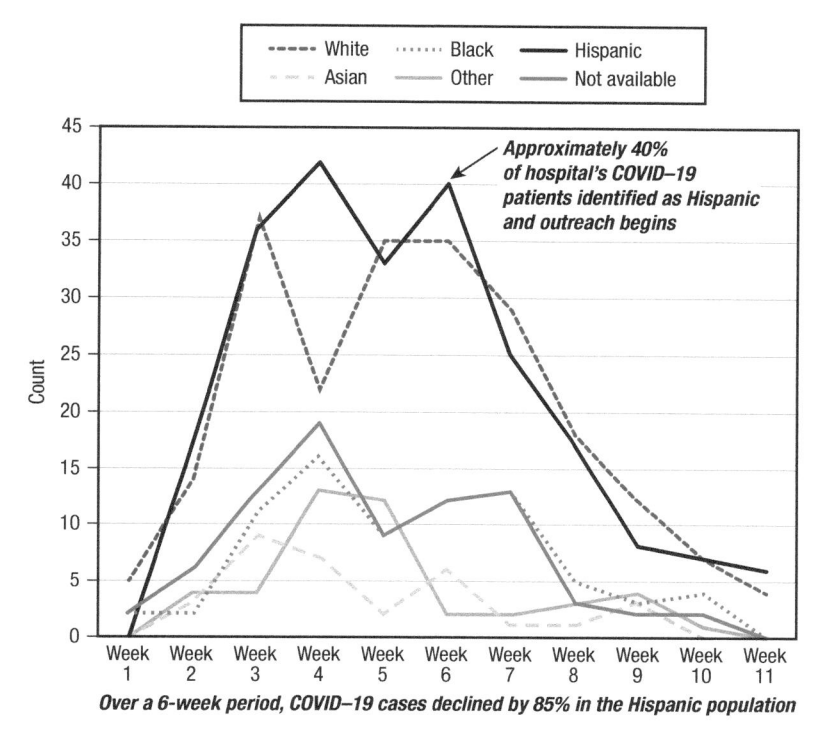

FIGURE 14.13 Race/Ethnicity Distribution of COVID-19 Cases at RWJUH Somerset. This graph is specific to the hospital

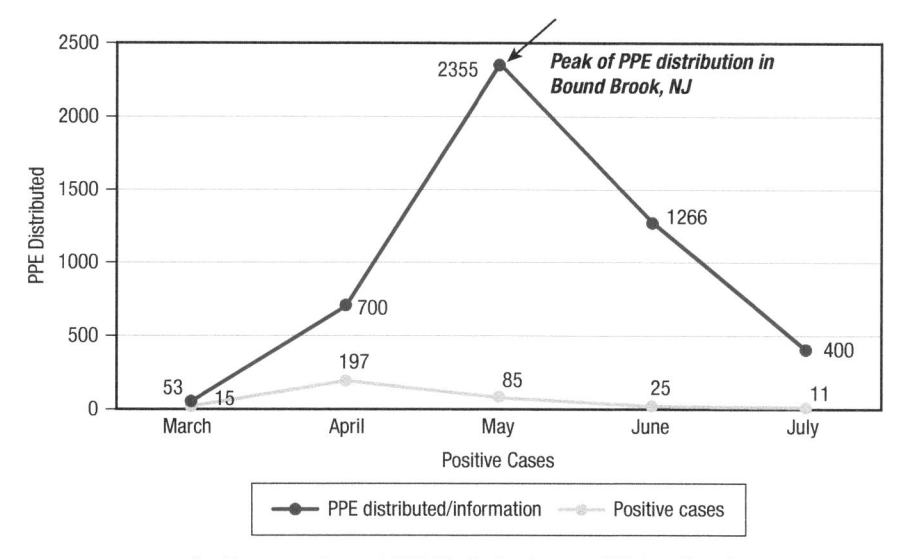

FIGURE 14.14 Decline in COVID-19 Cases in Bound Brook, New Jersey

Outcomes

The pandemic has shown that it takes nontraditional approaches to effectively reach vulnerable populations and address social determinants of health and health disparities in a time of crisis. This includes outreach into the communities to provide resources (food, masks, and hand sanitizers/soap), translation of materials for those with LEP, and engaging trusted community partners as well as leveraging staff from Community Health and Diversity & Inclusion's business resource groups to bridge cultural and communication gaps.

Because of the successful outreach, RWJUH Somerset formed a Latino Advisory Council (LAC). This council is comprised of over 20 representatives from local government, businesses, and organizations serving the Hispanic community. The goal of this council is to continue community outreach efforts including the development of educational webinars in Spanish to keep the community engaged in order to establish their trust and maintain their health and wellness. By continuing to work together with trusted community partners, we can keep the public healthier and achieve greater equity in our most vulnerable populations.

DISCUSSION QUESTIONS

1. Did this outreach improve patient outcomes? If so, how?
2. What does the data tell you about effective interventions?
3. Describe the importance of collaborating with community organizations.
4. Why is it important to engage culturally competent and bilingual staff in the outreach?
5. Can outreach be impactful without the use of culturally and linguistically appropriate materials?
6. By flattening the curve among the Hispanic community, how does this affect other sectors of the community? The County?

Case Study 4. Coproduction Leadership for the Future Health Sector

Patrick D. Shay and Edward J. Schumacher

INTRODUCTION

The executive leaders from Trinity Falls Children's Hospital thought they had a winning strategy. In their presentation to members of the Hornbeak community, they were sharing the plans they had spent months developing in order to address the alarming rates of pediatric diabetes within the neighborhood. The Hornbeak community was one of several areas in the city of Trinity Falls that was badly underserved, suffering from high poverty rates, poor health outcomes, and limited access to health resources. Over the past several years, Trinity Falls Children's Hospital had made an intentional effort to prioritize health needs in the underserved areas throughout the greater Trinity Falls market, such as the Hornbeak neighborhood. This included building numerous neighborhood pediatric clinics as well as the development of targeted programs to address specific children's health needs, and in the Hornbeak neighborhood, a critical need pertained to pediatric diabetes.

Community Presentation

Gathered together in the Hornbeak Community Center, the leaders from Trinity Falls Children's Hospital gave a thorough and convincing presentation to the community members. They walked through the epidemiologic numbers they had tracked and analyzed, including where specifically in the community the highest pediatric diabetes incidence rates were, and they provided clinical reasoning behind their efforts to address pediatric diabetes, centering on the development of a comprehensive pediatric diabetes program. As they progressed through their presentation, providing details on why they expected their proposed interventions would be effective particularly for children with undiagnosed diabetes and their family members, they reached the moment in which they explicitly asked for the community members' support and enrollment in their new program.

The response was not what the executive leaders had anticipated. They received a few polite nods and kind smiles scattered across the room, but the predominant reaction was silence. After an awkward minute or two, some questions and critical comments began to emerge from the audience, and it quickly became clear to the leaders of Trinity Falls Children's Hospital that their well-intentioned plans to address pediatric diabetes had been received with resistance and skepticism from the Hornbeak community. Some uncomfortable conversations quickly developed, until one executive—out of frustration that all of their work seemed to be for nothing—reacted with a question that would unintentionally but profoundly shift the discussion: "Well, if this isn't something you're interested in, then what would *you* like to see? We're here to help, so what are *your* priorities?"

The Solution

As that question sank in, the mood in the room suddenly shifted. Hands started to quickly go up, and in a short period of time, a common response emerged. One parent from the community stood and explained: "We have a terrible problem with feral dogs in the neighborhood—they're all over the place, and they're dangerous! I can't tell you how many times we've tried to call Animal Control to come take care of it, but it's just not working. Now *that's* something we'd like to see some help with!"

Following the meeting, the team at Trinity Falls Children's Hospital felt energized. They spent time carefully talking and listening to different members of the Hornbeak community to better understand their perspective and their experiences dealing with feral dogs. Within a few weeks, they had also had the opportunity to meet the leaders from the Trinity Falls city government, gaining their awareness of the feral dog problem as well as their commitment to support Trinity Falls Children's Hospital's efforts to find a meaningful solution. The city's Animal Care Services department agreed to devote an 8-week period toward prioritizing their assistance to the Hornbeak community, including a commitment to respond within 30 minutes to any animal control issue that they received from the neighborhood. Similarly, the City Council representative for the Hornbeak community committed to closely follow progress on the feral dog problem, demanding that when any of the neighborhood's calls to Animal Care Services were not adequately responded to within 30 minutes, she be personally notified in order to hold their team accountable. Additionally, Trinity Falls Children's Hospital printed hundreds of refrigerator magnets to distribute throughout the neighborhood, listing both the phone numbers for Animal Care Services and their community's City Council representative.

In 3 months' time, the Hornbeak community saw a noticeable difference. The community expressed strong support for the response that they saw from their local government, and the problems with feral dogs seemingly disappeared. Shortly after that, the leaders from Trinity Falls Children's Hospital noticed some other interesting changes. Driving through the Hornbeak neighborhood, they saw many more children playing outside than they could ever previously remember, riding their bikes, walking down the community streets, and playing in the neighborhood's parks and playgrounds. Physical activity rates rose dramatically, and when the hospital leaders visited with community members, they heard comments such as "Our kids aren't afraid to go outside anymore" and "This neighborhood is now a happier place!"

After a few more weeks had passed, the leaders of the Hornbeak neighborhood hosted another community meeting, and they invited the executive leaders from Trinity Falls Children's Hospital to attend. At the meeting, the Hornbeak community had a message they wanted to publicly share with the hospital leaders: "We've talked together as a community, and we want to thank you. You've helped us solve the problem with feral dogs, and we really appreciate that. A while ago you spoke with us about a pediatric diabetes program you wanted to offer, and now we'd be willing to talk with you more about that."

Needless to say, the Trinity Falls Children's Hospital leadership was thrilled, and they came away from that meeting with a critical insight. As their Senior Vice President and Chief Population Health Officer put it:

> "Our work to understand the problems they experienced, and our efforts to help solve their problems with feral dogs, was what made the difference. Not only did that help lead to increased physical activity, which is a great outcome in itself, but it allowed us to gain legitimacy and buy-in with the members of the Hornbeak community. It's changed our entire approach to solving problems moving forward. In the past, we always tended to figure out what we thought the community must need, collect and organize the necessary resources to carry out our research or intervention, and then go to the community with our solution and expect their full cooperation. But that never really worked! Time and time again we would roll out our 'cookie-cutter' interventions and expect community members to make it their priority, never thinking about the importance of asking them what *their* priorities were or what their experiences were like from their own perspectives. It's no wonder that our past efforts never seemed to have much lasting power. Now, that script has been flipped. First, we're working to know the community better and have them truly know us as well. We're no longer outsiders; we're partners in their health. We're learning from the community what problems *they* want prioritized and what solutions are truly desirable for *them*, and as a result we're co-creating solutions that have their confidence and their vested interest. It leads to solutions that are more meaningfully desired, more deeply needed, and ultimately more effective over time. Who knew that in order to make a positive difference in addressing pediatric diabetes, we had to start by addressing their problem with feral dogs!"

DISCUSSION QUESTIONS

1. Contrast the "top-down" approach to problem-solving initially employed by Trinity Falls Children's Hospital, to the community-organizing approach that they ended up employing. How does this connect with the concepts of human-centered design?

2. How did empathy play a key role in allowing the Trinity Falls Children's Hospital leadership to progress from addressing the problem of childhood diabetes to understand a much deeper problem of community trust?

3. Identify the insights that the leadership team at Trinity Falls Children's Hospital gained in the process of exploring the problem of pediatric diabetes in the Hornbeak community. What were the underlying factors not seen in their data that contributed to the health problems described in their community?

4. Imagine you are a member of the Trinity Falls Children's Hospital executive leadership team. How would you frame a message to the members

of the Hornbeak community that would meaningfully address their health situation and effectively connect with them to be "coproducers" of better health?

5. Moving forward, in addition to gaining empathy, how might the executive leaders at Trinity Falls Children's Hospital utilize the concepts of design thinking when working with the Hornbeak neighborhood and similar communities?

Glossary

Accountable care organizations (ACOs)—ACOs are networks of providers who come together to provide whole-patient-centered care to patients, with the primary care physician (PCP) at the center of the network

Alternative payment system—The alternative payment model outlines a four-level continuum, with eight subcategories that capture levels of clinical and financial risk for provider organizations as they move from volume to a fee-based system.

Artificial intelligence—An analysis based on sophisticated technologies that capture the complex process of human thought and intelligence.

Attack rate—A measure of disease occurrence used when a disease increases greatly within a population over a short period.

Behavioral economics—The incorporation of economic, cognitive, and social psychology disciplines to determine how individuals (and institutions) make economic decisions.

Biopsychosocial model—One of the first theoretical models to posit that biology alone does not influence health and that health is also a function of social determinants of health (SDOH) and psychological well-being.

Bridges Model of Change—A change process model composed of three important segments: ending, losing, letting go; the neutral zone; and new beginnings phase.

Bundled payments—Bundled payments include the total allowable acute and/or postacute expenditures (target price) for a predetermined episode of care (EOC).

Case and care management—Approaches to managing chronic diseases and other conditions in populations with care management focusing on ensuring coordinating patient's routine care, and case managers often tailoring care for individuals with complex needs.

Case definition, report, investigation, series—Refers to the various activities in assessing and validating disease outbreak.

Case fatality rate—The proportion of cases of a particular condition that are fatal within a specified time.

Chain of transmission—Pathway of disease transmission from reservoir, via agents through various modes of transition to susceptible host.

Change management—An approach and tools that can be used to help people understand, accept, move forward, and appreciate, and then act.

Chronic disease—Chronic disease is one lasting 3 months or more, which generally cannot be prevented by vaccines or cured by medication and does not disappear.

Clinical and randomized controlled trials—Refers to the gold standard of clinical trials when everyone is randomly assigned to test or control groups.

Cohort study—An observational study in which participants are classified according to their exposure status and then followed over time to ascertain the outcome.

Collaboration—Working with others.

Community benefit—Clinical, nonclinical programs and activities providing treatment and/or promoting health and healing that are responsive to identified community needs, not provided for marketing purposes.

Community health—Refers to the health status of a defined group of people and the actions and conditions, both private and public (governmental), to promote, protect, and preserve their health.

Community health assessment toolkit (CHAT)—A web-based tool offering a nine-step pathway to guide and support a robust, community-engaged health assessment process.

Community health improvement plan (CHIP)—A long-term, systematic effort to address public health problems based on the results of community health assessment activities and the community health improvement process.

Community health needs assessment (CHNA)—A systematic process, conducted by a hospital, involving the community to identify and analyze community health needs and assets, prioritize those needs, and then implement a plan to address significant unmet needs.

Community health workers—Frontline public health workers who serve as liaisons between the community and needed health and social services.

Comparative effectiveness research (CER)—A technique used to compare various population health programs and assess their viability and effectiveness with a focus on efficacy of the program intervention.

Components of health—Refers to the physical, mental, social, emotional, and spiritual well-being of an individual.

Comprehensive primary care plus (CPC+)—A national private–public partnership which currently supports 2,804 primary care practices and 52 aligned payers in 18 regions through a unique multipayer payment system.

Consumerism—People proactively using trustworthy, relevant information and appropriate technology to make better-informed decisions about their healthcare options.

Convener model—A coproduction of health model that involves a third party so that healthcare providers do not make direct investments in social needs services or forge direct partnerships with community-based organizations.

Coordinated care—Coordinated care implies an established health plan that ensures access to appropriate providers and health services when needed.

Coproduction decision-making pathway (CDMP)—A framework of eight specific steps for aligning the various health sector partners to produce a quality health outcome.

Coproduction of health—The idea that community organizations, clinicians, social services, government agencies, and the service recipients (patients) must be engaged and focused on the well-being of the population.

Cost–benefit analysis—A cost–benefit analysis (CBA) is the process used to measure the benefits of a decision or acting minus the costs associated with taking that action.

County Health Rankings and Road Maps—An interactive web-based program that compares the health of nearly all counties in the United States to others within its own state and supports coalitions tackling the social, economic, and environmental factors that influence health by revealing a snapshot of how health is influenced by where we live, learn, work, and play.

Crude, age-specific, cause-specific, and adjusted rates—Common types of epidemiological rates where the numerator represents a condition or disease, and the denominator reflects the population size.

Culture of Health—The Culture of Health: Action Framework combines essential components of community, public, global, and population health approaches by establishing 10 principles that provide a foundation for four action steps.

Design thinking—An approach to problem-solving that emphasizes empathy, innovation, collaboration, and continual experimentation.

Digital marketing—Any marketing strategy that uses an electronic device that may or may not be connected to the internet and is the best digital approach to reach the consumer.

Distribution and determinants—Refers to epidemiological considerations of spread (frequency and patterns) and causes and other factors of disease in a population.

Divergent thinking—Describes the process during ideation of developing multiple ideas; it is paired with convergent thinking, which sifts through those ideas to explore concepts of merit and leads to iteration and experimentation.

Diversity and inclusion—Diversity encompasses acceptance and respect. It means understanding that everyone is unique and recognizing individual differences. Inclusion is a state of being valued, respected, and supported.

Drexler/Sibbet High-Performing Teams Model—A seven stage process model focusing on teaching PHM teams how to implement new strategies sustaining the team.

Electronic health record—A universal repository of patient's information.

Empathy map—Mapping that includes the consumers perceptions of what they see, hear, think, feel, say, feel, and want in their environment.

Endemic, epidemic, pandemic—Distinguishes the different amounts of disease within a group or location; endemic—being expected or constant presence, epidemi—in excess of normal expectations, and pandemic—meaning worldwide distribution.

Epidemiology—analytic, descriptive, managerial—Refers to the various branches of epidemiology, the study of the distribution and determinants of disease in a population with analytic focusing on associations, descriptive answering questions of who, what, where, when and why, and managerial addressing decision-making processes by applying basic epidemiological tools and principles.

Fast healthcare interoperability resource (FHIR)—A protocol for ensuring that applications can be seamlessly used across EHRs and health information exchanges.

Fee for service (FFS)—Refers to the payment a healthcare provider receives for services a patient might need and is also known as volume-based care.

Frequency measures of disease—Refers to measures of the occurrence of a disease.

Global Health—Collaborative transnational research and action for promoting health for all.

Health—A state of complete physical, mental, and social well-being and not the merely the absence of disease or infirmity.

Health belief model—A health behavior model that suggests individuals are motivated to change their health behavior by examining three major components: expectations, threats, and cues to action.

Health data analytics—Focuses on the technologies and processes that measure, manage, and analyze healthcare data.

Health disparities—Preventable differences in the burden of disease, injury, violence, or opportunities to achieve optimal health that are experienced by socially disadvantaged populations.

Health equity and equality—Health equity is the absence of unfair and avoidable or remediable differences in health among population groups defined socially, economically, demographically, or geographically, and health equality is ensuring that every individual has an equal opportunity to make the most of their lives and talents.

Health in All Policies—A collaborative approach that brings together policymakers and practitioners from all sectors related to SDOH under the assumption that all multisectoral policies affect health outcomes.

Health informatics—A term used to describe the science of information management in healthcare.

Health information exchanges (HIE)—Access to patient data and treatment history across healthcare providers and organizations using a database repository of patient data that are easily accessible due to universal standards requirements.

Health Information Technology—Involves the processing, storage, and exchange of health information in an electronic environment.

Health risk assessment (HRA)—Formal questionnaires used to collect data from thousands of individuals that can be aggregated to determine various disease risks across a population.

Heuristics—Rule of thumb decisions based on short-cut thinking from past experiences.

High-level wellness—A desirable balance and integration between the five components of health—physical, mental, social, emotional, and spiritual.

High reliability program—Programs that serve as attainable examples for the value of quality improvement as an integrated strategy in achieving both positive health outcomes and cost savings.

Horizontal and vertical integration—Horizontal integration is between agencies on the same level (primary, secondary, or tertiary), while vertical integration is between agencies on different levels (primary to secondary, secondary to tertiary, etc.) and occurs when organizations at different levels of care delivery coordinate the provision of care.

Hotspotting—A strategy of identifying those at-risk patients with multiple comorbidities who overuse emergency treatment because of a lack of coordinated care and aligning them with doctors, other caregivers, and social service providers, in an attempt to prevent rehospitalizations and other intensive, expensive forms of care.

Incidence and prevalence rates—Indicators of rates of illness/disease within a population with the incidence rate referring to the number of new cases in a population for a given time period and prevalence rate being the total number of people having a condition at a particular time divided by the population at risk of having the condition.

Independent Practice Association (IPA)—A group of physicians participating as a network to contract with health insurance plans.

Influencers—Trusted individuals who promote an idea or a cause, such as wellness and encourage populations of followers to adopt suggested preferences with the purpose of shaping behaviors.

Innovation—Executing an idea which addresses a specific challenge and achieves value for both company and customer.

Integrated delivery networks (IDNs)—A single organization or group of organizations working together in an organized coordinated effort as a network or providers for population health.

Integrator—An entity that serves a convening role and works intentionally and systemically across various sectors to achieve improvements in health and well-being for an entire population in a geographic area.

Interlocking chain for health outcomes—A visual model that illustrates the codependency of various health sectors, such as medical care, population health, public health, and community stakeholders.

Interoperability—Ability of various systems and organizations to work together to exchange information.

Isolation and quarantine—Ways of separating infected people from other individuals to stop transmission of a disease with quarantine referring to a restriction of the activities of people who have been exposed to a communicable disease.

Lean—A type of quality improvement process that focuses on the elimination of waste.

Loss aversion—— Personal preference for loss avoidance as compared with acquiring gains when decision-making.

Machine learning—Uses artificial intelligence to repeatedly learn from large data sets and improve the identification of patterns in data.

Marketing—A multiphase essential process for creating value via planning and executing the conception, pricing, promotion, and distribution of ideas, goods, and services to create exchanges that satisfy individual and organizational objectives.

Marketing mix—Refers to marketing's four factors of product, place, price, and promotion.

Marketing SWOT—An analysis for marketing decision-making by identifying the organizations strengths, weaknesses, opportunities, and threats.

Meaningful consumerism—Refers to five communication requirements; shared decision-making; engagement in research and practice; transparency of information; communicating, disseminating, and implementing evidence and other information; and consumer participation and input as part of the value discussion.

Meaningful use—A term used to describe the requirement for providers to demonstrate performance on defined metrics and measures from their electronic health record.

Medicare Access and CHIP Reauthorization Act of 2015 (MACRA)—Legislation that created a national framework for financial rewarding health providers (clinicians) for adopting value over volume models.

Mental accounting—Involves weighing the pros and cons of a health action.

Merit-based incentive payment system—Refers to legislation that finalized alternative payment systems and innovative models, including ACOs.

Mobilizing for Action through Planning and Partnership Model (MAPP)—A recently revised multiphase model based on a community-driven strategic planning process.

Morbidity and mortality rates—Rates that represent the presence of illness in a population (morbidity) and death (mortality).

Multispecialty group practice (MSGP)—Either a horizontally integrated group through the coordination of care provided by specialists at the same level or a vertically integrated group through coordination of both primary and secondary providers.

Nontraditional competitors—New and diverse entrants into the population health sector include drug stores, retail, venture capitalists, e-commerce businesses, third-party vendors, and fortune 500 companies.

Nudges—Concept that targeted and tailored information can be used to engage consumers/patients to participate in healthy actions and activities.

Odds ratio and relative risk (risk ratio)—Risk ratios measure associations with relative risk (cohort study) showing the measure of association expressed as incidence of disease in the exposed group divided by the incidence of disease in the nonexposed group and odds ratio (case–control studies) representing the odds of exposure to a particular disease for the case group relative to the control group.

PAST Change Model—A linear change model featuring four stages: preparation, action, sustaining change, and transformation.

Patient-centered medical homes (PCMHs)—Multiple providers under one organizational banner created with the intention of reducing costs while improving patient outcomes.

Patient engagement—Described as activities or efforts to involve an individual in their own care.

Patient experience—A patient's perception of the total healthcare interaction experience.

Patient Protection and Affordable Care Act (PPACA)—The Affordable Care Act provides for numerous rights and protections that make health coverage fairer and easier to understand and more affordable.

Patient registries—Patient information repositories that store data related to a health condition or disease.

Patient satisfaction—Patient's feelings and attitude regarding their health expectations and outcomes.

Pay for performance—Alternative payment models that align performance (quality) with cost.

PDSA—Refers to plan, do, study, and act; it is a useful tool for documenting and piloting a change in the quality improvement process.

Physician-hospital organization (PHO)—An arrangement when hospitals purchase physician practices and gain linkage which results in an affiliation agreement that allows physicians and the hospital to work cooperatively while being governed independently.

PolicyMap—A geographical information system that is an interactive, visual resource that aligns multiple determinants of health metrics with pinpointed locations on a map.

Population health—The health outcomes of a group of individuals, including the distribution of such outcomes within the group.

Population Health Alliance Framework—Developed by industry's multistakeholder professional and trade association, conceptualizes healthcare delivery systems implementation activities for quality health outcomes.

Population health approaches—Frameworks such as the Triple Aim, the Culture of Health, Pathways to Population Health, and the Four Pillars of Health, among others.

Population health data—Information related to the health outcomes of specific groups of people, namely nations, communities, or ethnic groups.

Population health management (PHM)—The organization and management of the healthcare delivery system in a manner that makes it more clinically effective, cost-effective, and safer.

Population medicine—A branch of medicine concerned with clinical or healthcare determinants of health, but also acknowledges the vital role of multisector partnerships to influence more broadly.

Postacute care—All healthcare activities following acute (treatment) care.

Predictive modeling—The use of large databases to determine characteristics of vulnerable patients who may be at risk for infection, diseases, or other health needs.

Prevention—Primary, secondary, tertiary refer to the various levels of prevention with primary focusing on the elimination of risk factors for a disease, secondary efforts focus on the early detection and treatment of disease, and tertiary activities seek to minimize disability associated with advanced disease.

Proportional (population) mortality ratio (PMR)—Number of deaths within a population resulting from a specific cause or disease, divided by the total number of deaths in a population.

Prospective and retrospective cohort study—Prospective cohort student groups participants by past or current exposure and follows them going forward while retrospective cohort studies look at past exposure and outcomes of a cohort.

Protocol for Responding to and Assessing Patient Assets, Risks and Experiences (PRAPARE)—A systematic SDOH data collection and action tool and measures, developed by the National Association of Community Health Centers (NACHC), which aligns with EHR templates.

Public health—Science and art of preventing disease, prolonging life, and promoting physical health and efficiency through organized community efforts.

Quality—A high standard of health services.

Quality improvement—Processes and models that help provide frameworks and guide population health managers through the process of improving healthcare outcomes.

Radical collaboration—Organizational strategy of working with nontraditional or unexpected organizations or entities.

Relationship marketing—The concept of relationship marketing builds on seeking loyalty among consumers and can build a sense of trust and encourage patient engagement.

Risk— The probability that an event will occur.

Risk factor—It is an exposure that is associated with a disease or a condition, without certainty.

Risk management—An approach to developing and implementing safe and effective patient care practices, preserving financial services, and maintaining safe working environments.

Risk segmentation—Uses current and prospective medical costs, health status, attitudes, and level of healthcare engagement to select individuals from a population.

Risk stratification—A systematic process for identifying and predicting patient's risk levels relating to healthcare needs, services, and care coordination with the goal of identifying those at highest risk and managing their care to prevent poor outcomes.

Salerno and Brock's Cycle of Change—A change model that focuses heavily on the emotions of the individual experiencing change, such as feelings, thoughts, and behaviors.

Self-management education (SME)—Programs that educate patients in ways to help manage their chronic symptoms and diseases such as asthma, arthritis, diabetes, COPD, and chronic pain.

Shared savings—Risk associated with the positive health outcomes in alternative payment models can be shared between the health provider, health agency (hospital), and the payor (proprietary insurance companies or state and federal health agencies).

Shared Savings Program—A voluntary payment model, created by CMS, for eligible accountable care organizations.

Single specialty group practice—The most common type of practice management which uses shared resources to yield economies of scale, negotiation leverage and advantages with insurance companies, improved quality of care, and consolidated administrative responsibilities.

Six Sigma—A quality improvement process that emphasizes variation reduction and uses statistical data analysis, experimental design, and hypothesis testing.

Social determinants of health (SDOH)—Conditions in which people are born, grow, live, work, and age. These circumstances are shaped by the distribution of money, power, and resources at the global, national, and local levels

Social justice—The view that everyone deserves equal economic, political, and social rights and opportunities.

Social marketing—Application of proven concepts and techniques drawn from the commercial sector to promote changes in diverse socially important behaviors such as drug use, smoking, and sexual behavior.

Social media—Refers to many diverse electronic platforms selected to convey tailored population health messages.

Social networks—Groups of individuals who want to connect and build relationships.

Social Vulnerability Index—An index based on U.S. census variables at tract level to identify factors that are indicative of a community's resilience or ability to recover after disaster.

Spend—The cost for individual patients with known risk factors that would identify them for additional interventions.

Standardized (morbidity/mortality) ratio—The ratio of the number of deaths observed in a study population to the number that would be expected if that population had the same specific rates as the standard population.

Structural racism—Defined as the macrolevel systems, social forces, institutions, ideologies, and processes that interact with one another to generate and reinforce inequities among racial and ethnic groups.

Study—Common study types such as cross-sectional designed to estimate disease prevalence and examine the relationship between health outcomes and other variables in a defined population, experimental where the researcher determines the exposure for the subjects and then tracks the subjects to observe exposure effects, and observational studies where the researcher does not intervene.

Surveillance—The systematic collection, analysis, and interpretation of health data with active surveillance involve local public health practitioners collecting information via in-person interviews, phone calls, ad other methods, while passive surveillance relies submission of standardized reporting.

Tableau—It is a visual analytic software that helps people see and understand data.

Transitions of care—Transitions of care refer to the linkages between primary care, acute care, and multiple options for postacute care.

Transtheoretical (stages of change) Model—A model that focuses on the cycle of addictive behaviors and lifestyle behaviors needed for long term change.

Triple/Quadruple Aim—Addresses simultaneously the population health issues of access, quality, and cost.

Upstream, midstream, downstream—Upstream issues address the SDOH. Midstream issues refer to educating individuals to improve their condition and include factors related to individual-level behavior change such as promoting healthy eating, healthy family relationships, and exercise, and downstream issues include costs of treating and expenses such as treatment of chronic and relapsing conditions and related disease complications.

Value-based care—Requires, quality services, positive health outcomes, and cost reduction, and may use incentives as part of an alternative payment system.

Value stream mapping—A quality improvement process that relies on mapping the process visually to depict the steps necessary to produce a service as a starting point for process improvement.

Virtual care (telehealth)—Digital interactions between a health provider and patient.

Volume-based care—Care based on cost associated with single EOC with payment irregardles of quality.

Wicked problem—A problem that consists of challenges that have no easy solutions because they involve many interdependent, changing, and difficult to define factors.

Index

AAP. *See* American Academy of Pediatrics
AAPCHO. *See* Association of Asian Pacific Community Health Organization
Accountable Care Organizations (ACOs), 112, 125, 127–129, 143–146, 148, 156
   Atlantic ACO, 150–152
   coordination of care, 150
   criticisms of, 129
   eligibility criteria and requirements, 127
   one-sided risk and two-sided risk, 153
   Performance Improvement Incentive Program, 150
   quality indicators, 150–152
   savings of, 150
   Southwestern Health Resources (SWHR) Accountable Care network, 127–128
ACHI. *See* Association for Community Health Improvement
ACOs. *See* Accountable Care Organizations
ACP. *See* American College of Physicians
activity trackers, 167
ADI. *See* Area Deprivation Index
adjusted rate, 29
Advanced APMs, 146–147
advertising, 180, 185
Affordable Care Act. *See* Patient Protection and Affordable Care Act (PPACA)
Agency for Healthcare Research and Quality (AHRQ), 130, 165
age-specific rate, 30
AHA. *See* American Hospital Association
AHIMA. *See* American Health Information Management Association
AHRQ. *See* Agency for Healthcare Research and Quality
AI. *See* artificial intelligence
allostasis, 60
Alternative Payment Model (APM), 140, 141–142, 144
   Accountable Care Organizations, 143–146
   adopting and aligning for population health, 142
   Advanced APMs, 146–147
   alternative care delivery models, 142, 143
   basic and enhanced, 145–146
   benefits of value-based care, 141
   Medicaid Health Homes, 147
   Patient Centered Medical Homes, 146–147
   value-based *vs.* volume-based care, 140–141
AMA. *See* American Marketing Association

American Academy of Family Physicians, 129
American Academy of Pediatrics (AAP), 129
American College of Physicians (ACP), 129, 146
American Health Information Management Association (AHIMA), 81
American Hospital Association (AHA), 13, 44, 142
American Marketing Association (AMA), 179, 182
American Medical Informatics Association (AMIA), 81
American Osteopathic Association (AOA), 129
American Public Health Association (APHA), 57, 64
AMIA. *See* American Medical Informatics Association
analytic epidemiology, 26, 31
Annual Wellness Visits (AWVs), 271
AOA. *See* American Osteopathic Association
APHA. *See* American Public Health Association
API. *See* application programming interface
APM. *See* Alternative Payment Model
application programming interface (API), 84
Area Deprivation Index (ADI), 67
Area Resource File (ARF), 63
ARF. *See* Area Resource File
artificial intelligence (AI), 85, 86
Association for Community Health Improvement (ACHI), 44
Association of Asian Pacific Community Organization (AAPCHO), 73
asthma, 48
Atlantic ACO (AACO), 150–152
   key performance indicators, 152
Atrium Health, 220
attack rate, 29, 30
AWVs. *See* Annual Wellness Visits

Baby's First program, 255–261
   budget, 258
   care messages, 258–259
   challenges and success, 261
   milestone accomplishment data, 258
   mobile support, 259, 260
   outcomes, 259, 261
   stakeholders, 258
   surveys, 259
   timeline, 257
bandwagon effect, 233

behavior change models, 160–161
behavioral economics, 177–178
behavioral healthcare, 166, 168
Behavioral Risk Factor Surveillance Survey (BRFSS), 45–46
bias towards action, 239
big data, 85
biopsychosocial model, 58, 59
blinded experiments, 34
BRFSS. *See* Behavioral Risk Factor Surveillance Survey
Bridges Model of Change, 241

CABs. *See* Community Advisory Boards
care coordination financing, 147
care coordinators, 159, 165
care management, 164–165
case management, 164–165
case reports (counts), 29
case series, 29
case-control studies, 31–32
case-fatality rate, 30
catastrophic care management, 110
Catholic Health Association (CHA), 40
cause-specific rate, 30
CBA. *See* Cost Benefit Analysis
CBOs. *See* community-based organizations
CCC. *See* Connected Communities of Care
CDC. *See* Centers for Disease Control and Prevention
CDC Wonder, 45
CDMP. *See* Coproduction Decision-Making Pathway
Center for Medicare and Medicaid Innovation (CMMI), 42, 130
Centers for Disease Control and Prevention (CDC), 23, 36, 51, 56–57, 63, 67, 192, 220, 222
Centers for Medicare and Medicaid Services (CMS), 42, 64–65, 83, 147, 160
CER. *See* Comparative Effectiveness Research
certification, 202–203
CHA. *See* Catholic Health Association
change management, 240–241
    change models, 241–245
    skills, 245
    strategy, 248
    team's concerns, questions, and leadership responses, 246
CHAs. *See* community health assessments
CHATs. *See* Community Health Action Teams
CHIPs. *See* community health improvement plans
CHNAs. *See* community health needs assessments
Chronic Disease Self-Management Program, 158
chronic diseases/conditions, 156–158, 166, 192
CHRR. *See* County Health Rankings and Roadmap
CHWs. *See* community health workers

claims data, 88, 269
clinical data, 88
clinical trials, 34
cluster, definition of, 27
CMMI. *See* Center for Medicare and Medicaid Innovation
CMS. *See* Centers for Medicare and Medicaid Services
cohort studies, 31–32
collaboration, 212, 256. *See also* coproduction of health
    advancing, 216
    and coproduction of health, 215
    Health in All Policies approach, 64, 212–213
    Healthy Families, Healthy Communities, 222–223
    input requirements for inclusive community collaborations, 215
    radical, 240
    relationship continuums for business and community collaborative perspectives, 218
Commission on Accreditation for Health Informatics and Information Management Education, 90
Commonwealth Fund, 70, 220
community, 8, 40
    collaboration, 215, 218, 223–224
    and coproduction leadership, 279–281
    Healthy Families, Healthy Communities, 223–224
    ignored communities, 46
    and population health, alignment of, 41–42, 44–45
Community Advisory Boards (CABs), 50–51
community benefits, 40–41, 43
    objectives and criteria, 41
    Schedule H (IRS Form 990), 41
Community Care of North Carolina initiative, 126
community garden, 245
community health, 8
Community Health Action Teams (CHATs), 70
Community Health Assessment Toolkit, ACHI, 44–45
community health assessments (CHAs), 43, 48
Community Health Improvement Matrix, 48
community health improvement plans (CHIPs), 43, 45, 52
community health needs assessments (CHNAs), 43–45, 64, 216
    case study, 49–52
    Community Advisory Boards, 50–51
    core requirements, 43
    corporate planning, 50
    County Health Rankings and Roadmap, 46
    hospital leadership and corporate service lines, 51–52
    models, 45

INDEX

PolicyMap, 46
  primary data and role of community organizations, 51
  recent findings, impact of, 46–49
  secondary data options, 51
  stakeholder and components of, 50
  step-by-step community alignment, 44–45
  tools and applications, 45–46
community health workers (CHWs), 56
community organizations, 51
community relationships, 217
community-based organizations (CBOs), 220
Comparative Effectiveness Research (CER), 201–202
compliance of patients, 161–163
Comprehensive Primary Care Plus (CPC+) program, 131, 132, 147
confidentiality, 63
Connected Communities of Care (CCC), 220
consumer experience, 174–176
consumerism, 174
  case study, 185–187
  consumer and patient experience, 174–176
  consumer health decision-making, 176–177
  consumer marketing, 177–178
  and coproduction of health, 222
  health marketing strategies, 178–183
  meaningful, 174, 175
  SWOT analysis, 183–184, 185–186
continuous glucose monitors, 167
Continuum of Care framework, 16, 17
convener model, 219
coordinated care, 156–158, 165
Coproduction Decision-Making Pathway (CDMP), 216, 217
coproduction of health, 212–213
  aligning health sector relationships, 217–219
  alignment of stakeholders and organizations, 215
  atypical stakeholder relationships, aligning, 218
  case study, 223–224, 253, 255–261
  consumers as central to, 222
  engagement of stakeholders, 214
  examples, 220
  input requirements for inclusive community collaborations, 215
  and leadership, 279–281
  models, 216, 219–220
  non-traditional health partnership model, 220–222
  relationship continuums for business and community collaborative perspectives, 218
  strategies, 214–216
corporate planning, 50
corporate service lines, 51–52
Cost Benefit Analysis (CBA), 201–202

cost-effectiveness ratio, 202
cost-effectiveness research, 203
County Health Rankings and Roadmap (CHRR), 46, 87, 93–98
COVID-19 pandemic, 4, 16, 63, 92, 156–157, 230–231, 254
  application of Health Belief Model, 161
  case study, 36–37
  and consumer-oriented care, 174
  and coproduction of health, 220
  epidemiology, 26–27
  frequency of disease measures of, 31
  Garden State Regional Medical Center (GSRMC), 185–187
  health inequity during, 273–278
  integrated telehealth during, 88
  mass testing for, 220
  outbreak investigations, 35–36
  race/ethnicity distribution of, 277
  virtual care visits during, 166
  wicked problem, 231
CPC+. *See* Comprehensive Primary Care Plus program
creative problem solving, 233, 238, 240
cross-sectional studies, 29
crude birth rate, 30
crude mortality rate, 30
crude rate, 29
Culture of Health model, 8–9, 13
cumulative incidence, 29
cybersecurity, 88

DALYs. *See* disability adjusted life years
data. *See also* health data analytics
  CHNAs
    primary data, 51
    secondary data options, 51
  DIKW paradigm, 80
  external data that addresses SDOH, 63
  integration, 88–89
  SDOH, 86–87
  security and safety, 88
  volume/type, growth in, 91
demand management, 110
descriptive epidemiology, 26, 28–29
design thinking, 235–236
  experimentation for advancing meaningful solutions, 239–240
  ideation for generation of unexpected ideas, 238–239
  innovation process, 236
  observations, 237
determinants of health, 26, 47. *See also* social determinants of health (SDOH)
diabetes, 67, 68

digital applications, 166–167
digital marketing, 179, 180
DIKW paradigm, 80
disability adjusted life years (DALYs), 201
disability management, 110
disease management, 110
divergent thinking, 239
diversity, 59
double-blind studies, 34
DPP. *See* National Diabetes Prevention Program
Drexler/Sibbet High-Performing Teams Model, 245–246, 247

e-commerce, 174
effectiveness, and cost, 201
EHRs. *See* electronic health records
electronic health records (EHRs), 45, 61–62, 82, 84, 159, 164, 167, 231
electronic medical records. *See* electronic health records (EHRs)
emotional health, 6
empathy, 233, 236–237
  exercises, 237
  map, 237, 238, 248
endemic, definition of, 27
epidemic, definition of, 27
epidemiology, 26
  analytic, 26, 31
  COVID-19, 26–27
  definition of, 26
  descriptive, 26, 28–29
  determinants, 26
  distribution, 26
  frequency of disease, 27–28
  managerial, 27, 35–36
exercise, and physical inactivity, 94–98
experimental studies, 31, 34

Facebook, 182
Fast Healthcare Interoperability Resource (FHIR), 84, 85
Federal Medical Assistance Percentage (FMAP), 147
fee-for-service (FFS) model, 61, 140, 141
FFS. *See* fee-for-service model
FHIR. *See* Fast Healthcare Interoperability Resource
5 Whys, 199
FMAP. *See* Federal Medical Assistance Percentage
food deserts, 60
food insecurity, 115
food swamps, 60
Four Pillars of Health, 12–13
frequency of disease, 27–28
  measures of, 29–31

Gawande, Atul, 221
general fertility rate, 30
global health, 8
governance, and quality, 194
government facilitated networks, 126
Grady Health System, Atlanta, 84

HBM. *See* Health Belief Model
HCPLAN. *See* Health Care Payment Learning & Action Network
health, 5–6
  community health, 8
  components of, 6
  Culture of Health model, 8–9, 13
  definition of, 5
  global health, 8
  impact of SDOH on, 58
  population health, 7–9
  public health, 8
Health Belief Model (HBM), 160, 161
Health Care Payment Learning & Action Network (HCPLAN), 141
healthcare systems
  approaches towards SDOH, 64–65
  components of quality care, 193–194
health data analytics, 80–81, 106. *See also* value-based care, health data analytics for
  case study, 253, 263–272
  County Health Rankings, 93–98
  data categories, 87
  data integration, 88–89
  data security and safety, 88
  impact on PHM, 90–92
  PHM data analyst career opportunities, 90
  selection of PHM software, 89
  sources of PHM data and methods, 86–89
health disparities, 57, 60, 116, 156, 254
health equality, 59
health equity, 59, 254, 273–278
Health in All Policies (HiAP) approach, 64, 212–213
health informatics, 80
  strategies, 83–86
  tools, 82–83
Health Information Exchanges (HIEs), 83
health information literacy, 81
health information technology (HIT), 80, 81–82
Health Information Technology for Economic and Clinical Health (HITECH) Act of 2009, 81–82
Health Insurance Portability and Accountability Act (HIPAA), 82, 88
health maintenance organizations (HMOs), 122–123, 126, 143
health risk assessments (HRAs), 105, 117

health sector relationships, aligning, 217–219
Healthcare Information and Management System Society (HIMSS), 90
healthcare prevention approaches, 24–25
HealthEASE e-newsletter, 42–43, 159
Healthy Families, Healthy Communities, 222
Healthy People 2020, 11, 56, 254
heuristic, 178
HiAP. *See* Health in All Policies approach
HIEs. *See* Health Information Exchanges
high reliability programs, NCQA, 204–205
HIMSS. *See* Healthcare Information and Management System Society
HIPAA. *See* Health Insurance Portability and Accountability Act
Hispanics
    and COVID pandemic, 273–278
    population, systemic health barriers in, 273
histograms, 200
HIT. *See* health information technology
HITECH. *See* Health Information Technology for Economic and Clinical Health Act of 2009
HMOs. *See* health maintenance organizations
horizontal integration, 123–125, 126–127
hospice care, 159
Hospital Without Walls program, 160
hospital-at-home, 167
Hospitals' Benefit to the Community: Research, Policy and Evaluation, 41
hotspotting, 104
HRAs. *See* health risk assessments

IAF. *See* Institute for Alternative Futures
ICD. *See* International Classification of Diseases
ICPSR. *See* Inter-University Consortium for Political and Social Research
identifiable victim effect, 193
IDNs. *See* integrated delivery networks
IHI. *See* Institute for Healthcare Improvement
incidence rate, 29, 30
inclusion, 59
income inequality, 115
Independent Practice Association (IPA), 125
infant mortality rate, 30
infection control measures, 28
Influencer Model for Change, 243–245
influencers, 181–182
influenza pandemic (1918), 4
informed consent, 34
innovation, 233–235
    barriers, 234
        individual, 234
        organizational, 234
        system level, 234
    definition of, 233
    search for innovative ideas, 235
    and success, 238–239
    understanding problems, 236–238
Institute for Alternative Futures (IAF), 73
Institute for Health Metrics and Evaluation, 87
Institute for Healthcare Improvement (IHI), 11, 13, 64, 122
integrated delivery networks (IDNs), 122–123
    horizontal integration, 123–125
    vertical integration, 123, 124, 125–126
Integrated Service Lines, 143
integration, data, 88–89
integrators, 122, 126, 219
Interlocking Chain Model of Outcomes, 216, 217
Internal Revenue Service (IRS), 40
International Classification of Diseases (ICD), 45
    ICD-10 SDOH Z-codes, 63
interoperability, 84–85, 88, 231
Inter-University Consortium for Political and Social Research (ICPSR), 87
IPA. *See* Independent Practice Association
IRS. *See* Internal Revenue Service
isolation, 28

Kaizen, 198–199

LCP. *See* lifestyle change program
leadership, 216
    case study, 254, 279–281
    change management, 240–241
        change models, 241–245
        skills, 245
    design thinking, 235–240
    hospital, 51–52
    and innovation, 233–235
    mini scenarios, 248
    and quality, 194
    role of healthcare leaders, 230–231
    SDOH leadership competencies, 65
    team building, 245–246, 247
    transformation of health sector, 231–232
Lean, 194–197
    5 Whys, 199
    Kaizen, 198–199
    Plan-Do-Study-Act cycle, 200
    project failures, 197
    value stream maps, 197–198
Lean Six Sigma, 194
lifestyle behaviors, 6, 178
    Health Belief Model, 160
    Transtheoretical Model, 160–161
lifestyle change program (LCP), 67
lifestyle management, 110
long haulers, 108
loss aversion, 178

machine learning, 85
MACRA. *See* Medicare Access and CHIP Reauthorization Act of 2015
managed care organizations (MCOs), 65, 255
managerial epidemiology, 27, 35–36
MAPP. *See* Mobilizing for Action through Planning and Partnerships model
marketing
  application of Four Ps on population health management, 180
  concepts, skills and competencies useful for PHM, 184
  consumer, 177–178
  definition of, 179
  digital, 180
  health marketing strategies, 178–183
  relationship marketing, 183
  segmentation by generational differences, 183
  social marketing, 180–181
  social media marketing, 181–183
  SWOT analysis, 183–184, 185–186
  telemarketing, 186
  traditional health marketing advertising options, 180
marketing mix, 179
maternal mortality rate, 30
MCOs. *See* managed care organizations
meaningful consumerism, 174, 175
meaningful use, 81, 83
measures of association between exposure and disease, 31–32
  odds ratio, 32–33
  relative risk, 33–34
Medicaid, 65, 146, 147, 264
Medicaid Health Homes (MHHs), 147
Medical Home Model, 147
Medical Neighborhoods, 129
Medicare, 156, 167
  ACOs, 145
  MSSP — 33 quality indicators, 150–152
Medicare Access and CHIP Reauthorization Act of 2015 (MACRA), 122, 144, 145, 146–147
Medicare and Medicaid Act of 1965, 125
Medicare Shared Savings Program (MSSP), 145, 149
  MSSP — 33 quality indicators, 150–152
medication adherence, 178
mental health, 6
Merit-based Incentive Payment System (MIPS), 144–145
  vs. Advanced APMs, 146
  scoring criteria, 144
m-health, 164, 166
MHHs. *See* Medicaid Health Homes
MIPS. *See* Merit-based Incentive Payment System
Mobilizing for Action through Planning and Partnerships (MAPP) model, 44
MSGP. *See* Multispecialty Group Practice

MSSP. *See* Medicare Shared Savings Program
multihospital systems, 125
Multispecialty Group Practice (MSGP), 126

NACCHO. *See* National Association of County and City Health Officials
NACHE. *See* National Association of Community Health Centers
National Academy of Medicine, 22
National Association of Community Health Centers (NACHE), 62, 73
National Association of County and City Health Officials (NACCHO), 44, 47
National Center on Shaken Baby Syndrome, 255
National Committee for Quality Assurance (NCQA), 130, 203
  high reliability programs, 204–205
  PCMH recognition process, 131
  population health program assessment criteria, 204
  quality improvement framework, 204
National Diabetes Prevention Program (DPP), 67–69
  availability by diabetes incidence, 68
  availability for socioeconomic disadvantage status, 69
National Ehealth Collaborative, 164
National Institute of Science and Technology, 88
National Library of Medicine, 201
National Priorities Partnership (NPP), 12, 13
NCQA. *See* National Committee for Quality Assurance
net cost savings, 202
neurobiology of change, 241–242
New Jersey, County Health Rankings, 94–98
nontraditional health organizations, 221–222
nontraditional health partnership model, 220–222
not-for-profit hospitals, 64, 216
NPP. *See* National Priorities Partnership
nudges, 178

OCR. *See* Office of Civil Rights
odds ratio, 32–33
ODPHP. *See* Office of Disease Prevention and Health Promotion
Office of Civil Rights (OCR), 88
Office of Disease Prevention and Health Promotion (ODPHP), 57
Office of the National Coordinator (ONC), 88
ONC. *See* Office of the National Coordinator
outbreak, definition of, 27

P2PH. *See* Pathways to Population Health
palliative care, 159

pandemic, definition of, 28
Pareto charts, 200
Pareto principle, 200
PAST Change Model, 241–242
Pathways to Population Health
    (P2PH), 13
Patient Activation Measure, 163
Patient centered care coordination, 127
Patient Centered Medical Homes (PCMHs),
    129–132, 143, 146–147, 156, 219
  certification options, 130–131
  characteristics of, 130
  functions and attributes, 130
  and MACRA, 146–147
  models, comparison of, 132
  NCQA recognition of, 131
  recognition options for, 133
  three-part model, 146
patient engagement, 161–163, 168, 178, 222
  aligning technological advances with, 164
  definition of, 163
  framing capacity for, 162
  phases of, 164
  programs, role and components of, 163–164
Patient Engagement Capacity Model, 162
patient experience, 163, 174–176
Patient Protection and Affordable Care Act
    (PPACA), 15–16, 41–42, 43, 47, 61–62, 64,
    125, 127, 130, 143, 144, 216, 233
patient registries, 82
patient satisfaction, 163
pay for performance systems, 140
PCMHs. *See* Patient Centered Medical Homes
PDSA. *See* Plan-Do-Study-Act cycle
personal health records, 80
PHA. *See* Population Health Alliance
PHM. *See* population health management
PHOs. *See* physician-hospital organizations
PHQ-9, 117
physical health, 6
physician-hospital organizations (PHOs), 125–126
Plan-Do-Study-Act (PDSA) cycle, 200
PMR. *See* proportional (population) mortality ratio
PolicyMap, 46
population health, 7–9, 81
  alignment, 43–45
  data, additional sources of, 86–87
  definition of, 7, 25
  four portfolios of, 13
  Healthy People 2020, 11
  impact of SDOH on, 57–58
  process, 149
  projected U.S. healthcare expenditures, 149
  risk, 108–109
  status factors, 7
Population Health Alliance (PHA), 212
  PHM Framework, 13–15, 140, 157
  step-by-step risk segmentation and stratification, 105
population health analytics
  benefits, 92
  data stream, 91
  intermingling of challenges and opportunities, 91
  operational drivers, 92
population health management (PHM), 4, 25, 65
  approaches and frameworks, 10–11
  case study, 18–19, 36–37
  categories and recent innovations, 109–111
  challenges for, 17–18
  conceptual progression of, 5
  data/methods, sources of, 86–89
  Four Pillars of Health, 12–13
  health, 5–6
  health informatics strategies for, 83–86
  health informatics tools for, 82–83
  health information technology for, 81–82
  impact of health data analytics on, 90–92
  impacts and outcomes, 15–17
  implementation of, 13–18
  leveraging digital applications for, 166–167
  manager accountability, 64
  National Priorities Partnership, 12, 13
  Pathways to Population Health, 13
  PHA's framework of, 13–15, 140, 157
  and PPACA, 15–16
  program evaluation/certification, 202–203
  role of, 9–10
  Triple Aim, 11–12, 13, 122
  types of, 110
  workflows, impacting, 167–168
population health management, models of, 122, 156
  Accountable Care Organizations, 127–129, 148–153
  behavior change models, 160–161
  coordinated care, 156–158
  horizontal and vertical integration, 123–127
  Hospital Without Walls program, 160
  integrated delivery networks, 122–123
  leveraging digital applications, 166–167
  Patient Centered Medical Homes, 129–132, 133
  patient engagement, 161–163
    aligning technological advances with, 164
    programs, role and components of, 163–164
  post-acute care, 159
  self-management education, 158–159
  strategic decision-making, 169
  telehealth, 165–166, 167, 168, 186
  transitions of care model, 158
  virtual care, 165–166, 167–168
  wearables, 167
population medicine, 25
post-acute care, 159
PPACA. *See* Patient Protection and Affordable
    Care Act

PRA Screening Instrument, 117
PRAPARE. *See* Protocol for Responding to and Assessing Patient Assets, Risks and Experiences
prediabetes, 67
predictive analytics, 84
predictive modeling, 83–84
prevalence rate, 29, 30
prevention, 24–25
   primary, 25
   secondary, 25
   tertiary, 25
Primary Care First Act, 144
primary data for CHNAs, 51
primary prevention, 25
process control charts, 200
process models of quality improvement, 194, 195
program models of quality improvement, 194, 195
proportional (population) mortality ratio (PMR), 31
Protocol for Responding to and Assessing Patient Assets, Risks and Experiences (PRAPARE), 62, 71–73
prototypes, 239
Provider-Sponsored Health Plans, 143
public health, 8
   activities, 24
   core functions of, 24
   definition of, 22–23
   essential public health services, 23, 24
   and healthcare prevention approaches, integration of, 24–25
Public Health Agency of Canada, 25
public health system, 23, 35
   assessment, 23
   assurance, 23
   policy development, 23
public trust, 40

QALYs. *See* quality adjusted life years
QI. *See* quality improvement
QPP. *See* Quality Payment Program
Quadruple Aim, 12, 13
quality, 192–193
   care, components of, 193–194
   definition of, 193–194
   and leadership/governance, 194
   measures, value-based care, 265–266
quality adjusted life years (QALYs), 201
quality improvement (QI)
   Comparative Effectiveness Research, 201–202
   Lean, 194–197
      tools, 197–200
   National Committee on Quality Assurance, 203–205
   process models of, 194, 195
   program evaluation and certification, 202–203
   program models of, 194, 195
   Six Sigma, 194–197
      statistical tools, 200–201
   tools for, 194–197
quality of life, 5, 6, 40, 93
Quality Payment Program (QPP), 132–133, 143, 144
quarantine, 28

racism, 60
radical collaboration, 240
randomized controlled trials (RCTs), 34
RCTs. *See* randomized controlled trials
REACH 2010 initiative, 222
readmissions, 62, 156
reimbursement, 61, 64–65, 144, 146
relationship marketing, 183
relative risk, 33–34
remote health monitoring (RHM) system, 166
remote patient monitoring (RPM), 166
return on investment (ROI), 112, 259
RHM. *See* remote health monitoring system
risk
   definition of, 106
   fundamentals, 104–108
   identification, patient data used for, 107
   one-sided risk/two-sided risk ACOs, 153
   PHM risk-based intervention strategies, 111–113
   population health risk, 108–109
risk adjustment, 83
risk factors, 106
risk management, 109
   categories, 110
risk matrix, 108–109, 112
risk score, 106, 117–118
risk segmentation, 104, 106, 140, 167, 254
   case study, 114–119
   patient data used for, 107
   Population Health Alliance, 105
   and population management intervention, 111, 112
risk stratification, 104, 108, 140, 167, 256, 268
   case study, 114–119
   Population Health Alliance, 105
   and population management intervention, 111, 112
Robert Wood Johnson University Hospital Somerset (RWJUH Somerset), 273–274
   Community Health and Diversity & Inclusion, 274, 276
   Latino Advisory Council (LAC), 278
   outreach methods and strategies, 275
   outreach participants and events, 275
   SALUD business resource group, 274
ROI. *See* return on investment
root cause analysis, 199
RPM. *See* remote patient monitoring

RWJBarnabas Health (RWJBH), 273

Salerno and Brock's cycle of change model, 242–243
SAS, 87
Schedule H (IRS Form 990), 41
SDOH. *See* social determinants of health
SEC. *See* socioeconomic factors
secondary data sources for CHNAs, 51
secondary prevention, 25
Security Risk Assessment (SRA), 88
Security Rule, HIPAA, 82
SEER. *See* Surveillance, Epidemiology and End Results Program
self-efficacy, 160
self-management education (SME), 158–159
self-management programs (SMPs), 42–43, 158–159
SF-36. *See* 36 Item Short Form Health Survey
shaken baby syndrome. *See* abusive head trauma (AHT)
single specialty group practices, 124–125
Six Sigma, 194–196
    curve of variation, 196
    statistical tools, 200–201
smartwatches, 167
SME. *See* self-management education
SMPs. *See* self-management programs
SMR. *See* standardized morbidity (mortality) ratio
Snapchat, 182
SNP. *See* Special Needs Plan
SOC. *See* Stages of Change Model
social associations, 115
social determinants of health (SDOH), 6, 16, 47–48, 56–57, 115, 231, 274
    biopsychosocial model, 58, 59
    case study, 67–70
    data, 86–87
    external data that addresses, 63
    healthcare systems approaches, 64–65
    Health in All Policies approach, 64
    impact on health status, 58
    impact on population health, 57–58
    leadership competencies, 65
    measurement and monitoring of, 61–63
    and patient engagement, 164
    population health management, 65
    and social needs, 60–61
    upstream/downstream parable, 57–58
    and vulnerable populations, 58–60
social health, 6
social justice, 60
social marketing, 180–181
social media marketing, 181–183
social needs, 60–61
social networks, 181
Social Vulnerability Index, 63

socioeconomic (SEC) factors, 6
Somerset County (New Jersey), COVID-19 infections in, 273
    case elements, context, and supporting materials, 274–276
    case problem statement and description, 274
    decline in cases, 277
    guiding conceptual models, 276–277
    local organizations donating masks, 276
    outcomes, 278
Southwestern Health resources (SWHR) Accountable Care network, 127–128
Special Needs Plan (SNP), 114–119
specific rate, 29
spiritual health, 6
SRA. *See* Security Risk Assessment
Stages of Change Model (SOC), 160–161
standardized morbidity (mortality) ratio (SMR), 31
structural racism, 60
Summit Medical Group-City MD, 263–264
surveillance, 28
Surveillance, Epidemiology and End Results Program (SEER), 45
surveillance cycle, 28
SWOT analysis, 183–184, 185–186

TCMS. *See* transitional care management visits
team building, 245–246, 247
technology, 168
    advances, aligning with patient engagement, 164
    health information technology, 80, 81–82
    virtual care/telehealth, 165–166
telehealth, 88, 165–166, 167, 168, 186, 231, 256
telemarketing, 186
telemedicine, 16, 166, 168, 185–187
tertiary prevention, 25
36 Item Short Form Health Survey (SF-36), 105
transformation of health sector, 231–232
transitional care management visits (TCMS), 271
transitions of care model, 158
Transtheoretical Model (TTM), 160–161
Trinity Falls Children's Hospital, 279–281
Triple Aim, 11–12, 13, 64, 122
TTM. *See* Transtheoretical Model
12-item Short Form Survey, 105
Twitter, 182
2 × 2 table, 32, 33

upstream/downstream parable, 57–58
urgent optimism, 235
U.S. Department of Health and Human Services, 51

value stream maps (VSM), 197–198
value-added analytics, 90–91

value-based care, 140–141. *See also* alternative payment systems
    alternative care delivery models, 142, 143
    arrangements, 143
    benefits of, 141
value-based care, health data analytics for, 264
    attribution of appropriate population, 264, 265
    choosing meaningful outcomes measures/appropriate benchmarks, 265–266
    cost performance, 266
    development of and investment in comprehensive clinical model, 267–268
    effective use of data, 272
    intervention planning and implementation, 268–271
    negotiation of value-based contracts, 264, 265
    operation strategy, 268
    organizational alignment of PHM components, 270
    quality and utilization measures, 266
    timeframe for building data analytics platform, 270
value-based reimbursement, 61, 146
varicella (chickenpox), 34
vertical integration, 123, 124, 125–127
VES. *See* Vulnerable Elder Survey
Veterans Health Administration (VHA), 123
VHA. *See* Veterans Health Administration
virtual care, 165–166, 167–168
volume-based care, 141
VSM. *See* value stream maps
Vulnerable Elder Survey (VES), 117
vulnerable populations
    chronic care in, 156–158
    and SDOH, 58–60
    Special Needs Plan, 117–118
Vulnerable Populations Footprint Tool, The, 63

Walgreens, 221, 222
walking groups, 245
wearables, 167
wellness, 5, 6
WHO. *See* World Health Organization
World Health Organization (WHO), 64, 160, 213

Z-codes, ICD-10 SDOH, 63